Essential Psychopharmacology explains the neurobiological concepts underlying the drug treatment of psychiatric disorders, with particular emphasis on the principles of chemical neurotransmission. For the student learning psychopharmacology for the first time, this book provides an easily readable introduction to the subject. For the physician or scientist with prior background in the field, the book is organized to provide a quick review of the key dimensions of psychopharmacology and the drug treatment of mental illness.

The clearly written text is supplemented by a wealth of high-quality color graphics that are both instructive and entertaining. These illustrations and their captions may be used independently of the main text for a rapid introduction to the field, or for review. Covering both the neurobiology of drug action, and the range of psychiatric disorders and their treatments, this book will indeed be an essential text for students, scientists, psychiatrists, and other mental health professionals.

ESSENTIAL PSYCHOPHARMACOLOGY

ESSENTIAL
PSYCHOPHARMACOLOGY

Neuroscientific Basis and
Clinical Applications

STEPHEN M. STAHL, M.D., Ph.D.

Director
Clinical Neuroscience Research Center
and
Adjunct Professor of Psychiatry
University of California, San Diego

With Illustrations by
Nancy Muntner

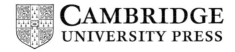
CAMBRIDGE
UNIVERSITY PRESS

PUBLISHED BY THE PRESS SYNDICATE OF THE UNIVERSITY OF CAMBRIDGE
The Pitt Building, Trumpington Street, Cambridge CB2 1RP, United Kingdom

CAMBRIDGE UNIVERSITY PRESS
The Edinburgh Building, Cambridge CB2 2RU, UK   http: //www.cup.cam.ac.uk
40 West 20th Street, New York, NY 10011-4211, USA   http: //www.cup.org
10 Stamford Road, Oakleigh, Melbourne 3166, Australia

First published 1996
Reprinted 1996, 1997 (thrice), 1998

Printed in the United States of America

This book is dedicated to the memory of Daniel X. Freeman.

Typeset in Garamond

A catalogue record for this book is available from the British Library

Library of Congress Cataloguing-in-Publication Data is available

ISBN 0-521-56011-X hardback
ISBN 0-521-42620-0 paperback
ISBN 0-521-62659-5 paperback/CD-ROM Set

Prepublication Reviews of *Essential Psychopharmacology*

"*Essential Psychopharmacology* is a superb book and there is nothing quite like it available in our field today. It is an extraordinarily complete compendium of the relevant basic and clinical information necessary to have a full understanding of how psychotropic drugs work and how to use them. The author has been able to describe state-of-the-science concepts of complex brain mechanisms, which underlie drug action in the brain, and to do so with a very clear, highly readable and easy-to-understand style. Further, it is very practical, filled with solid clinical information on the effects and use of drugs from every psychopharmacological class. The book is beautifully and intelligently illustrated and many very technical concepts are reduced to very comprehensible illustrations. *Essential Psychopharmacology* will appeal to a wide readership. It will be particularly useful, perhaps even essential, for psychiatric practitioners and primary care physicians who prescribe psychotropic agents on a regular basis. I recommend the book without reservations and with high praise to the author for his meticulous and complete scholarship in the rapidly expanding field of psychopharmacology and for his presentation and organization of the material in a manner that is very easy to assimilate and understand."

Lewis L. Judd, M.D.
Mary Gilman Marston Professor
Chairman, Department of Psychiatry
University of California, San Diego
Former Director of National Institute of Mental Health
President, International College of Neuropsychopharmacology (CINP)

"*Essential Psychopharmacology* is a modern masterpiece by a master clinical and basic neuroscientist with a broad understanding of clinical disorders in psychiatry and neurology, and the actions and sound clinical use of the medicinal agents used to treat them. This textbook is unusually lucid, while retaining an authoritative representation of sound scientific principles and findings. As such, it should appeal to those who know the field of contemporary psychopharmacology well or are responsible for teaching it. Its use of cartoons and simplified diagrams is charming and should be helpful to students unfamiliar with this field. It looks like a 'gottahaveit' book for my own professional library."

Ross J. Baldessarini, M.D.
Professor, Psychiatry and Neuroscience
Harvard Medical School
Director, Laboratories for Psychiatric Research
Mailman Research Center
Director, General Adult Psychiatry and the Bipolar and Psychotic Disorders Program
McLean Division of Massachusetts General Hospital
Boston, Massachusetts

PREFACE

This book is the outgrowth of lectures given over many years and frequent requests from students, physicians, and mental health professionals for copies of lecture slides, as well as text materials which present the fundamentals of psychopharmacology in simplified and readily readable form. Thus, this text attempts to prepare the reader to better consult more sophisticated books, as well as the professional literature. The whimsical approach at times may be off-putting to some (especially experts) but is intended to make the journey into psychopharmacology more enjoyable. This book also attempts to apply principles of programmed learning for the reader, namely, repetition and interaction.

Therefore, it is suggested that novices first approach this text by going through it from beginning to end and reviewing only the color graphics and the legends for these graphics. Virtually everything covered in the text is also covered in the approximately 300 pictures in this textbook. Once having gone through all of the color graphics in the book, it is recommended that the reader then go back to the beginning of the book and read the text, reviewing the graphics at the same time. Finally, after the text has been read, the entire text can be rapidly reviewed once again by merely referring to the various graphics of the book. This mechanism of using the materials will create a certain amount of programmed learning by incorporating the elements of repetition, as well as interaction with visual learning through graphics. Hopefully, the visual concepts learned via the graphics will reinforce the written concepts learned from the text.

For those who are already familiar with psychopharmacology, this book should provide easy reading from beginning to end. Going back and forth between the text and the graphics should provide interaction. Following review of the complete text, it should be simple to review this entire field by going through just the graphical pictures once again.

The text is purposely written at a conceptual level rather than a pragmatic level and includes ideas which are simplifications and rules, while sacrificing precision and discussion of exceptions to rules. Thus, this is not a text for the sophisticated sub-specialist in psychopharmacology.

One other limitation of the text is that it is not extensively referenced to original papers but rather just to textbooks and reviews, including several of the author's. Best wishes for your first step on the journey into this fascinating field of psychopharmacology.

STEPHEN M. STAHL, M.D., Ph.D.
January 1996

CONTENTS

CHAPTER 1

PRINCIPLES OF CHEMICAL NEUROTRANSMISSION

Modern psychopharmacology is largely the story of chemical neurotransmission. To understand the actions of drugs on the brain, to grasp the impact of diseases upon the central nervous system (CNS), and to interpret the behavioral consequences of psychiatric medicines, one must be fluent in the language and principles of chemical neurotransmission. The importance of this fact cannot be overstated for the student of psychopharmacology. What follows in this chapter will form the foundation for the entire book, and the roadmap for one's journey through one of the most exciting topics in science today, namely the neuroscience of how drugs act upon the CNS.

1

The Synapse

Chemical neurotransmission occurs at synapses, specialized sites that connect two neurons. Neurons are organized so that they can both send synaptic information to other neurons, as well as receive synaptic information from other neurons. Figure 1–1 is an artist's concept of how a neuron is organized in order to *send* synaptic information. This is accomplished by a long *axon* branching into terminal fibers ready to make synaptic contact with other neurons. Figure 1–2, by contrast, shows how a neuron is organized to *receive* synaptic information, on its dendrites, cell body, and axon. The synapse itself is enlarged conceptually in Figure 1–3, showing its specialized structure, which enables the chemical neurotransmission to occur.

Three Dimensions of Neurotransmission

Chemical neurotransmission can be described in three dimensions: space, time, and function.

Space: The Anatomically Addressed Nervous System

Classically, the CNS has been envisioned as a series of "hard-wired" connections between neurons, not unlike millions of telephone wires within thousands upon thousands of cables (see Fig. 1–4). This idea has been referred to as the "anatomically addressed" nervous system. The anatomically addressed brain is thus a complex wiring diagram, ferrying electrical impulses to wherever the "wire" is plugged in (i.e., at a synapse).

Neurons send electrical impulses from one part of the cell to another part of the same cell via their axons, but these electrical impulses do not jump directly to other neurons. Neurons communicate by one neuron hurling a chemical messenger, or neurotransmitter, at the receptors of a second neuron. This happens only at the sites of synaptic connections between them (Fig. 1–3). Communication *between* neurons is therefore chemical, not electrical. That is, an electrical impulse in the first neuron is converted to a chemical signal at the synapse between it and a second neuron, in a process known as chemical neurotransmission. This occurs only in one direction, from the presynaptic axon terminal, to any of a variety of sites on a second post-synaptic neuron.

Space: The Chemically Addressed Nervous System

Recently, it has been discovered that the chemical messenger sent by one neuron to another can spill over to sites distant to the synapse by diffusion. Thus, neurotransmission can occur at any compatible receptor within the diffusion radius of the neurotransmitter, not unlike modern communication with cellular telephones that function within the transmitting radius of a given cell (Fig. 1–5). This concept is called the "chemically addressed" nervous system, where neurotransmission occurs in chemical "puffs." The brain is thus not only a collection of wires, but also a sophisticated "chemical soup." The chemically addressed nervous system is particularly important to understanding the actions of drugs that act at various neurotransmitter receptors, since such drugs will act wherever there are relevant receptors,

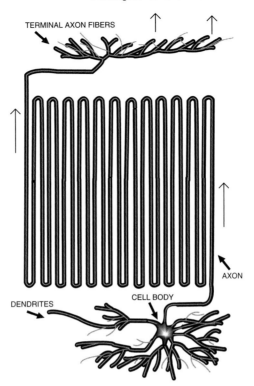

TERMINAL AXON FIBERS

AXON

DENDRITES

CELL BODY

FIGURE 1–1. This is an artist's concept of how a neuron is organized in order to **send** synaptic information. It does this via a long **axon** that sends its information into numerous branches called **terminal axon fibers**. Each of these axon terminals can potentially make presynaptic contacts with other neurons. Also shown is the **cell body**, which is the command center of the nerve, contains the nucleus of the cell, and processes both incoming and outgoing information. The **dendrites** are organized largely to capture information from other neurons (see also Fig. 1–2).

and not just where such receptors are innervated by the anatomically addressed nervous system.

Time: Fast versus Slow Signals

Some neurotransmitter signals are very brief, lasting only milliseconds. Two of the best examples of fast signals are the neurotransmitters glutamate and gamma-amino-butyric acid (GABA). Glutamate is a neurotransmitter that universally stimulates almost any neuron, whereas GABA is a messenger that inhibits almost any neuron (Fig. 1–6). Both of these neurotransmitters act by fast signals.

On the other hand, signals by other neurotransmitters can be longer, lasting many milliseconds, or even several full seconds of time. Sometimes these longer acting neurotransmitters are called neuromodulators, since slow signals may last long enough to carry over and modulate a subsequent neurotransmission by another neurotransmitter (Fig. 1–6). Thus, a long-acting neuromodulating signal can set the tone of a neuron, and can influence it not only by a primary action of its own but also by a modifying action on the neurotransmission of a second chemical message

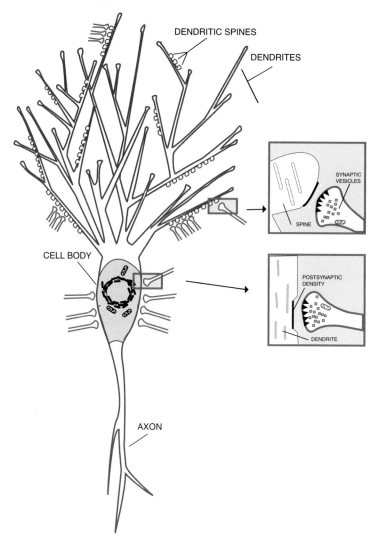

FIGURE 1–2. This figure shows how a neuron is organized to **receive** synaptic information. Presynaptic input from other neurons can be received postsynaptically at many sites, but especially upon **dendrites**, often at specialized structures called **dendritic spines**. Other postsynaptic neuronal sites for receiving presynaptic input from other neurons include the **cell body** and **axon**.

sent before the first signal is gone. Examples of slow-signaling neurotransmitters are norepinephrine, serotonin, and various neuropeptides.

Function

The third dimension of chemical neurotransmission is function, namely that cascade of molecular and cellular events set into action by the chemical signaling process. An electrical impulse in the first neuron is converted to a chemical signal at the synapse by a process known as excitation-secretion coupling. Once an electrical im-

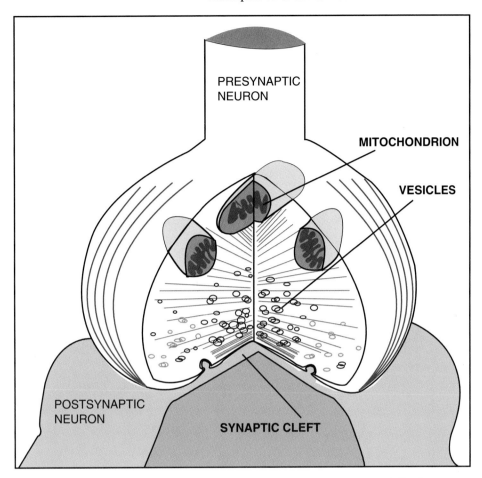

FIGURE 1–3. The synapse is enlarged conceptually in Figure 1–3, showing its specialized structures, which enable chemical neurotransmission to occur. Specifically, a **presynaptic neuron** sends its **axon terminal** to form a synapse with a **postsynaptic neuron**. Energy for this process is provided by **mitochondria** in the presynaptic neuron. Chemical neurotransmitter is stored in small **vesicles** ready for release upon firing of the presynaptic neuron. The **synaptic cleft** is the connection between the presynaptic neuron and the postsynaptic neuron. Receptors are present on both sides of this cleft, and are key elements of chemical neurotransmission.

pulse invades the presynaptic axon terminal in the first neuron, it causes the release of chemical neurotransmitter stored there (Fig. 1–3). The way is paved for chemical communication by previous synthesis and storage of neurotransmitter in the first neuron's presynaptic axon terminal. Enzymes (Fig. 1–7), receptors (Fig. 1–8), and various other chemical supplies are sent there from the nucleus, the neuronal "command center" or headquarters in the cell body, being transported down the axon to the terminals, which act as "field offices" for that neuron throughout the brain (see Figs. 1–1 through 1–3, 1–7, and 1–8). Neurotransmitter is packaged and stored in the presynaptic neuron in vesicles, like a loaded gun, ready to fire.

Once neurotransmitter has been fired from the presynaptic neuron, it shoots across the synapse where it seeks out and hits target sites on receptors very selective for

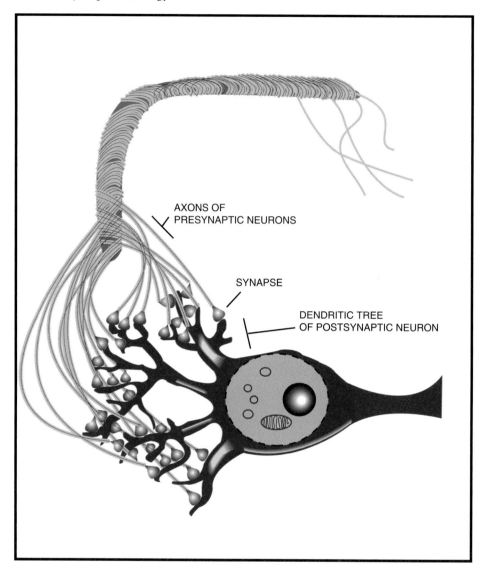

FIGURE 1−4. This figure shows the **anatomically addressed nervous system**. This is the concept that the brain is a series of hard-wired connections between neurons, not unlike millions of telephone wires within thousands and thousands of cables. Shown in this figure is a cable of axons from many different neurons all arriving to form synaptic connections with the dendritic tree of the postsynaptic neuron shown.

that neurotransmitter. (This will be discussed in much greater detail in Chapters 2, 3, and 4). Receptor occupancy by neurotransmitter binding to highly specific sites is very similar to enzymes binding substrates at their active sites. The neurotransmitter acts as a key fitting the receptor lock quite selectively. This opens a process that converts the chemical message back into an electrical impulse in the second nerve. It also sets into motion numerous biochemical consequences in the second neuron.

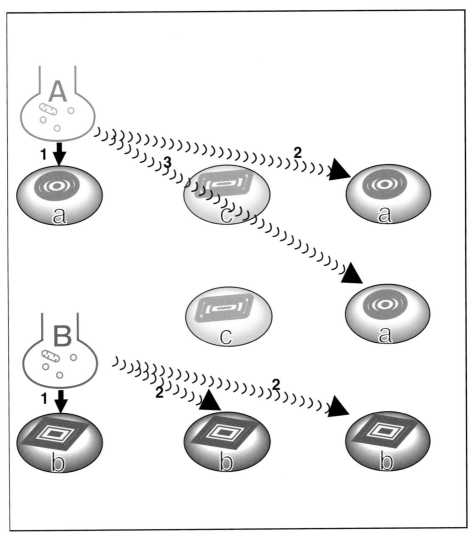

FIGURE 1−5. This figure shows a conceptualization of the **chemically addressed nervous system**. Two anatomically addressed synapses are shown (neurons *A* and *B*) communicating (*arrow 1*) with their corresponding postsynaptic receptors (*a* and *b*). However, there are also receptors for neurotransmitter *a*, neurotransmitter *b*, and neurotransmitter *c* that are distant from the synaptic connections of the anatomically addressed nervous system. If neurotransmitter *A* can diffuse away from its synapse before it is destroyed, it will be able to interact with other receptor-*a* sites distant to its own synapse (shown in *arrow 2*). If neurotransmitter *A* encounters a different receptor not capable of recognizing it (receptor *c*), it will not interact with that receptor even if it diffuses there (*arrow 3*). Thus, chemical messenger sent by one neuron to another can spill over by diffusion to sites distant to its own synapse. Neurotransmission can occur at a compatible receptor within the diffusion radius of the matched neurotransmitter. This is analogous to modern communication with cellular telephones that function within the transmitting radius of a given cell. This concept is called the "chemically addressed" nervous system in which neurotransmission occurs in chemical "puffs." The brain is thus not only a collection of wires (Fig. 1−2 and the anatomically addressed nervous system), but also a sophisticated "chemical soup," (Fig. 1−3 and the chemically addressed nervous system).

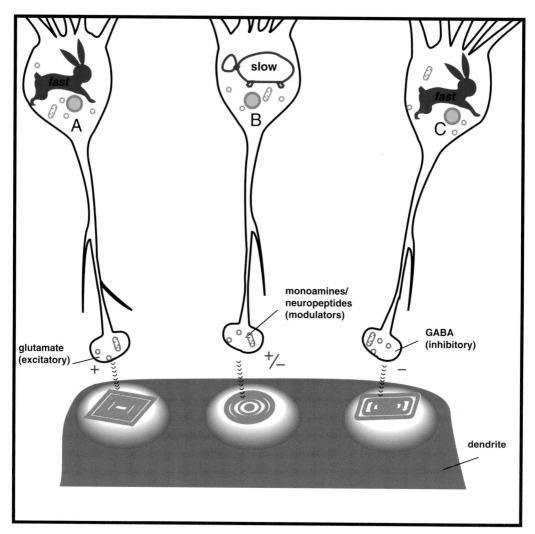

FIGURE 1–6. Some neurotransmitter signals are **fast** (rabbit/hare neurons *A* and *C*), whereas other transmitter signals are **slow** (tortoise neuron *B*). The neurotransmitter **glutamate** (neuron *A*) is both fast and **excitatory** (+), whereas the neurotransmitter **GABA** (neuron *C*) is both fast and **inhibitory** (−). In contrast to the fast glutamate and GABA signals, neurotransmission following those neurotransmitters known as **monoamines** or **neuropeptides** tends to be slow (neuron *B*), and either excitatory (+) or inhibitory (−). "Fast" in this context is a few milliseconds, whereas "slow" signals are many milliseconds or even several full seconds of time. Slower acting neurotransmitters are sometimes called **neuromodulators**, since they may modulate a different signal from another neurotransmitter. In this figure, three neurons (*A*, *B*, and *C*) are all transmitting to a postsynaptic dendrite on the same neuron. If the slow signal from *B* is still present when a fast signal from *A* or *C* arrives, the *B* signal will modulate the *A* or *C* signal. Thus, a long-acting neuromodulating signal of neuron *B* can set the tone of the postsynaptic neuron not only by a primary action of its own by also by modifying the action of neurons *A* and *B*.

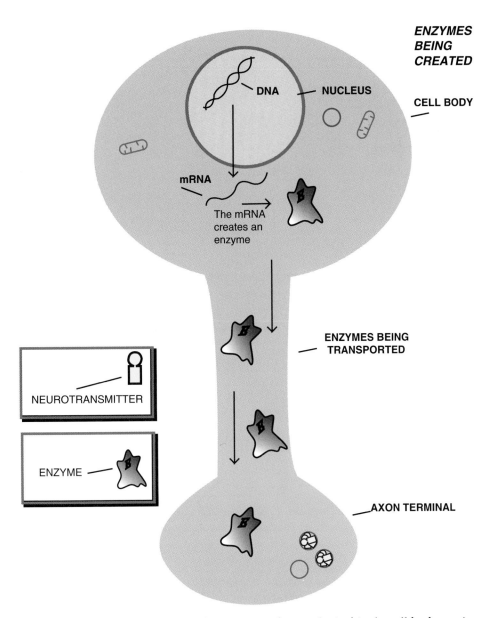

FIGURE 1–7. Enzymes are protein molecules that are **created** or synthesized in the **cell body** starting in the cell **nucleus**. Once synthesized, enzymes may be **transported** down the axon to the **axon terminal** to perform functions necessary for neurotransmission, such as making neurotransmitter molecules or destroying neurotransmitter molecules. **DNA** in the cell nucleus is the "command center" where orders to carry out the synthesis of enzyme proteins are executed. DNA is a template for **mRNA** synthesis, which in turn is a template for protein synthesis in order to form the enzyme by classical molecular rules.

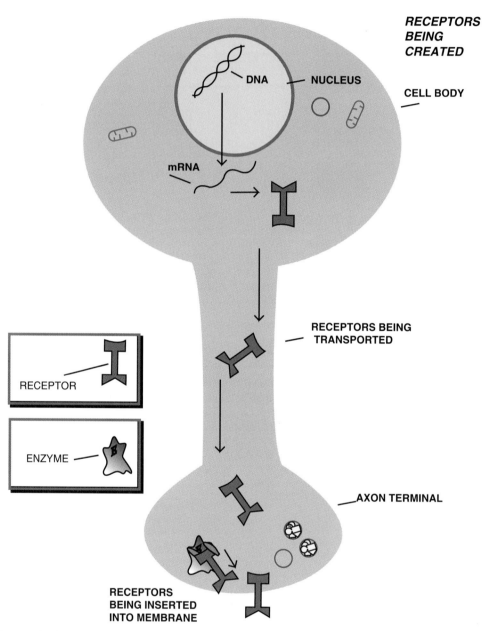

RECEPTORS
BEING
CREATED

DNA   NUCLEUS

CELL BODY

mRNA

RECEPTOR

ENZYME

RECEPTORS BEING
TRANSPORTED

AXON TERMINAL

RECEPTORS
BEING INSERTED
INTO MEMBRANE

FIGURE 1–8. Analogous to the process just shown in Figure 1–8, **receptors** are also protein molecules **created** (i.e., synthesized) in the **cell body** of the neuron. Receptors can also be **transported** to various parts of the neuron, including the **axon terminal**, where they can be **inserted** into neuronal membranes to perform various functions during neurotransmission such as capturing and reacting to neurotransmitters released from incoming signals sent by neighboring neurons.

10

Receptor occupancy by the neurotransmitter – the first messenger – causes various intracellular events to occur, starting with additional messengers within the cell (Fig. 1–9). The "second messenger" is an intracellular chemical that is created by the first messenger neurotransmitter occupying the receptor outside of the cell, in the synaptic connection between the first and the second neuron. The best examples of second messengers are cyclic adenosine monophosphate (AMP) and phosphatidyl inositol (PI). Some receptors are linked to one type of second messenger, and others to different second messengers.

The second-messenger intracellular signal tells the second neuron to change its ionic fluxes, to propagate or disrupt neuronal electrical impulses, to phosphorylate intracellular proteins, and many, many other events. Most of these events are still mysteries to neuroscientists. Our best contemporary knowledge is that part of the process starting from the manufacture and storage of neurotransmitter, through the release of neurotransmitter, interaction with synaptic receptors, and triggering of second messengers intracellularly in the second neuron.

The drugs known to work in the central nervous system affect nearly every conceivable component of this process of chemical neurotransmission. Also, mental and neurological illnesses are known or suspected to affect these same aspects of chemical neurotransmission. Therapeutic drugs are thought to exert their therapeutic effects by interacting with these processes, as are caffeine and the drugs of abuse, including alcohol and nicotine.

Multiple Neurotransmitters

The number of known or suspected neurotransmitters in the brain already number several dozen (Table 1–1). Based upon theoretical considerations of the amount of genetic material in neurons, there may indeed ultimately prove to be several hundred to several thousand unique brain chemicals. Originally, about half a dozen "classical" neurotransmitters were known. In recent years, an ever-increasing number of neurotransmitters are being discovered as new members. That is, the classical neurotransmitters were relatively small-molecular-weight amines or amino acids. Now we know that strings of amino acids called peptides can also have neurotransmitter actions, and many of the newly discovered neurotransmitters are peptides.

God's Pharmacopoeia

Some of the naturally occurring neurotransmitters may be similar to drugs we use. For example, it is well known that the brain makes its own morphine (i.e., beta-endorphin). The brain may even make its own antidepressant, its own anxiolytic, and its own hallucinogens. Drugs often mimic the brain's natural neurotransmitter. Often, drugs are discovered prior to the natural neurotransmitter. Thus, we knew about morphine before the discovery of beta-endorphin, the benzodiazepine Valium (diazepam) before the discovery of benzodiazepine receptors, and the antidepressant Elavil (amitriptyline) before the discovery of the serotonin transporter site. This underscores the point made above that the great majority of drugs that act in the central nervous system, act upon the process of neurotransmission. Indeed, this apparently occurs at times in a manner that often replicates or mimics the actions of the brain itself, when the brain uses its own chemicals.

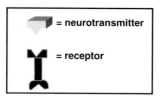

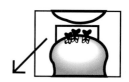

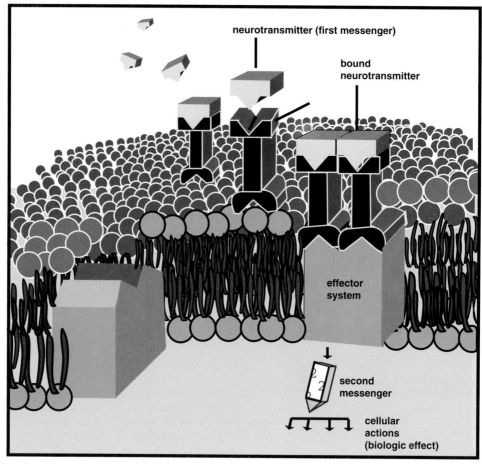

FIGURE 1–9. The functional outcome of neurotransmission is depicted here in the postsynaptic neuron. **Neurotransmitter** released from the presynaptic neuron is considered the **first messenger**. It binds to its **receptor** and the **bound neurotransmitter** causes an **effector system** to manufacture a **second messenger**. That second messenger is inside the cell of the postsynaptic neuron. It is this second messenger that then goes on to create **cellular actions** and **biological effects**. Examples of this are to have the neuron begin to synthesize a chemical product, or to change its firing rate. Thus, information in the presynaptic neuron is conveyed to the postsynaptic neuron by a chain of events. This is how the brain is envisioned to do its work: thinking, remembering, controlling movement, etc., through the synthesis of brain chemicals and the firing of brain neurons.

12

Table 1–1. *Neurotransmitters in brain*

Amines	*Amino Acids*
Serotonin (5HT)	Gamma aminobutyric acid (GABA)
Dopamine (DA)	Glycine
Norepinephrine (NE)	Glutamic acid
Epinephrine (E)	Aspartic acid
Acetylcholine (ACh)	
Pituitary Peptides	*Gut Hormones*
Corticotropin (ACTH)	Cholecystokinin (CCK)
Growth hormone (GH)	Gastrin
Lipotropin	Motilin
α-Melanocyte–stimulating hormone (α-MSH)	Pancreatic polypeptide
Oxytocin	Secretin
Vasoporessin	Substance P
	Vasoactive intestinal peptide
Circulating Hormones	*Opioid Peptides*
Angiotensin	Dynorphin
Calcitonin	β-Endorphin
Glucagon	Met-enkephalin
Insulin	Leu-enkephalin
	Kyotorphin
Hypothalamic-Releasing Hormones	*Miscellaneous Peptides*
Corticotropin-releasing factor (CRF)	Bombesin
Luteinizing-hormone-releasing hormone (LHRH)	Bradykinin
Somatostatin	Carnosine
Thyrotropin-releasing hormone (TRH)	Neuropeptide Y
	Neurotensin
	Prolactin
	Substance K

Co-transmitters

Each neuron was originally thought to use one neurotransmitter only, and to use it at all of its synapses. Today, we now know, however, that many neurons have more than one neurotransmitter (Table 1–2). Thus, the concept of co-transmission has arisen.

Incredibly, the neuron therefore uses a certain "polypharmacy" of its own. The rationale behind the use and action of many drugs, however, grew up in the era of thinking about one neuron using only one neurotransmitter, so that the more selective a drug, perhaps the better it could modify neurotransmission. This may be true only to a point. That is, the physiological function of many neurons is now known to be that of communicating by using more than one neurotransmitter.

To replace or influence abnormal neurotransmission, it may therefore be necessary to use multiple drug actions. If the neuron itself uses polypharmacy, maybe occasionally so should the psychopharmacologist. Today we still lack a rationale for specific multiple drug uses based upon the principle of co-transmission, so much polypharmacy is empiric or even irrational. As understanding of co-transmission

Table 1–2. *Co-transmitter pairs*

Amine/Amino Acid	*Peptide*
Dopamine	Enkephalin
Dopamine	Cholecystokinin
Norepinephrine	Somatostatin
Norepinephrine	Enkephalin
Norepinephrine	Neurotensin
Epinephrine	Enkephalin
Serotonin	Substance P
Serotonin	Thyrotropin-releasing hormone
Serotonin	Enkephalin
Acetylcholine	Vasoactive intestinal peptide
Acetylcholine	Enkephalin
Acetylcholine	Neurotensin
Acetylcholine	Luteinizing-hormone-releasing hormone
Acetylcholine	Somatostatin
Gamma aminobutyric acid (GABA)	Somatostatin
Gamma aminobutyric acid (GABA)	Motilin

increases, the scientific basis for multiple drug actions may well become established for clinical application.

Molecular Neurobiology

Enzymes (Fig. 1–7) and receptors (Fig. 1–8) are synthesized as proteins in the cell body by the neuron's cell nucleus (see also Fig. 1–10). The code for this synthesis of receptor protein is obviously the cell's DNA. Understanding receptor function fully involves knowledge of the exact structure of the receptor protein, and its amino acid sequence. This can be derived from cloning the receptor by standard molecular techniques. In this manner, subtle differences in receptor structure can be keys to

---

FIGURE 1–10. As in Figure 1–8, **DNA** in the cell nucleus is the "command center" where orders to carry out the synthesis of receptor proteins are executed. DNA is a template for **mRNA** synthesis, which in turn is a template for protein synthesis in order to form the receptor by classical molecular rules. Shown in this figure is the molecular neurobiology of receptor synthesis. The process begins in the **cell nucleus** when **DNA** is transcribed into messenger **RNA** (*arrow 1*). Messenger RNA then travels to the **endoplasmic reticulum** (*arrow 2*), where **ribosomes** cause the messenger RNA to be translated into **partially formed receptor protein** (*arrow 3*). The next step is for partially formed receptor protein to be transformed into **complete receptor** molecules in the **Golgi** apparatus (*arrow 4*). Completely formed receptor molecules are proteins and these are transported to the cell membrane (*arrow 5*) where they can interact with **neurotransmitters** (*arrow 6*). Neurotransmitters can bind to the receptor as shown in Figure 1–9. In addition to causing second-messenger systems to be triggered as shown in Figure 1–9, the bound neurotransmitter may also reversibly cause the membrane to form a pit (*arrow 7*). This process takes the bound receptor out of circulation in cases when the neuron wants to decrease the numbers of receptors available. This can be reversed or it can progress into lysosomes (*arrow 8*), where receptors are destroyed (*arrow 9*). This helps to remove old receptors so that they can be replaced by new receptors coming from DNA in the cell nucleus.

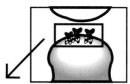

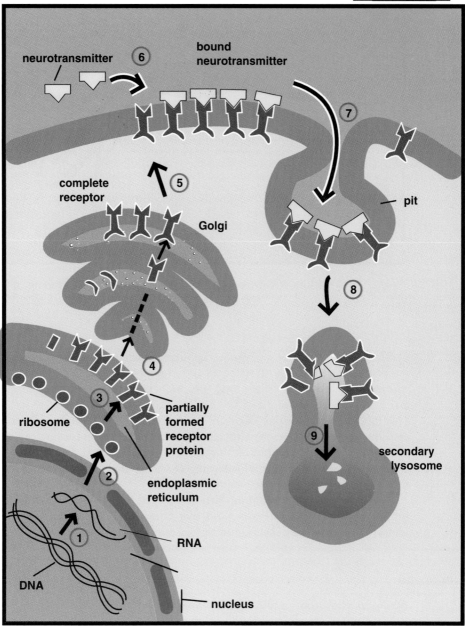

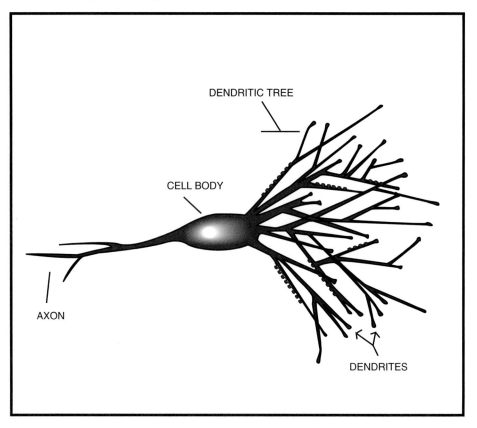

FIGURE 1–11. The neuron is composed of a **cell body**, an **axon**, and a **dendritic tree** (literally a tree of branching dendrites). The dendritic tree is in constant flux and revises its synaptic connections throughout life.

differences in species (e.g., man versus experimental animals), diseases (i.e., "sick" receptors), and subtypes of receptors (i.e., receptors that bind the same neurotransmitters, but do so quite differently, and with vastly different pharmacological properties). This will be amplified in Chapter 2.

Molecular neurobiology not only helps to clarify receptor functioning in neurotransmission by giving scientists the structure of the receptor but can also assist in comparing receptor families of similar structure, in describing changes in receptor structure caused by inherited diseases, and in documenting changes in receptor synthesis caused by drugs or by acquired diseases.

The conceptual point to grasp here is that the genome (i.e., DNA) is responsible for the production of receptors, and this production can be modulated by physiological adaptations, by drugs, and by diseases.

Plasticity

Analogies of neurons to telephone cables sometimes inaccurately imply that the brain is "hard-wired" at the beginning of life, and stays that way forever. Nothing could

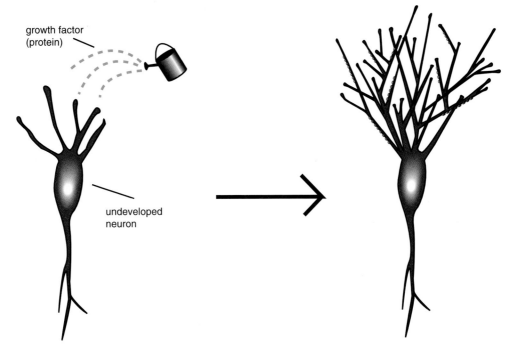

FIGURE 1–12. The dendritic tree of a neuron can sprout branches, grow, and establish a multitude of new synaptic connections throughout its life. The process of making dendritic connections upon an **undeveloped neuron** may be controlled by various **growth factors** that act to promote the branching process and thus the formation of synapses on the dendritic tree.

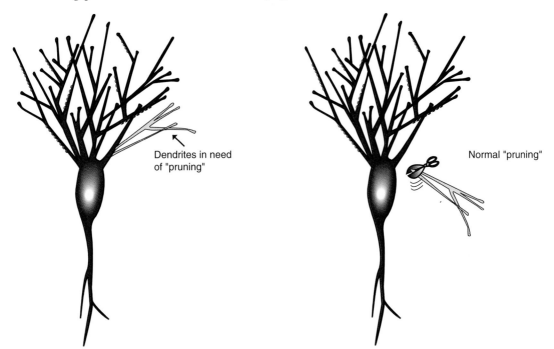

FIGURE 1–13. The dendritic tree of a neuron not only sprouts branches, grows, and establishes a multitude of new synaptic connections throughout its life as shown in Figure 1–12 but can also remove, alter, trim, or destroy such connections when necessary. The process of dismantling synapses and dendrites may be controlled by removal of growth factors, or by a naturally occurring destructive process sometimes called excitotoxicity. Thus, there is a **normal "pruning"** process for removing **dendrites in need of "pruning."**

be further from the truth. The neuron is quite "plastic," changeable and malleable. This process begins prenatally during gestation and continues throughout the life of the neuron. It is true that neurons do not replicate after birth and that new neurons do not grow when other neurons die, as is the case with most other cells. However, the axons and dendrites of each neuron are constantly changing, establishing new connections and removing old connections, in a manner reminiscent of the branches of a tree (see Fig. 1–11). Indeed, the "arborization" of neuronal terminals and the "dendritic tree" are terms implying a constant branching (Fig. 1–12) and pruning (Fig. 1–13) process throughout the lifetime of that neuron.

It is suspected that neurons elaborate various growth factors that promote their synaptic connections (Fig. 1–12) or eliminate them (Fig. 1–13), allowing for constant revision throughout the lifetime of that neuron.

Summary

The reader should now appreciate that chemical neurotransmission is the foundation of psychopharmacology. It has three dimensions: space, time, and function. The *spatial* dimension is both that of "hard-wiring" as the anatomically addressed nervous system, and that of a "chemical soup" as the chemically addressed nervous system. The *time* dimension reveals that neurotransmission can be fast (milliseconds) or slow (up to several seconds), depending upon the neurotransmitter or neuromodulator, of which there are dozens. The *functional* dimension of chemical neurotransmission is the process whereby an electrical impulse in one neuron is converted into a chemical message at the synaptic connection between two neurons, and then reconverted into an electrical impulse in the second neuron.

This chapter has also emphasized a few additional points: Chemical neurotransmission sometimes occurs with more than one neurotransmitter in a single neuron. Naturally occurring neurotransmitters are often mimicked by drugs (e.g., morphine and Valium). Molecular neurobiology and its techniques demonstrate that the genetic materials of a neuron are responsible for the production of neurotransmitter receptors and that this can be modulated by physiological adaptations, by drugs, and by diseases. Finally, the neuron is dynamically modifying its synaptic connections throughout its life, in response to learning, life experiences, genetic programming, drugs, and diseases.

CHAPTER 2

RECEPTORS AND ENZYMES AS THE TARGETS OF DRUG ACTION

Chapter 1 discussed how modern psychopharmacology was essentially the study of chemical neurotransmission at the synapse. This chapter will become more specific and discuss how virtually all central nervous system (CNS) drugs act in one of two general ways upon chemical neurotransmission: first, and most prominently, as stimulators (agonists) or blockers (antagonists) of neurotransmitter receptors; or second, and less commonly, as inhibitors of regulatory enzymes.

Given the far-reaching importance of receptors and enzymes in current thinking about how drugs work in the brain, this chapter will explore the properties of these targets of CNS drug action. This chapter will first explore the organization of single receptors, and how they form binding sites for neurotransmitters and drugs. Next, this chapter will describe how receptors work as members of a synaptic neurotransmission team including ions, ion channels, transport carriers, and second-messenger systems. Finally, this chapter will discuss how enzymes and receptors are sites of drug actions, and how such drug actions in turn modify chemical neurotransmission.

The Organization of a Single Receptor: Three Parts of a Receptor

Receptors are long chains of amino acids and, therefore, a type of protein (Fig. 2–1). Receptors reside partially within neuronal membranes (Figs. 2–1 and 2–2). In fact, neurotransmitter receptors can be thought of as containing three portions: extracellular segments, transmembrane segments, and intracellular segments (Fig. 2–2). The chain of amino acids constituting the receptor is not arranged in a straight line as might be implied by oversimplified representations in diagrams such as those in Figures 2–1 and 2–2, but rather in an alpha helical manner in the transmembrane segments, as a spiral around a central core (Figs. 2–3 and 2–4). The binding site for the neurotransmitter is inside the central core for many receptors (i.e., inside the ring of transmembrane helices of Figs. 2–3 and 2–4; also represented as a simplified icon in Fig. 2–5).

The *extracellular binding portion* of a receptor is the part of the receptor located outside the cell. It was originally believed that this portion of the receptor contained the selective binding site for its neurotransmitter; this is why chemical neurotransmission is so often pictorially represented by receptors binding their neurotransmitter extracellularly (e.g., see Figs. 1–9 and 2–5). However, as mentioned above,

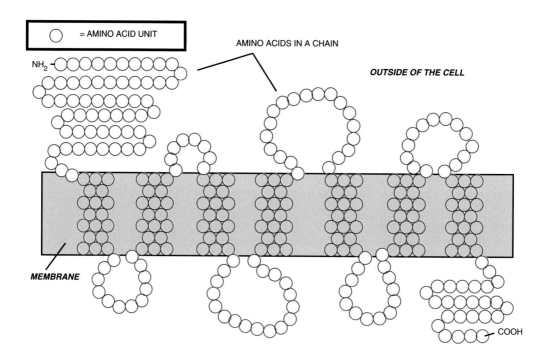

FIGURE 2–1. This figure is a schematic diagram of a receptor showing that it is a protein arranged essentially as a long **chain of amino acids**. The chain of amino acids winds in and out of the cell several times. This creates three regions of the receptor: first, the extracellular portions are those parts of the chain entirely **outside** the neuron; second, the intracellular portions is those bits of the chain entirely **inside** the neuron; and third, the transmembrane portion, which are the regions of the receptor that reside within the **membrane** of the neuron.

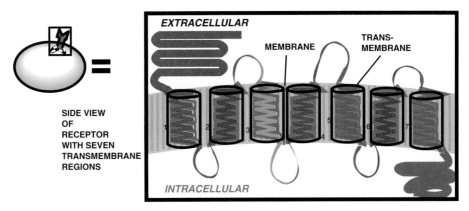

FIGURE 2–2. A side view of a receptor with seven **transmembrane regions** is shown here. This is a common structure of many receptors for neurotransmitters and hormones. That is, the string of amino acids goes in and out of the cell several times to create three portions of the receptor: first, the part that is outside of the cell (called the **extracellular** portion); second, the part inside the receptor that is inside the cell (called the **intracellular** portion; and finally, the part already mentioned that traverses the membrane several times (called the **transmembrane** portion). Throughout the text, this receptor will be represented in a simplified schematic manner with the icon shown in the small box.

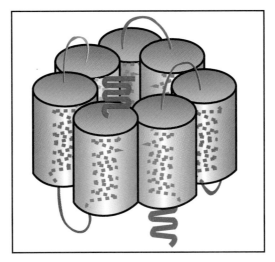

FIGURE 2–3. The **seven-transmembrane regions** are not arranged in a line, but rather in a circle. In the middle of this circle is a **central core** where neurotransmitters find their **binding sites**. This figure depicts each transmembrane region as a spiral, since each is actually an alpha helix. Also shown is how these spirals are arranged so that the seven of them form a circle. In the middle of the circle is the binding site for the neurotransmitter.

it is now known that the selective binding site for neurotransmitter is often located within the second portion of the receptor, its transmembrane regions (Figs. 2–3 through 2–5).

Some drugs may compete with the neurotransmitter for its own binding site, attempting to mimic the neurotransmitter that normally binds there, or to block that neurotransmitter. Drugs may also act at totally separate and unique binding

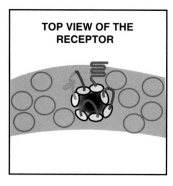

FIGURE 2–4. This figure shows a top view of the receptor. All that is seen in this figure are the **extracellular portions** of the receptors sticking out of the membrane. These extracellular regions of the receptor connect the various transmembrane regions to each other. In the center of the bits of receptor is the **central core** where the neurotransmitter for that receptor binds.

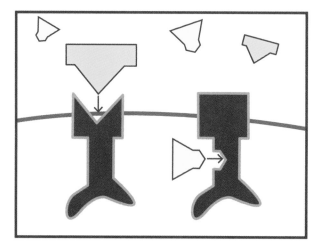

FIGURE 2–5. Some receptors have their neurotransmitter binding site located **extracellularly** (left), and others in the **transmembrane** region (right).

sites at other locations on the receptor to change the actions of the neurotransmitter upon its receptor. The locations of such binding sites are still under intense investigation, but may also be located in the transmembrane regions, yet separate from the neurotransmitter's binding site. This recognition site for the neurotransmitter receptor is quite unique from one receptor to the next, and indeed may be one of the major distinguishing characteristics of one receptor versus another.

The *transmembrane regions* (Figs. 2–2 and 2–3) probably also serve in part a structural purpose, holding the entire receptor in place, or allowing a certain movement of the receptor relative to the membrane itself. Transmembrane regions of one neurotransmitter receptor are often similar to those of other neurotransmitter receptors, forming large families of receptors (sometimes called superfamilies) that are structurally similar but which use different neurotransmitters.

One example of this is the superfamily of receptors organized with seven transmembrane regions. This is a structure common to many neurotransmitter receptors that use second-messenger systems and are "slow" (e.g., serotonin-2 receptors, and beta adrenergic receptors). The "seven-transmembrane region" superfamily of receptors is linked to second-messenger systems.

Another example of the organization of receptor structure shared by many different neurotransmitter receptors is that of five transmembrane regions common to many other neurotransmitter receptors that interact with ion channels and are "fast."

The third part of a neurotransmitter receptor is *intracellular* (Fig. 2−3). These intracellular sections of the receptor − sometimes termed "cytoplasmic loops" − can interact with other transmembrane proteins or with intracellular proteins in order to trigger second messenger systems (as shown in Fig. 1−9). The great majority of neurotransmitter and hormone receptors interact with second-messenger systems to modify the transition of molecular information from the neurotransmitter first messenger to the second-messenger system, and on to the genetic machinery (i.e., DNA) of the cell nucleus.

Synaptic Teamwork

Much importance and emphasis is given to the selective interaction of neurotransmitter with its unique binding site on its *receptor* because this is how information is encoded and decoded, both by neurotransmitters and by drugs mimicking neurotransmitters. Indeed, the majority of psychopharmacological agents are thought to act at such sites on various receptors. However, this is far from a complete description of chemical neurotransmission, nor certainly of all the sites where drugs can potentially modulate neurotransmission.

Chemical neurotransmission can be described more completely as a *team* of molecular players. The neurotransmitter may be the captain of the team, but it is only one key player. Other molecular players on the synaptic transmission team include ion channels (Fig. 2−6), ions themselves (Fig. 2−7), enzymes (Fig. 2−8), transport carriers (Fig. 2−9), active transport pumps (Fig. 2−10), and second messengers (Fig. 2−11). In addition to the role of these players in chemical neurotransmission, each molecule is a known or potential site of drug interactions. Each is also a theoretical

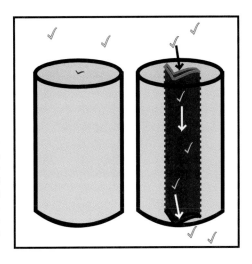

FIGURE 2−6. An **ion channel** is depicted here, with the channel **closed** on the left, and **open** on the right. Ion channels traverse the membrane, forming a lane for ions to get from the outside of the neuron to the inside of the neuron. A channel is required because the ion has a charge, which prevents it from getting through the membrane without the use of a channel.

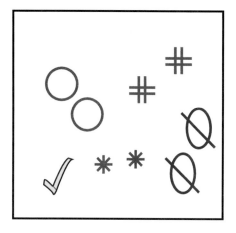

FIGURE 2–7. Various **ions** are represented. Channels for one ion are unique from channels for other ions. Ions include **sodium, potassium, chloride, and calcium**.

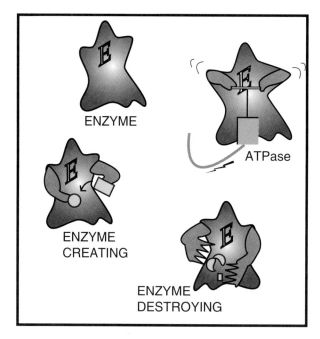

FIGURE 2–8. **Enzymes** are very important to the functioning of the cell. Some enzymes **create** molecules (i.e., build them up) and some enzymes **destroy** molecules (i.e., tear them apart). One enzyme responsible for using energy is **ATPase**.

site of malfunction that could possibly lead to a nervous or mental disorder, as will be discussed in general terms in Chapter 4 and in specific relationship to various psychiatric disorders in Chapters 5 through 10.

The spatial arrangement of these different molecules relative to one another facilitates their mutual interactions. These various elements of chemical neurotransmission (represented as icons in Figs. 2–5 through 2–11) can be arranged to cooperate on teams to accomplish various aspects of chemical neurotransmission.

Ion Channels

Some transmembrane proteins form channels across the neuronal membrane to enable charged ions to cross the membrane (Figs. 2–6, 2–12, and 2–13). Channels exist

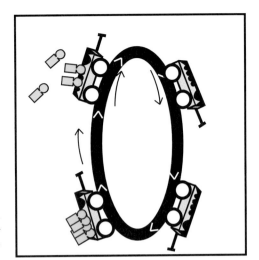

FIGURE 2–9. A **transport carrier** is used to shuttle molecules into cells that otherwise would not be able to get into the cell through the membrane.

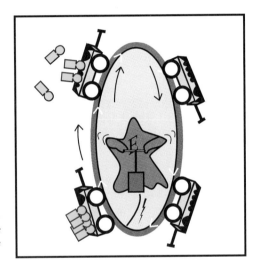

FIGURE 2–10. If a **transport carrier** is coupled with an energy-providing enzyme such as **ATPase**, it is called an **active transport pump**.

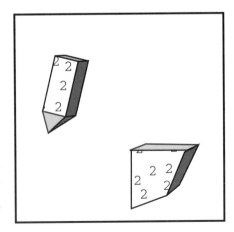

FIGURE 2–11. **Second messengers** are intracellular chemicals produced when some neurotransmitters bind to their receptors. Such receptors are capable of converting the binding information of their neurotransmitter into the synthesis of these second messengers.

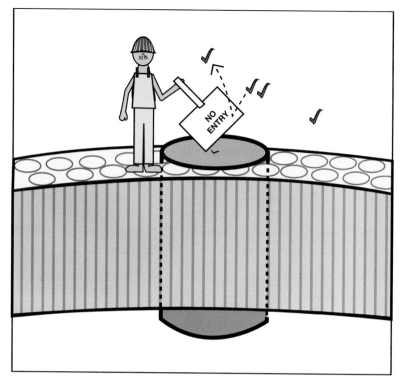

FIGURE 2–12. This schematic shows an **ion channel** that is **closed**. It has a molecular **gatekeeper**, shown here keeping the channel closed so that ions cannot get into the cell.

for many ions including, for example, sodium, potassium, chloride, and calcium (see Fig. 2–7). Ion channels in the CNS can be modulated such that the channel may be open or permeable at times (Fig. 2–13) and closed or impermeable at other times (Fig. 2–12). Some channels accomplish this by means of a molecular "gate" (Figs. 2–12 and 2–13).

Transport Carriers and Active Transport Pumps

Membranes normally serve to keep the internal milieu of the cell constant by acting as a barrier to the intrusion of outside molecules and to the leakage of internal molecules. However, selective permeability of the membrane is required to allow uptake as well as discharge of specific molecules to respond to the needs of cellular functioning. This has already been mentioned as regards ions, but also applies to other specific molecules. For example, glucose is transported into the cell in order to provide energy for cellular functions that include neurotransmission. Neurotransmitters are also transported into neurons as a recapture mechanism following their release and use during neurotransmission. This is done in order for neurotransmitter to be repackaged and reused in a subsequent neurotransmission.

In order to accomplish selective shuttling of certain molecules across an otherwise impermeable membrane, other transmembrane proteins known as *transport carriers* or *transporters* work to bind that molecule needing a trip inside the cell (Figs. 2–9,

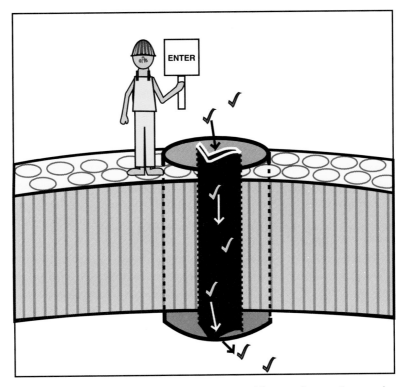

FIGURE 2–13. Here the **ion channel** of Figure 2–12 is **open**. The **gatekeeper** has acted – perhaps upon instruction from some neurotransmitter – to open the channel and allow ions to travel into the cell.

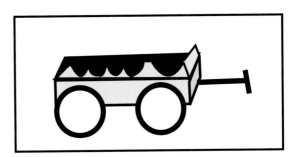

FIGURE 2–14. The **transport carrier** for neurotransmitter reuptake is like a box car with reserved seats for molecules of neurotransmitter. Here the transport carrier is **empty**.

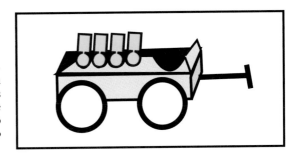

FIGURE 2–15. The neurotransmitter reuptake **transporter** can bind neurotransmitter molecules at specific binding sites. Here the neurotransmitter is bound to transporter sites, ready for a trip inside the neuron.

and 2–14 through 2–16). The transport carrier is thus itself a type of receptor. In order for some transport carriers to concentrate the shuttling molecules within the cell, they require energy.

An important example of molecular transport requiring energy is the reuptake of neurotransmitter into its presynaptic neuron. In this case, the energy comes from linkage to an enzyme known as sodium-potassium adenosine triphosphatase (ATPase) (Fig. 2–8). An *active transport pump* is the term for this type of organization of two neurotransmitter players, namely a transport carrier and an energy-providing system, as a team to accomplish transport of a molecule into the cell (Fig. 2–10).

Neurotransmitter Synaptic Reuptake as an Example of Molecular Transport Using an Active Transport Pump

In the case of the active transport pump for presynaptic transport of neurotransmitter, the job is to sweep synaptic neurotransmitter molecules out of the synapse and back into the presynaptic neuron. The reuptake pump is comprised of a carrier for neurotransmitter (Fig. 2–14) that can bind synaptic neurotransmitter molecules (Fig. 2–15). This reuptake pump can also be inhibited so that neurotransmitter molecules can no longer bind to the reuptake carrier (Fig. 2–16). This is how many antidepressants act.

In the neurotransmission process, the first event is the firing of the presynaptic neuron, which releases neurotransmitter (Fig. 2–17). This neurotransmitter diffuses across the synapse, binds its neurotransmitter receptor selectively, and triggers all the subsequent events in the postsynaptic neuron which translate that chemical message into another neuronal impulse in the postsynaptic neuron. This process has already been discussed in Chapter 1 and shown pictorially in Figure 1–9. The neurotransmitter then diffuses off its receptor, and can be destroyed by enzymes or transported back into the presynaptic neuron.

When neurotransmitter successfully diffuses back to the presynaptic neuron, a transport carrier is waiting there for it (Figs. 2–14 and 2–17), binds it (Figs. 2–15 and 2–17), and with the help of its teammate energy-providing enzyme system sodium-potassium ATPase, shuttles the neurotransmitter back into the neuron for

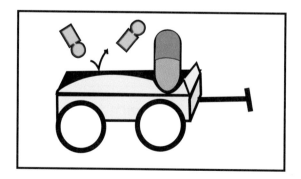

FIGURE 2–16. If an **inhibitor** of the **transport carrier** binds to its own binding site, it **prevents** neurotransmitter molecules from being able to bind to their sites. This figure shows an antidepressant, fluoxetine (Prozac), binding to the serotonin transporter. When this drug binds to the serotonin transporter, it essentially bumps serotonin neurotransmitter molecules out of their seats on the transport carrier. This causes **inhibition or blockade** of neurotransmitter transport into the neuron.

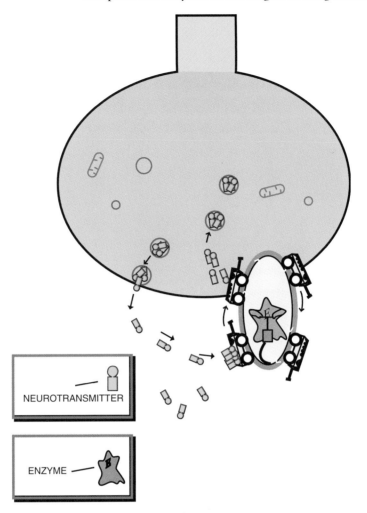

NEUROTRANSMITTER

ENZYME

FIGURE 2–17. This figure shows how the box cars of neurotransmitter transporters are arranged on a track to act as a **neurotransmitter shuttle system**. Once the neurotransmitter molecules are released by the neuron, they can be snatched by the transport carrier, given a seat on the shuttle, and driven into the cell on the track created by the **transport carrier** using energy provided by **ATPase**. Once inside the cell, the neurotransmitter gets out of its seat on the shuttle and is stored again in synaptic vesicles so it can be reused in a subsequent neurotransmission.

repackaging and reuse (Fig. 2–17). Several molecules therefore cooperate to make this reuptake complex function so as to transport neurotransmitter back into the neuron. The most important of these are the transport carrier (Figs. 2–9 and 2–14) and the enzyme sodium-potassium ATPase (Fig. 2–8). Inhibiting this transport of monoamine neurotransmitters is the mechanism of action of most antidepressant drugs (Figs. 2–16 and 2–18).

Reuptake of synaptic neurotransmitter is thus another example of how molecules cooperate with each other as players on a team in order to accomplish a complex but elegant dimension of chemical neurotransmission.

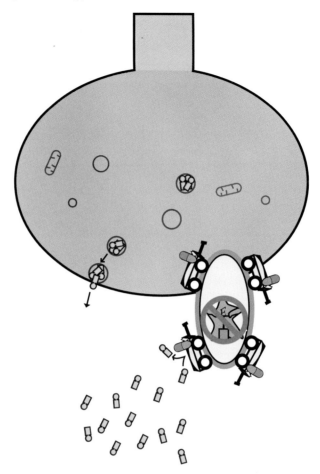

FIGURE 2–18. Shown here is how the antidepressant fluoxetine (Prozac) disrupts neurotransmitter from shuttling into the neuron. In this case, binding of the transport carrier by fluoxetine prevents serotonin neurotransmitter molecules from taking a seat on the shuttle. Thus, there is no ride for the serotonin into the neuron. This means that the neurotransmitter serotonin remains in the synapse until it diffuses away or is destroyed by enzymes.

Second-Messenger Systems

A neurotransmitter receptor can also cooperate with a team of specialized molecules comprising what is known as a second-messenger system (Figs. 2–19 through 2–22). The *first* messenger is the neurotransmitter itself (Fig. 2–19). It hands off its message to a second messenger, which is intracellular (see Figs. 1–9, and 2–19 through 2–22). It does this via two proteins that cooperate with each other (Figs. 2–19 through 2–22). These two proteins are the neurotransmitter receptor itself, and another class of transmembrane proteins known as a G protein. Once these two molecules have interacted (Figs. 2–20 and 2–21), this permits yet another interaction with an enzyme (Figs. 2–21 and 2–22). The enzyme manufactures a second messenger in response to its interactions with the cooperating receptor and G protein (Fig. 2–22), but cannot do this by interaction with either the receptor or G protein separately.

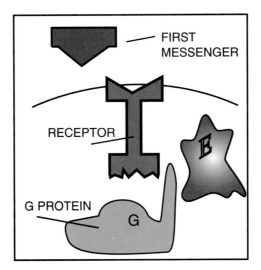

FIGURE 2–19. Shown here is a **second-messenger system**. It is comprised of four elements. The first element is the neurotransmitter itself, sometimes also referred to as the **first messenger**. The second element is the neurotransmitter **receptor**. The third element is a connecting protein called a **G protein**. The fourth element of the second-messenger system is an **enzyme**, which can synthesize a second messenger.

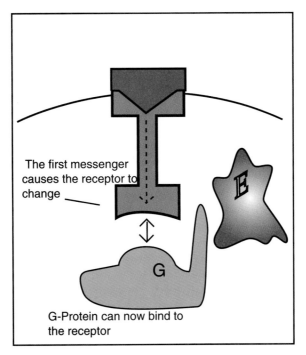

FIGURE 2–20. In this figure, the neurotransmitter has docked into its receptor. The first messenger does its job by **transforming** the receptor – indicated here by turning the same color as the neurotransmitter – in order to make it **capable of binding to the G protein**. This requires a **conformational change** of the receptor shown here as a change in shape of the bottom of the neurotransmitter receptor.

31

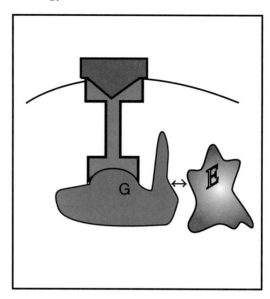

FIGURE 2–21. The next stage in producing a second messenger is for the transformed neurotransmitter receptor to **bind to the G protein**, depicted here as the G protein turning the same color as the neurotransmitter and its receptor. Binding of the binary neurotransmitter–receptor complex to the G protein causes yet another **conformational change**, this time in the G protein, represented here as a change in the shape of the right-hand side of the G protein. This gets the G protein ready to bind to the enzyme capable of synthesizing the second messenger.

A second-messenger system thus includes several elements (Figs. 2–19 through 2–22): (1) the first messenger (neurotransmitter); (2) the neurotransmitter's receptor; (3) a collaborating G protein interacting with the neurotransmitter receptor; (4) an enzyme triggered into action by the interaction of receptor and G protein; and (5) a second-messenger molecule manufactured by this enzyme. The two best known examples of second messengers are cyclic adenosine monophosphate (AMP) and phosphatidyl inositol (PI); the systems that produce these second messengers are also sometimes known as the cAMP second-messenger system and the PI second-messenger system, respectively.

Thus, the handoff of first messenger to second messenger is accomplished by means of a molecular cascade: neurotransmitter to neurotransmitter receptor (Fig. 2–19); neurotransmitter receptor to G protein (Fig. 2–20); binary complex of two proteins to an enzyme (Fig. 2–21); and enzyme to second-messenger molecule (Fig. 2–22).

As if this were not complex enough, the cascade put into motion by the first messenger and continued by the second messenger in fact does not stop here. The exact molecular events of this continuing cascade are the subject of intense current investigation and are just beginning to be unraveled. The cascade continues as second messengers change various cellular activities. For example, the second messenger can activate enzymes (Fig. 2–23) that are capable of altering virtually any function within the cell. One of the most important functions triggered by enzymes activated by second messengers is to change the membrane's permeability to ions such as calcium (Fig. 2–24). Altering fluxes of ions in the neuron is one of the key ways

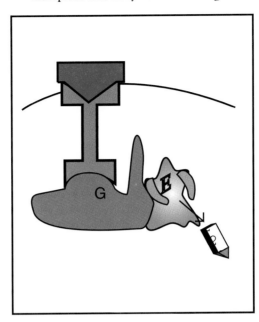

FIGURE 2–22. The final step in formation of the second messenger is for the ternary complex of neurotransmitter–receptor–G protein to bind to a **messenger synthesizing enzyme**, depicted here as the enzyme turning the same color as the ternary complex. Once the enzyme binds to this ternary complex, it becomes activated and capable of **synthesizing the second messenger**. Thus, it is the cooperation of all four elements, wrapped together as a quaternary complex, that leads to the production of the second messenger. Information from the first messenger thus passes to the second messenger through use of receptor–G protein–enzyme intermediaries.

to modify the excitability of the neuron that the second messenger is trying to influence (Fig. 2–24).

Alternatively, in some neurons, second messengers can activate yet another enzyme to phosphorylate proteins and enzymes inside the cell (Figs. 2–25 through 2–27). This process can alter the synthesis of various molecules in the cell that the second messenger wishes to regulate in order to modify the functioning of that neuron. Eventually, the message is passed along via messenger after messenger until the information reaches the cell nucleus and the DNA (genes) that is there (Figs. 2–25 and 2–26). Once the message has been received at this site, virtually any biochemical change conceivable is possible, since the DNA is the command center of the cell and has all the know-how and power to change any and all biochemical events of which the cell is capable.

The biochemical changes that are directed by messages from DNA are alterations in the synthesis of proteins. Since such proteins are often receptors themselves, the neurotransmission process can therefore come full circle (Figs. 2–25 and 2–26). Drugs and neurotransmitters first influence receptors directly by interacting with a binding site. The complex, multistep biochemical cascade set in motion by this simple event of drug or neurotransmitter binding to receptor, however, can lead to changes in the synthesis of its own receptor. When a neurotransmitter receptor's synthesis is decreased, it is sometimes called down-regulation (see Figs. 2–26 and 2–28). When a neurotransmitter receptor's synthesis is increased, it is sometimes

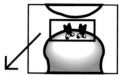

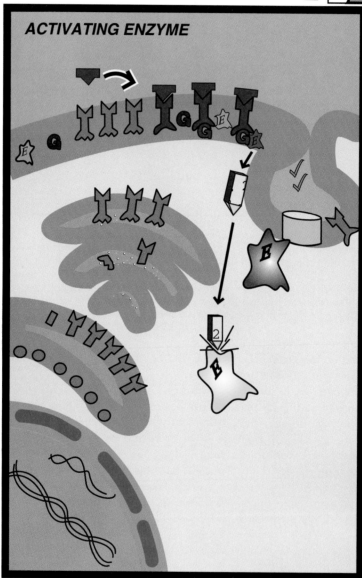

ACTIVATING ENZYME

FIGURE 2–23. Once second messenger has been synthesized, it can continue the information transfer by further molecular conversations. Shown here is second-messenger synthesis, depicted as blue neurotransmitter binding extracellularly, cascading the transfer of blue information through receptor, G protein, and enzyme, to produce a second messenger just as indicated in Figures 2–19 through 2–22. However, this figure goes past second-messenger synthesis to depict second messenger **activating** an intracellular **enzyme**. Note that the ion channel is closed in this figure and that no information is being directed at the cell's DNA here.

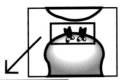

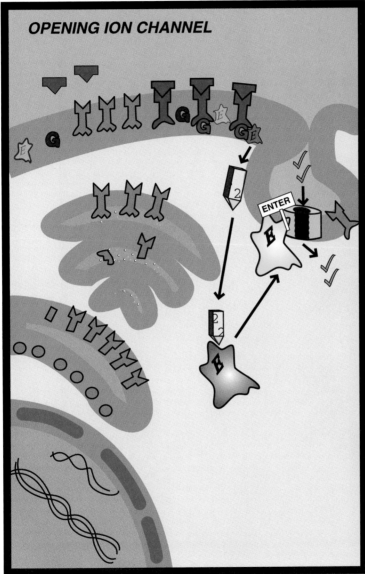

The second messenger tells the enzyme to open an ion channel, allowing Calcium to enter the cell.

FIGURE 2–24. One of the consequences of activating an intracellular enzyme by a second messenger is that some activated enzymes can instruct **ion channels to open**. This may be mediated by a complicated molecular cascade set in motion by a second messenger activating an intracellular enzyme, which itself creates still further molecular instructions to an ionic gatekeeper to **open the ion channel**.

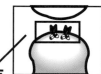

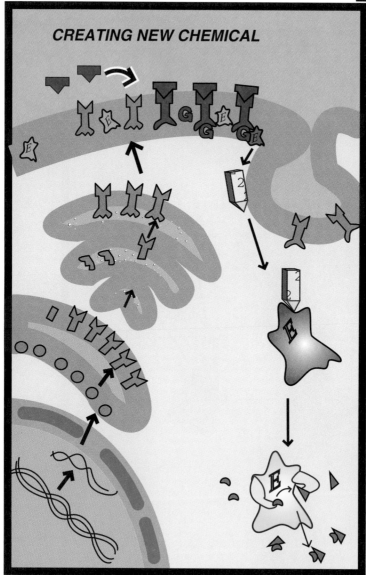

CREATING NEW CHEMICAL

The second messenger tells the enzyme to start making a new or altered chemical inside the cell.

FIGURE 2–25. One intracellular enzyme activated by a second messenger can in turn activate additional intracellular enzymes. Such an activation of a **sequence of intracellular enzymes** leads to the production of a sequence of intracellular molecules by these enzymes. Thus, one could say that there is the production of third, fourth, fifth, etc., messengers. Such additional intracellular messengers can potentially instruct the cell to perform a wide array of functions, some of which are represented in the next two figures.

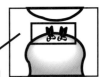

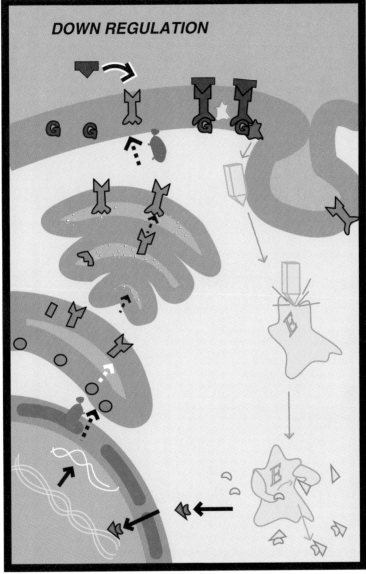

DOWN REGULATION

The new chemical affects the cell's DNA. Here, it causes DOWN-REGULATION of receptors.

FIGURE 2–26. The production of chemical instructions by intracellular enzymes can include orders for the cell's DNA. Shown here is the blue neurotransmitter cascade leading to second-messenger formation, and then second messenger activating an intracellular enzyme, which in turn has triggered yet another intracellular enzyme to produce red molecules. These red molecules contain instructions for the cell's DNA that order it to **slow down** the synthesis of the neurotransmitter receptor. Thus, fewer blue neurotransmitter receptors are being formed, as represented by the tortoise on the arrows of neurotransmitter receptor synthesis. Such slowing of neurotransmitter receptor synthesis is called **down-regulation**.

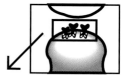

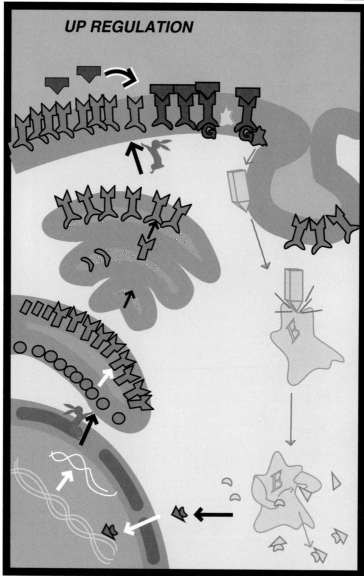

UP REGULATION

FIGURE 2−27. The production of chemical instructions by intracellular enzymes can also include orders for the cell's DNA to speed up the synthesis of neurotransmitter receptors. Thus, the blue neurotransmitter cascade leads to second-messenger formation, and then second messenger activating an intracellular enzyme, which in turn has triggered yet another intracellular enzyme to produce red molecules. In contrast to the molecules of Figure 2−26, the red molecules depicted here contain instructions for the cell's DNA that order it to **speed up** the synthesis of the neurotransmitter receptor. Thus, a greater number of blue neurotransmitter receptors are being formed, as represented by the hare on the arrows of neurotransmitter receptor synthesis. Such an increase in neurotransmitter receptor synthesis is called **up-regulation**.

38

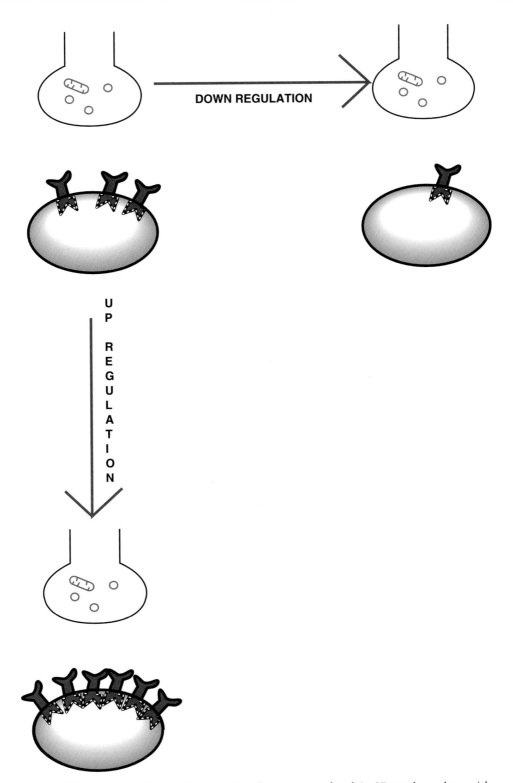

FIGURE 2–28. The complicated molecular cascades of Figures 2–26 and 2–27 are shown here with simplified icons. Thus, when **fewer** neurotransmitter receptors are formed, it is called **down-regulation**. When **more** neurotransmitter molecules are formed, it is called **up-regulation**.

39

called up-regulation which can mediate increased function ("supersensitivity") (Figs. 2–27 and 2–28). Neurotransmitter-induced molecular cascades into the cell nucleus can also lead not only to changes in the synthesis of the transmitter's own receptors but also to changes in the synthesis of other proteins, including enzymes and receptors for other neurotransmitters.

In summary, second-messenger systems (Figs. 2–19 through 2–22) have a general theme of using neurotransmitter first messengers occupying their receptors in order to precipitate a cascade of molecular events, carried out by a team of molecular players that interact with one another cooperatively, handing off the message from one molecule to another. This accomplishes the transfer of information sent via a transmitting neuron's neurotransmitter outside of the receiving neuron (Fig. 2–19) to inside that receiving neuron (Figs. 2–20 through 2–22) with many potential effects upon intracellular processes (Figs. 2–23 through 2–27).

Once the extracellular first messenger from the transmitting neuron has handed off to an intracellular second messenger of the receiving neuron, the message then penetrates deep inside the recipient cell in a complex molecular cascade until it reaches enzymes, receptors, ion channels, and DNA in order to carry out the message of how the neurotransmitter from the transmitting neuron wants to alter cellular function in the receiving neuron (Figs. 2–23 through 2–27).

The further one gets from the first messenger and its actions on its receptor, the less well understood are the nature and functions of the subsequent molecular events. At each point along the way, there are potential sites of action for psychotropic drugs or for malfunctions that may cause psychiatric and neurological diseases.

Changes in the rates of receptor or enzyme synthesis can powerfully modify chemical neurotransmission at the synapse; that is, decreased rate of receptor synthesis results in less receptor being made and less transported down the axon to the terminal for insertion into the membrane (see Figs. 1–8, 2–26, and 2–28). This would theoretically diminish the sensitivity of neurotransmission.

On the other hand, receptors may also be synthesized in excess under some conditions (Figs. 2–27 and 2–28). Too much receptor synthesis might not only increase the sensitivity of neurotransmission but may also produce a disease. Exactly this is suspected to be the case for the condition known as tardive dyskinesia (see Chapter 9 and Fig. 9–5), which is apparently caused when dopamine receptor blocking drugs cause an abnormally increased number or sensitivity of dopamine receptors.

Finally, altering the rates of synthesis of enzymes that can either create or destroy neurotransmitters can also affect the amount of chemical neurotransmitter available for neurotransmission, and can thereby alter the chemical neurotransmission process itself.

Enzymes as Sites of Drug Action

Enzymes are involved in multiple aspects of chemical neurotransmission, as discussed earlier in this chapter. Every enzyme is also a potential target for drugs acting as enzyme inhibitors. However, in practice, only a minority of currently known drugs are enzyme inhibitors.

Enzymes most important in the neurotransmission process are those that make and destroy the neurotransmitters. Thus, precursors are transported into the neuron with the aid of an enzyme-assisted transport pump, and converted into neurotrans-

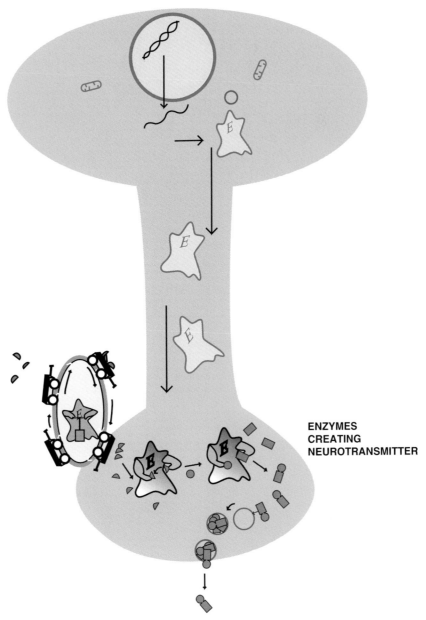

ENZYMES
CREATING
NEUROTRANSMITTER

FIGURE 2–29. Depicted here is the **synthesis of neurotransmitter molecules**. Specific enzymes are involved in the **creation of neurotransmitter**. This process begins with **transport** of molecular **precursors** into the cell by means of an active transport pump. This active transport pump is unique for the precursor and unrelated to the transport pump for the neurotransmitter itself. Once inside the cell, this precursor is handed off to an assembly line of enzymes, each modifying the precursor until the neurotransmitter is completely formed, and then stored in the synaptic vesicles until released during neurotransmission. Enzymes for the **synthesis** of one neurotransmitter differ from those for the synthesis of another neurotransmitter.

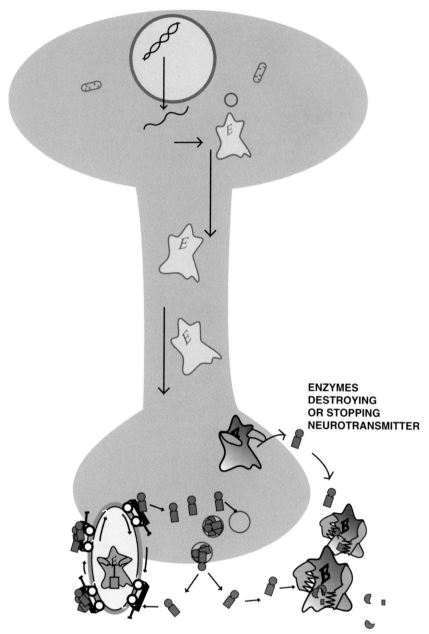

**ENZYMES
DESTROYING
OR STOPPING
NEUROTRANSMITTER**

FIGURE 2–30. Depicted here is the manner in which **neurotransmitter action can be terminated**, either by **transport** or by **enzymatic destruction**. Thus, neurotransmitter actions in the synapse can be stopped by the transport of neurotransmitter molecules out of the synapse for re-storage. This removal of synaptic neurotransmitters, like a vacuum cleaner, is performed by an **active transport pump** selective for the neurotransmitter. It differs from the active transport pump for neurotransmitter precursors involved in the synthesis of neurotransmitter. A variety of **neurotransmitter-destroying enzymes** are also capable of terminating the action of neurotransmitter. Such enzymes break down the neurotransmitter into inactive molecules.

42

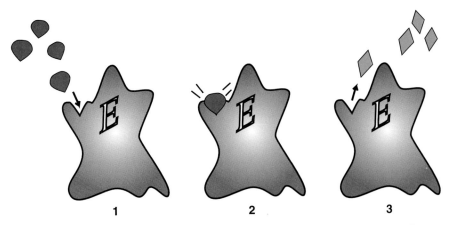

FIGURE 2−31. **Enzyme activity** is conversion of one molecule into another. Thus, a **substrate** is said to be turned into a **product** by enzymatic modification of the substrate molecule. The enzyme has an active site where the substrate can bind specifically (*1*). The substrate then finds the active site of the enzyme, and binds to it (*2*) so that a molecular transformation can occur, changing the substrate into the product (*3*).

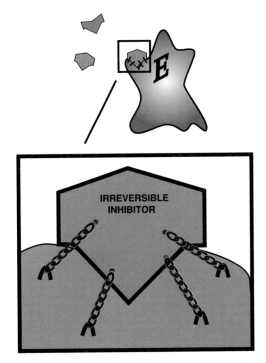

FIGURE 2−32. Some drugs are **inhibitors of enzymes.** Shown here is an **irreversible inhibitor** of an enzyme, depicted as binding to the enzyme with chains. The binding is locked so permanently that such irreversible enzyme inhibition is sometimes called the work of a "suicide inhibitor," since the enzyme essentially commits suicide by binding to the irreversible inhibitor. Enzyme activity cannot be restored unless another molecule of enzyme is synthesized by the cell's DNA. The enzyme molecule that has bound the irreversible inhibitor is permanently incapable of further enzymatic activity and therefore is essentially "dead."

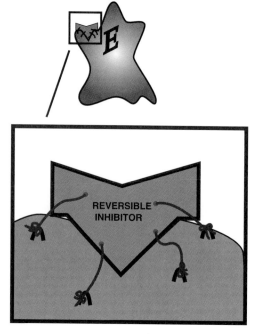

FIGURE 2–33. Other drugs are **reversible enzyme inhibitors,** depicted as binding to the enzyme with a string. It is possible for the inhibitor to be chased off the enzyme under the right circumstances, in which case the inhibition is reversed and the enzyme becomes fully functional again.

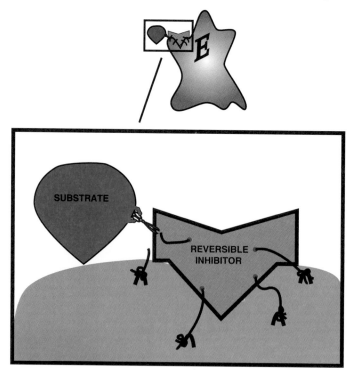

FIGURE 2–34. This **reversible enzyme inhibitor** is being challenged by the **substrate** for this same enzyme. In the case of a reversible inhibitor, the molecular properties of the substrate are such that it can get rid of the reversible inhibitor, depicted as scissors cutting the string that binds the reversible inhibitor to the enzyme.

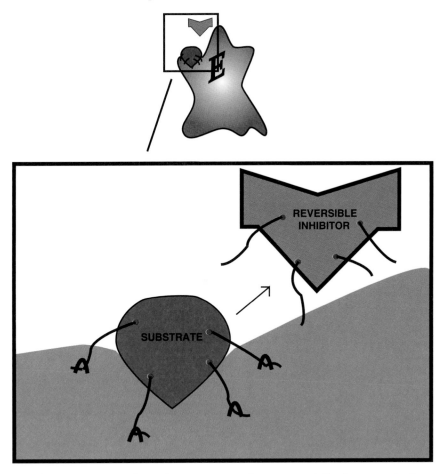

FIGURE 2–35. The consequence of a **substrate competing successfully** for reversal of enzyme inhibition is for the substrate essentially to **displace** the inhibitor and **shove it off**. Because the substrate has this capability, the inhibition is said to be **reversible**.

mitters by a series of neurotransmitter synthesizing enzymes (Fig. 2–29). Once synthesis of the neurotransmitter is complete, it is stored in vesicles, where it stays until released by a nerve impulse. In the vesicle, the neurotransmitter is also protected from enzymes capable of breaking it down. Once released, however, the neurotransmitter is not only free to diffuse to its receptors for synaptic actions but also to enzymes capable of destroying it (Fig. 2–30), or to the reuptake pump already discussed above and represented in Figures 2–14 through 2–18.

Enzyme activity is thus the conversion of one molecule into another, namely a substrate into a product. The substrates for each enzyme are very selective, as are the products. The inhibitors of an enzyme are also very selective for one enzyme compared to another. Enzymes doing their normal work bind their substrate prior to converting them into products (Fig. 2–31). However, in the presence of an enzyme inhibitor, the enzyme can also bind to the inhibitors, which prevents the binding of substrate and the making of products (Figs. 2–32 and 2–33). The binding of inhibitors can be either reversible (Fig. 2–32) or irreversible (Fig. 2–33).

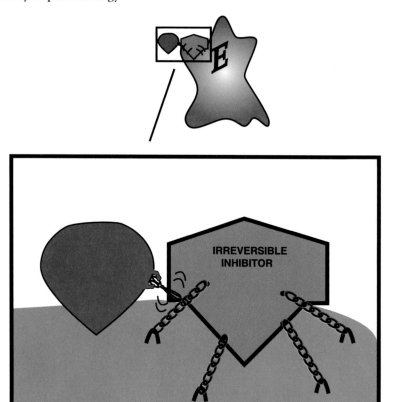

FIGURE 2–36. The consequence of a **substrate competing unsuccessfully** for reversal of enzyme inhibition is for the substrate to be **unable to displace** the inhibitor. This is depicted as scissors unsuccessfully attempting to cut the chains of the inhibitor. In this case, the inhibition is **irreversible**.

In the case of reversible enzyme inhibitors, an enzyme's substrate is able to compete with that reversible inhibitor for binding to the enzyme (Fig. 2–34), and literally shove it off the enzyme (Fig. 2–35). Whether the substrate or the inhibitor "wins" or predominates depends upon which one has the greater affinity for the enzyme or is present in the greater concentration. Such an interaction is called "reversible."

However, when an irreversible inhibitor binds to the enzyme, it cannot be displaced by the substrate, that inhibitor binds irreversibly (Fig. 2–36). The irreversible type of enzyme inhibitor is sometimes called a "suicide inhibitor" because it covalently and irreversibly binds to the enzyme protein, permanently inhibiting it and therefore essentially "killing" it by thus making the enzyme nonfunctional forever (Fig. 2–36). Enzyme activity in this case is only restored when new enzyme molecules are synthesized.

These concepts can be applied potentially to any enzyme system. Given the rapid clarification of increasing numbers of enzymes, we should expect to see an ever-growing number of enzyme inhibitors entering psychopharmacology in future years.

Summary: How Drugs Modify Chemical Neurotransmission

In summary, this chapter has discussed the role of receptors and enzymes in the fascinating and dynamic processes of chemical neurotransmission. Understanding the fundamentals of how receptors and enzymes affect neurotransmission cannot be underestimated, and help to remind the reader that much of contemporary neuropharmacology is predicated upon the premise that most of the drugs – and many of the diseases – that affect the CNS do so at the level of the synapse, and upon the process of chemical neurotransmission.

This chapter has specifically reviewed how receptors and enzymes are the targets of drug actions in psychopharmacology. We have explored the components of individual receptors and discussed how receptors function as members of a synaptic neurotransmission team that has the neurotransmitter as captain, and receptors as major team players interacting with other players on this team including ions, ion channels, transport carriers, active transport pumps, second messenger systems, and enzymes. The reader should also have an appreciation for the elegant if complex molecular cascade precipitated by a neurotransmitter, with molecule-by-molecule transfer of that transmitted message inside the neuron receiving that message, eventually altering the biochemical machinery of that cell in order to carry out the message that was sent to it.

SPECIAL PROPERTIES OF RECEPTORS

The study of receptor psychopharmacology involves understanding not only that receptors are the targets for most of the known drugs but also that they have some very special properties. This chapter will build upon the discussion of the general properties of receptors introduced in Chapter 2 and introduce the reader to some of the special properties of receptors that help explain how they participate in key drug interactions. Specifically, this chapter will discuss three important psychopharmacological principles of receptors: first, that they are organized into multiple subtypes; second, that their interactions with drugs can define not only agonists and antagonists but also partial agonists and inverse agonists; and finally, that allosteric modulation is an important theme of receptor modulation by drugs.

Multiple Receptor Subtypes

Definition and Description

There are at least two ways to categorize receptors. One is based upon describing all the receptors that share a common neurotransmitter. This is sometimes called pharmacological subtyping. The other organizational scheme for receptors is to clas-

sify them according to their common molecular interactions, a classification sometimes called receptor superfamilies.

Pharmacological Subtyping

To increase the options for brain communication, each neurotransmitter can act on
more than one neurotransmitter receptor. That is, there is not a single acetylcholine
receptor, nor a single serotonin receptor, nor a single norepinephrine receptor. In
fact, multiple subtypes have been discovered for virtually every known neurotransmitter receptor.

It is as though the neurotransmitter keys in the brain can open many receptor
locks. Thus, the neurotransmitter is the master key. Whereas some drugs act like
duplicates of master keys, others can be made more selective and act at only one of
the receptors, like a submaster key for a single lock (Fig. 3–1).

This makes for clever engineering of the communications that occur via the brain's
neurotransmitters and receptors. Because the system of chemical neurotransmission
uses *multiple* neurotransmitters each working as well through *multiple* receptors,
chemical signaling provides the features of both selectivity and amplification. That
is, while there is *selectivity* of a receptor family for a single neurotransmitter, there
is nevertheless *amplification* of receptor communication due to the presence of a great

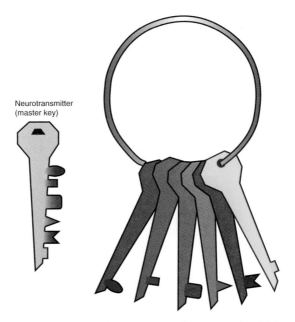

Neurotransmitter
(master key)

FIGURE 3–1. Neurotransmitters have multiple **receptor subtypes** with which to interact. It is as
though the **neurotransmitter** is the **master key** capable of unlocking each of the multiple receptor
subtype locks. Drugs can be made that mimic the neurotransmitter. The most selective drugs are
capable of mimicking the natural neurotransmitter's action at just one of the receptor subtypes. Thus,
such drugs act as submaster keys at only one of the receptor locks. This figure shows a neurotransmitter
capable of interacting with six different receptor subtypes (i.e., the master key). Also shown are six
different drugs on a key chain. Each of these drugs is selective for a different single subtype of the
neurotransmitter receptors.

variety of neurotransmitter receptors. Thus, each neurotransmitter not only has the property of selectivity compared to other neurotransmitters but the redundancy of receptor subtypes for every different neurotransmitter simultaneously allows for the amplification of each chemical's signaling capacity.

Receptor Superfamilies

There are two major superfamilies of receptors. The first is the superfamily whose members all have seven transmembrane regions, all use a G protein, and all use a second-messenger system (represented as an icon in Fig. 3–2). This was extensively discussed in text and figures in Chapter 2. Individual member receptors within this class may, however, use various different neurotransmitters and still be a member of this same superfamily. What makes one member of the family use one neurotransmitter and another member of this same family use another neurotransmitter is probably the molecular make-up of that portion of the transmembrane region that binds the neurotransmitter (see Figs. 2–3 and 2–5). The molecular configuration of the neurotransmitter binding site is different from one receptor to the next in the same family, and in fact is the reason one receptor uses a different transmitter from another receptor in the same family. The differences in binding sites between receptors are generally based upon substitution of different amino acids at a few critical places in the receptor's chain of amino acids (see Fig. 2–1). Precise substitution of amino acids in just a few key places can thus transform a receptor with binding characteristics for one neurotransmitter into a receptor with vast changes in its binding characteristics so that it now recognizes and binds an entirely different

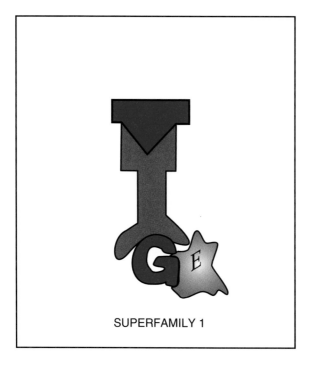

SUPERFAMILY 1

FIGURE 3–2. Represented here is one of the two major **superfamilies** of neurotransmitter receptors. This superfamily is called the **G protein–linked receptor superfamily**. Each member of this family has a receptor containing **seven transmembrane regions** (shown in Figs. 2–1 and 2–2) but given here as a simple receptor icon. Each receptor in this family is linked to a **G protein**, and also uses a **second-messenger system** triggered by a cooperating **enzyme**. A more detailed breakdown and explanation of this superfamily with a series of icons is shown in Figures 2–19 through 2–22.

neurotransmitter. This has been previously discussed in Chapter 2 and represented in earlier figures including Figures 2–1, 2–2, and 2–3.

A second superfamily of receptors share the common molecular make-up of every member having five transmembrane regions, and with several versions of each receptor configured around an ion channel (represented as icons in Figs. 3–3 and 3–4). The ion channel may differ from one receptor in this superfamily of receptors to another family member, and the neurotransmitter may also differ from one family member to another. However, all are arranged in a similar molecular form, concentrically around the ion channel.

Another common feature of this superfamily is that there are not only multiple copies of each receptor, but there are many different types of receptors present. Thus, the ion channel is surrounded by *multiple* copies of *many* different receptors (Fig. 3–3). This allows the critical passage of ions into the cell via the ion channel to be

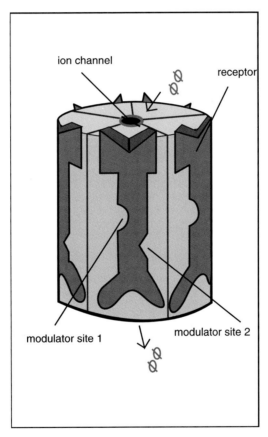

FIGURE 3–3. The second major superfamily of neurotransmitter receptors is represented in this figure. This superfamily is called the **ligand-gated ion channel receptors.** Each receptor has five transmembrane regions, not explicitly shown, but represented here as a simple receptor ion. Multiple copies of each such receptor are arranged as columns in a circle, and serve as **molecular gatekeepers** for an **ion channel.** The ion channel is located in the middle of the circle of receptors. On each receptor, there is not only the **receptor binding site** but also various different **modulatory sites** for additional neurotransmitters and drugs. In this figure, the ion channel is partially open.

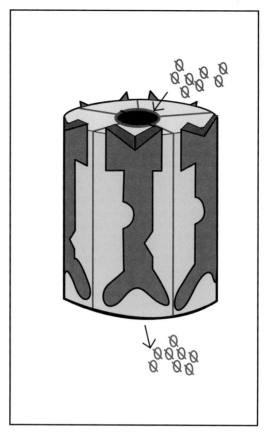

FIGURE 3–4. Another version of the ligand-gated ion channel receptor superfamily is shown here with the **ion channel opened** to a greater extent than in Figure 3–3. The **opening and closing of the ion channel** is controlled by the various ligands, which can bind to the different binding sites on the receptors in this family. That is why this superfamily is called "ligand-gated."

regulated by multiple neurotransmitters and drugs, and not just a single neurotransmitter. It seems that regulating an ion channel is too important a job to be left up to a single neurotransmitter. Thus, the brain has arranged for many different gatekeepers to watch over the passage of ions into the neuron. Sometimes the various gatekeepers that have a say in the regulation of the channel compete with each other to neutralize each other. Sometimes they cooperate to boost each other's actions.

The ion channel itself is essentially a column of columns. By neurotransmitter binding to the binding sites in the receptor columns, it causes the opening and closing of the ion channel column in the center of all the columns (i.e., within the column of columns) (Fig. 3–3). This arrangement is best documented for the nicotinic acetylcholine receptor, and for the gamma-amino-butyric acid (GABA) – benzodiazepine receptor, but is hypothesized as a general theme for several types of ligand-gated ion channel-mediated fast signaling.

As mentioned in Chapter 1 and as represented pictorially in Figure 1–6 on slow and fast neurotransmission, the superfamily of seven-transmembrane regions linked to second messenger systems utilizes *slow*, modulatory neurotransmission processes, and the superfamily of five-transmembrane regions linked to ion channels utilizes *fast* excitatory or inhibitory neurotransmission.

Agonists and Antagonists

Naturally occurring neurotransmitters stimulate receptors. These are called agonists. By contrast, the portfolio of options for drugs is far greater than just stimulating receptors. In fact, a whole spectrum of possibilities exists, sometimes called the agonist spectrum (Fig. 3–5). Some drugs do stimulate receptors just like the natural neurotransmitter, and are therefore agonists. Other drugs actually block the actions of the natural neurotransmitter at its receptor, and are called antagonists.

Antagonists only exert their actions in the presence of agonists, but have no activity of their own in the absence of agonists. Still other drugs do the opposite of agonists, and are called inverse agonists. Thus, drugs acting at a receptor exist in a *spectrum* from full agonist to antagonist to inverse agonist (Fig. 3–5).

Examples of the actions of agonists can be taken from each of the two major molecular superfamilies. For the slow-signaling family of seven-transmembrane-region receptors linked to G proteins and enzymic second-messenger systems, the agonist would turn on the synthesis of second messenger to the greatest extent possible (i.e., the action of a *full* agonist). The full agonist is generally represented by the naturally occurring neurotransmitter itself, although some drugs can also act in as full a manner as the natural neurotransmitter itself. Often the term "agonist" is therefore imprecise, and the better term is "full agonist."

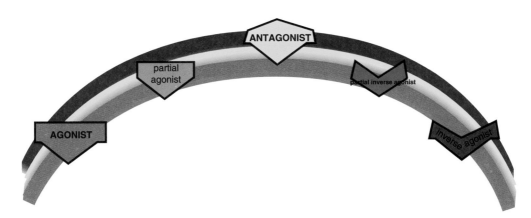

FIGURE 3–5. Shown here is the **agonist spectrum**. This spectrum reaches from **agonists** through **antagonists** to **inverse agonists**. Naturally occurring neurotransmitters are agonists. It is a common misconception that antagonists are the opposite of agonists, because antagonists block the actions of agonists. However, inverse agonists are the opposite of agonists. Antagonists can block anything in the agonist spectrum, including inverse agonists. If an agonist is partial and not as strong as the full agonist, it is called a **partial agonist**. Similarly, if an inverse agonist is partial an not as strong as a full inverse agonist, it is called a **partial inverse agonist**. Examples of the psychopharmacological actions of an agonist would be to **reduce** anxiety or to reduce pain. An inverse agonist, by analogy, would **cause** anxiety or cause pain. A partial agonist would weakly reduce anxiety or pain. A partial inverse agonist would weakly produce anxiety or pain. An antagonist would block the full and partial agonists from reducing any anxiety or pain, and would also block the full and partial inverse agonists from causing any anxiety or pain. However, an antagonist would neither reduce nor cause pain in itself.

For the fast-signaling family of five-transmembrane-region receptors, with multiple copies of each arranged as individual columns in a circle of columns forming an ion channel in the center, a full agonist acts by multiple molecules of the agonist each finding the transmembrane binding site for it within the receptor columns surrounding the ion channel column of columns. This in turn opens the ion channel column more completely; thus, the "full agonist" action (Fig. 3—6). At baseline, the ion channel is only partially open, and a full agonist therefore opens it much more (Fig. 3—6).

Antagonists

Antagonists block the actions of everything in the agonist spectrum (Fig. 3—5). By themselves, antagonists have no activity (Fig. 3—7). However, in the presence of an agonist, an antagonist will block the actions of that agonist (Fig 3—8).

Inverse Agonists

Inverse agonists do the *opposite* of agonists. An example of the action of inverse agonists can also be taken from receptors linked to an ion channel. By contrast to agonists and antagonists, an *inverse agonist* neither opens the ion channel like an agonist (Fig. 3—6) nor blocks the agonist from opening the channel like an antagonist (Fig. 3—8); rather, it binds the neurotransmitter receptor in a fashion so as to provoke an action opposite to that of the agonist, namely causing the receptor to *close* the ion channel (Fig. 3—9).

It might seem at first look that there is no difference between an inverse agonist and an antagonist. There is, however, a very important distinction between them. Whereas an antagonist blocks an agonist (Fig. 3—8), it has no particular action in the absence of the agonist (Fig. 3—7). An inverse agonist has the *opposite* action of an agonist (Fig. 3—9). Furthermore, an antagonist will actually block the action of an inverse agonist (Fig. 3—10), just like an antagonist will block the action of a full agonist (Fig. 3—7).

Partial Agonists

To add even more options to the actions of drugs at neurotransmitter receptors, and to influence neurotransmission in even more ways, there is a class of agents known as *partial agonists*. The partial agonists exert an effect similar to the full agonist, but weaker than the full agonist. Thus, in the example of the neurotransmitter system controlling an ion channel, a partial agonist would open the ion channel to a certain extent (Fig. 3—11), but only partially when compared to the full agonist (Fig. 3—6). Partial agonists are also blocked by antagonists (Fig. 3—12). It is even possible for the inverse agonists to be partial (Fig. 3—13). In this case, the partial inverse agonist closes the ion channel, but to a lesser extent (Fig. 3—13) than a full inverse agonist (Fig. 3—9).

This means that there is a spectrum of degree to which a receptor can be stimulated (Fig. 3—14). At one end of the spectrum, there is the full agonist, which elicits the same degree of physiological receptor-mediated response as the natural neurotransmitter agonist itself. At the other end of the spectrum is a full inverse

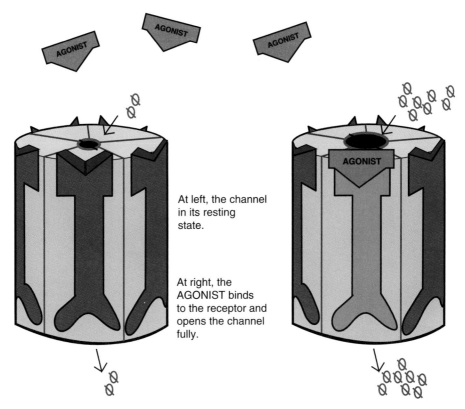

FIGURE 3–6. Actions of an agonist. On the left, the **ion channel** is in its resting state, a balance between being opened and closed. On the right, the **agonist** occupies its binding site on the ligand-gated ion channel receptor, and as gatekeeper, **opens the ion channel**. This is represented as the red agonist turning the receptor red and opening the ion channel as the agonist docks into its binding site.

agonist, which in concept does the opposite of the agonist. In the middle is the antagonist, which blocks the effects of all participants in the spectrum, but has no properties itself in changing the ion channel.

The spectrum thus goes from full agonist to partial agonist, to antagonist, to partial inverse agonist, to full inverse agonist (Fig. 3–14). Although this concept of agonists and antagonists and partial agonists is well developed for several neurotransmitter systems, there are relatively few examples of inverse agonists.

Light and Dark as an Analogy for Partial Agonists

It was originally conceived that a neurotransmitter could act at the receptor like a light switch to turn it on or off. We now know that the synapse and its receptors can function rather more like a rheostat. That is, a full agonist will turn the lights all the way on (Fig. 3–15), but a partial agonist will only turn the light on partially (Fig. 3–16). If neither full agonist nor partial agonist is present, the room is dark (Fig. 3–17).

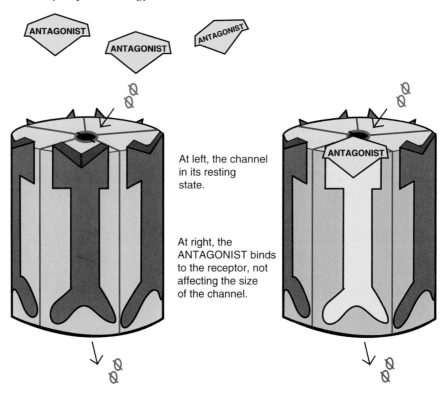

At left, the channel
in its resting
state.

At right, the
ANTAGONIST binds
to the receptor, not
affecting the size
of the channel.

FIGURE 3–7. Actions of an antagonist acting alone. On the left, the **ion channel** is in its resting state, a balance between being open and closed. On the right, the **antagonist** occupies the binding site normally occupied by the agonist on the ligand-gated ion channel receptor. However, there is **no consequence** to this and the **ion channel neither opens further nor closes**. This is represented as the yellow antagonist turning the receptor yellow and neither opening nor closing the ion channel as the antagonist docks into the binding site.

Each partial agonist has its own set point engineered into the molecule, such that it cannot turn the lights on brighter with a higher dose. No matter how much partial agonist is given, only a certain degree of brightness will result. A series of partial agonists will differ one from the other in the degree of partiality, so that theoretically all degrees of brightness can be covered within the range from "off" to "on," but each partial agonist has its own unique degree of associated brightness.

What is so interesting about partial agonists, is that they can appear as a net agonist, or as a net antagonist, depending upon the amount of naturally occurring full agonist neurotransmitter that is present. Take, for example, the case of neurotransmitters controlling an ion channel. When a full agonist neurotransmitter is absent, a partial agonist will be a net agonist (Fig. 3–18); that is, it *opens* the channel from its resting state. However, when full agonist neurotransmitter agonist is present, the same partial agonist will become a net antagonist (Fig. 3–18); that is, it *closes* the channel from its full agonist state. Thus, a partial agonist can simultaneously *boost* deficient neurotransmitter activity yet *block* excessive neurotransmitter activity (Fig. 3–18).

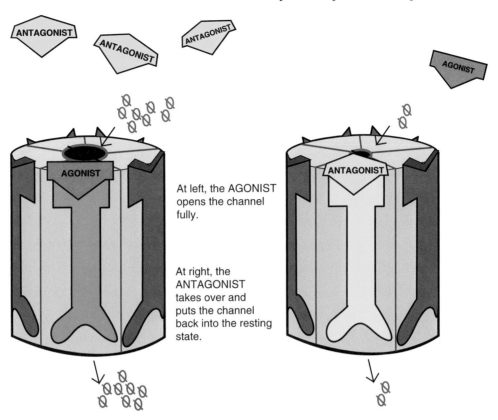

FIGURE 3−8. Actions of an antagonist acting in the presence of an agonist. On the left, the **ion channel** has been opened by the agonist occupying its binding site on the ligand-gated ion channel receptor, and acting as the gatekeeper, **opens the ion channel,** just as previously shown in Figure 3−6. This is represented as the red agonist turning the receptor red and opening the ion channel as it docks into its binding site, as in Figure 3−6. On the right, the yellow **antagonist prevails** and shoves the red agonist off the binding site, **reversing the agonist's actions.** Since the agonist had opened the ion channel, the antagonist reverses this opening by closing the ion channel back to the resting state. This causes the ion channel to return to how it was before the agonist acted.

Returning to the light-switch analogy, a room will be dark when agonist is missing and the light switch is off (Fig. 3−17). A room will be brightly lighted when it is full of natural full agonist and the light switch is fully on (Fig. 3−15). Adding partial agonist to the dark room where there is no natural full agonist neurotransmitter will turn the lights up, but only as far as the partial agonist works on the rheostat (Fig. 3−16). Relative to the dark room as a starting point, a partial agonist acts therefore as a net agonist.

On the other hand, adding a partial agonist to the fully lighted room will have the effect of turning the lights down to the level of lower brightness on the rheostat (Fig. 3−16). This is a net antagonistic effect relative to the fully lighted room.

Thus, after adding partial agonist to the dark room and to the brightly lighted room, both rooms will be equally lighted. The degree of brightness is that of being partially turned on as dictated by the properties of the partial agonist. However, in

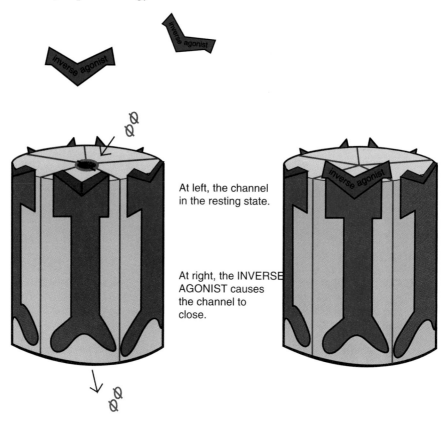

At left, the channel in the resting state.

At right, the INVERSE AGONIST causes the channel to close.

FIGURE 3–9. Actions of an inverse agonist. On the left, the **ion channel** is in its resting state, a balance between being opened and closed. On the right, the **inverse agonist** occupies the binding site on the ligand-gated ion channel receptor, and acting as gatekeeper, **closes the ion channel.** This is the **opposite** of what the agonist does (compare to Fig. 3–6). Inverse agonist action is represented as the light blue inverse agonist turning the receptor light blue and closing the ion channel as the inverse agonist docks into its binding site.

the dark room, the partial agonist has acted as a net agonist, whereas in the brighly lighted room, the partial agonist has acted as a net antagonist.

An agonist and an antagonist in the same molecule is quite a new dimension to therapeutics. This concept has led to proposals that partial agonists could treat not only states that are theoretically deficient in full agonist, but also states that are theoretically in excess of full agonist. An agent such as a partial agonist may even be able to treat simultaneously states that are mixtures of both excess and deficiency in neurotransmitter activity.

Allosteric Modulation

By now, it should be clear that a neurotransmitter and its receptor act as members on a team of specialized molecules, all working together in numerous ways to carry out the specialized functions necessary for the chemical neurotransmission of neuronal information. Another specific example of molecular interactions during chem-

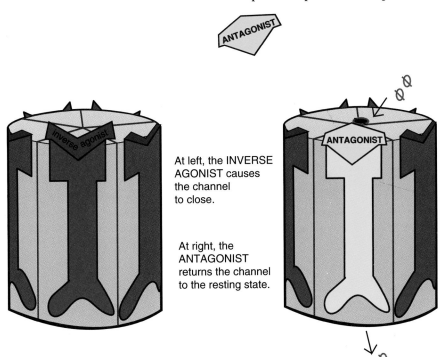

At left, the INVERSE AGONIST causes the channel to close.

At right, the ANTAGONIST returns the channel to the resting state.

FIGURE 3−10. Actions of an antagonist acting in the presence of an inverse agonist. On the left, the **ion channel** has been closed by inverse agonist occupying the binding site on the ligand-gated ion channel receptor and, acting as gatekeeper, **closes the ion channel,** just as shown in Figure 3−9. This is represented as the light blue inverse agonist turning the receptor light blue and closing the ion channel as it docks into its binding site, as in Figure 3−9. On the right, the yellow antagonist prevails and shoves the light blue inverse agonist off the binding site, **reversing the inverse agonist's actions.** Since the inverse agonist had previously closed the ion channel, the antagonist reverses this closing by opening the ion channel back to the resting state. This causes the ion channel to return to how it was before the agonist acted. In this way, the antagonist acts similarly on an inverse agonist's actions as it does on an agonists actions, namely by **returning the ion channel to its resting state** (compare to Fig. 3−8). However, in the case of an inverse agonist, the antagonist **opens** the channel but in the case of an agonist, the same antagonist **closes** the channel (compare Figs. 3−8 and 3−10). Thus, an antagonist can **reverse either an agonist or an inverse agonist** despite the fact that it does nothing on its own (Fig. 3−7).

ical neurotransmission is the configuration of two or more neurotransmitter receptor sites such that one can boost or blunt the activities of the other. In some instances, the two interacting receptor binding sites may be located on the same receptor molecule; in other cases, the binding sites may be on neighboring receptors of different classes.

When two different receptor sites utilizing different neurotransmitters are arranged so as to influence a single receptor, there is generally considered to be a primary neurotransmitter receptor site that influences its receptor in the usual manner (i.e., it turns on a second messenger or alters an ion channel). In this example, furthermore, there is also a second receptor site that can influence the receptor, but generally only when the primary neurotransmitter is binding at the primary receptor

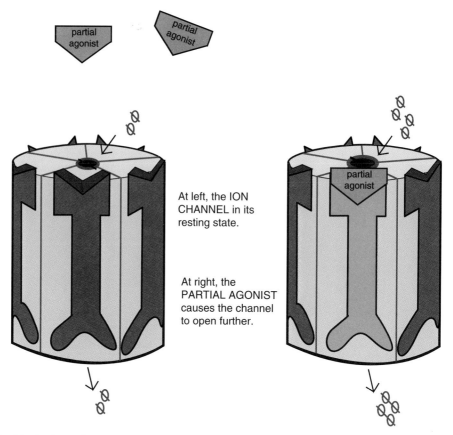

At left, the ION CHANNEL in its resting state.

At right, the PARTIAL AGONIST causes the channel to open further.

FIGURE 3–11. Actions of a partial agonist. On the left, the **ion channel** is in its resting state, a balance between being opened and closed. On the right, the **partial agonist** occupies its binding site on the ligand-gated ion channel receptor, and acting as gatekeeper, **partially opens the ion channel**. This is represented as the orange agonist turning the receptor orange and partially – but not fully – opening the ion channel as the partial agonist docks into its binding site. The ion channel is thus more open than it was in the resting state once a partial agonist acts, but less open than after the full agonist acts (compare with Fig. 3–6).

site. Thus, this second neurotransmitter interacting at the secondary site only acts *indirectly* and through an interaction with the receptor when the primary neurotransmitter is simultaneously binding at its primary (and different) receptor site. Since the binding of the secondary neurotransmitter to its secondary receptor site is influencing the receptor by a mechanism other than direct binding to the primary receptor site, it is said to be modulating that receptor *allosterically* (literally, "other site"). The "other site" is the second receptor binding site which utilizes a second neurotransmitter yet influences the same receptor as the primary neurotransmitter does at its primary receptor binding site, but only when the primary neurotransmitter is present at that primary binding site. As mentioned earlier, this allosteric modulation can either be amplifying or blocking of the actions of the primary neurotransmitter at the primary receptor binding site.

This allosteric cooperation among synaptic transmission teammates – in which one player interacts with a second player in order to modify or control it – is another

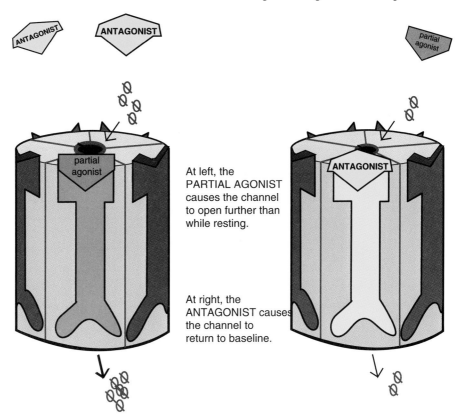

FIGURE 3–12. Actions of an antagonist acting in the presence of a partial agonist. On the left, the **ion channel** has been opened by the partial agonist occupying its binding site on the ligand-gated ion channel receptor and, acting as gatekeeper, **partially opens the ion channel,** just as shown in Figure 3–11. This is represented as the orange agonist turning the receptor orange and partially opening the ion channel as the partial agonist docks into its binding site, as shown in Figure 3–11. On the right, the yellow antagonist prevails and shoves the orange partial agonist off the binding site, reversing the partial agonist's actions. Since the partial agonist had partially opened the ion channel, the antagonist reverses this partial opening back to the resting state of the ion channel prior to the partial agonist's actions.

example of a common recurring theme in chemical neurotransmission: a cascade of molecular interactions is triggered by the neurotransmitter–receptor binding site events.

Positive Allosteric Interactions

An example of positive allosteric modulation is shown by the influence of modulatory sites upon the gatekeepers at ligand-gated ion channels. In this case, the primary neurotransmitter is the gatekeeper, which opens the ion channel as discussed previously. To explain allosteric modulation, we will introduce a second receptor binding site that can interact with the gatekeeper and its receptor.

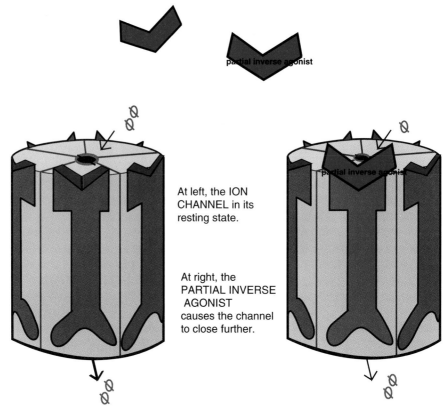

FIGURE 3–13. Actions of a partial inverse agonist. On the left, the **ion channel** is in its resting state, a balance between being opened and closed. On the right, the **partial inverse agonist** occupies its binding site on the ligand-gated ion channel receptor and, acting as gatekeeper, **partially closes** the ion channel. This is represented as the green inverse agonist turning the receptor green and partially closing the ion channel as the partial invese agonist docks into its binding site.

Thus, following occupancy of the gatekeeper receptor by the primary gatekeeper, that receptor in turn interacts with an ion channel to open it a bit as previously discussed for agonist actions (Fig. 3–19).

Nearby the gatekeeper's receptor site is not only the ion channel but also another neurotransmitter receptor binding site, namely a receptor capable of allosterically modulating the gatekeeper's receptor (Fig. 3–19). Allosteric modulatory sites do not directly influence the ion channel. They do so indirectly by influencing the gatekeeper receptor, which in turn influences the ion channel. Thus, the allosteric modulatory site acts literally at "another site" to influence the ion channel. Since the meaning of allosteric is other site, one can easily understand why this term is applied to such modulatory receptor sites and their neurotransmitters. The allosteric modulatory site thus has a knock-on effect upon the conductance of ions through the ion channel.

The mechanism of allosteric modulation is such that when an allosteric modulator binds to its own receptor site, which is a neighbor of the gatekeeper receptor binding site, nothing happens if the gatekeeper is not also binding to its own gatekeeper

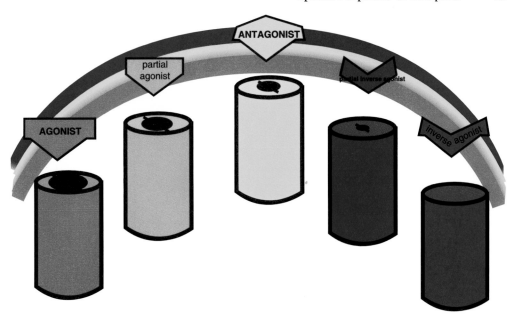

FIGURE 3–14. The agonist spectrum and its effects on the ion channel. Shown again is the **agonist spectrum**, this time with the corresponding effects of each agent upon the ion channel. This spectrum ranges from **agonists**, which fully open the ion channel, through **antagonists**, which retain the resting state between open and closed; to **inverse agonists**, which close the ion channel. Between the extremes are **partial agonists**, which partially open the ion channel; and **partial inverse agonists**, which partially close the ion channel. Antagonists can block anything in the agonist spectrum, returning the ion channel to the resting state in each instance.

receptor. On the other hand, when the gatekeeper is binding to its receptor site, the simultaneous binding of the allosteric modulator to its binding site causes a large amplification in the gatekeeper's ability to increase the conductance of ion through the channel (Fig. 3–19).

Why is this necessary? It turns out that most gatekeepers can increase ionic conductance through ion channels only a certain extent by themselves. Allosteric modulators cannot alter ionic conductance at all when working by themselves. However, allosteric modulation is a formula to maximize ionic conductance beyond that which the gatekeeper alone can accomplish. Thus, the gatekeeper can increase ionic conductance through an ion channel much more dramatically when an allosteric modulator is helping than it can when it is working to modulate an ion channel by itself.

Evident in this discussion of allosteric modulation of one receptor binding site by another receptor binding site is the possibility of *numerous* allosteric sites for a single receptor. As will be developed in greater detail in subsequent chapters, it is hypothesized that the anxiolytic, hypnotic, anticonvulsant, and muscle relaxant properties of numerous drugs, including the benzodiazepines, barbiturates, and anticonvulsants, are all mediated by **allosteric interactions** at molecular sites around the GABA receptor and the chloride channel. It is possible that a variety of allosteric sites, analogous to the benzodiazepine sites, modulate GABA-induced increases at chloride channels by a wide variety of drugs, even including alcohol.

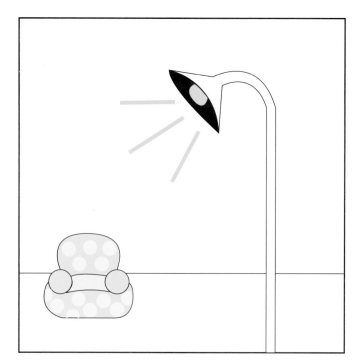

FIGURE 3–15. Light as an analogy for the agonist spectrum: actions of a full agonist. Light will be **brightest** after a full agonist turns the light switch **fully on**. When a **partial agonist** is added to the fully lighted (i.e., full agonist) room, it will "dim" the lights; thus, the partial agonist in this case acts as a **net antagonist**.

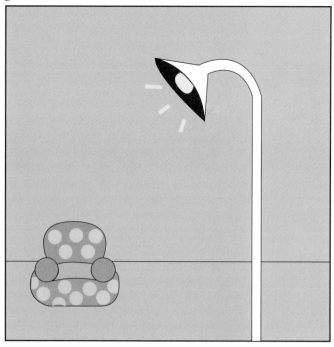

FIGURE 3–16. Light as an analogy for the agonist spectrum: actions of a partial agonist. By itself, a partial agonist neither turns the light fully on nor fully off. Rather, a **partial agonist** acts like a rheostat, or dimming switch, which turns on the light, but only **partially**.

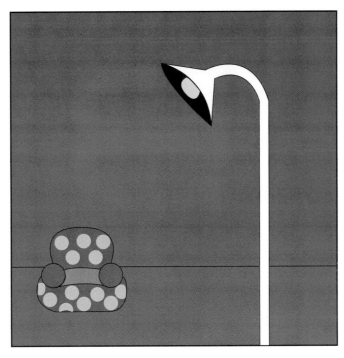

FIGURE 3–17. Light as an analogy for the agonist spectrum: actions when no agonist is present. When **no agonist** is present, the situation is analogous to the light switch being off. Adding the **partial agonist** when the lights are off has the effect of turning the lights partially "on," to the level preset in the partial agonist rheostat. Thus, in the **absence of a full agonist**, adding a partial agonist will "turn up" the lights. In this case, the **partial agonist acts as a net agonist**.

Negative Allosteric Interactions

An example of negative allosteric modulation is the case of the antidepressants, which act as neurotransmitter reuptake blockers for the neurotransmitters norepinephrine and serotonin. This has already been discussed in Chapter 2. When the neurotransmitters norepinephrine or serotonin bind to their own selective receptor sites, they are normally transported back into the presynaptic neuron as shown previously in Figure 2–17. Thus, the empty reuptake carrier (Fig. 2–14) binds to the neurotransmitter (Fig. 2–15) to begin the transport process (Figs. 2–9, 2–10, and 2–17). However, when certain antidepressants bind to an allosteric site close to the neurotransmitter transporter (represented as an icon in Fig. 2–16), this causes the neurotransmitter to no longer be able to bind there, thus blocking synaptic reuptake transport of the neurotransmitter (Fig. 2–18). Therefore, norepinephrine and serotonin cannot be shuttled back into the presynaptic neuron.

An antidepressant drug – which blocks norepinephrine and serotonin reuptake – can be said to modulate in a *negative allosteric* manner the presynaptic neurotransmitter transporter and thereby block neurotransmitter reuptake (Figs. 2–16 and 2–18). As will be developed in detail in later chapters, this action may have therapeutic implications for a number of disorders including depression, panic disorder, and obsessive compulsive disorder.

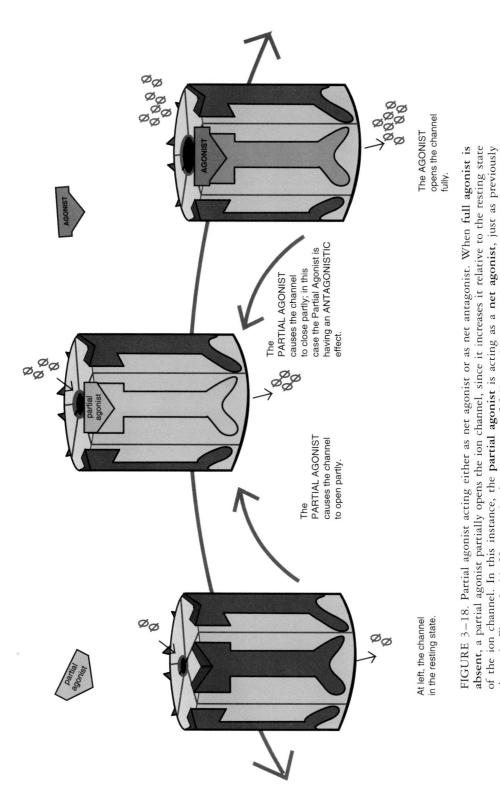

FIGURE 3–18. Partial agonist acting either as net agonist or as net antagonist. When **full agonist is absent**, a partial agonist partially opens the ion channel, since it increases it relative to the resting state of the ion channel. In this instance, the **partial agonist** is acting as a **net agonist**, just as previously shown in Figure 3–11. However, in the **presence of full agonist**, a partial agonist partially closes the ion channel, since it decreases it relative to the open state of the ion channel. In this instance, the **partial agonist** is acting as a **net antagonist**.

At left, the channel in the resting state.

The PARTIAL AGONIST causes the channel to open partly.

The PARTIAL AGONIST causes the channel to close partly; in this case the Partial Agonist is having an ANTAGONISTIC effect.

The AGONIST opens the channel fully.

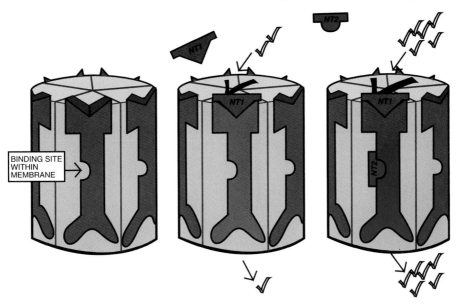

FIGURE 3–19. Allosteric modulation of the ligand-gated ion channel receptor. On the left, the receptor is shown not only with its agonist binding site for neurotransmitter 1 (NT1), but also with a **second binding site** within the membrane for neurotransmitter 2 (NT2). The ion channel is shown on the left to be **closed** in the absence of binding of either NT1 or NT2. When neurotransmitter full agonist (**NT1**) binds to its binding site, it of course **opens the ion channel**, as shown in the middle of the figure and has previously been shown in Figure 3–6. This is represented in the middle of the figure as purple NT1 binding to its agonist site, turning the receptor purple, and opening the ion channel to the greatest extent possible by a full agonist. If allosteric modulator (**NT2**) binds to the second binding site in the **absence** of neurotransmitter binding to its own binding site, it has **no particular effect**. However, if neurotransmitter (**NT1**) is already binding to its binding site, the addition of allosteric modulator (**NT2**) binding to the second membrane site is to **dramatically open the ion channel** even further than a full agonist can do on its own, as shown on the right. This is graphically represented as purple NT1 binding to the receptor, and turning it partially purple; as green NT2 binding to the receptor, and turning it partially green; and as the ion channel opening to an extent much greater than can be achieved by the action of a full agonist alone.

It should now be clear from these numerous examples that when neurotransmitter receptor binding sites are arranged as neighbors, they can interact with each other allosterically to promote or control some aspect of neurotransmission. This theme is amplified over and over again throughout psychopharmacology, with varying receptors, transmitters, ion channels, and allosteric modifying receptors and their transmitters. The exact architecture of specific sites is being discovered at a fast pace. It is only well worked out for a few specific neurotransmitters, such as the benzodiazepine complex, nicotinic cholinergic receptors, and glutamate receptors, for example. However, the most important thing to remember is the concept, and not necessarily the details, of allosteric modulation.

In summary, allosteric modulation is a specific concept in which neurotransmitters and their receptors may cooperate with each other to work much more powerfully and through a much greater range of action than they can by themselves. This may be mediated in many instances by the guarding of ion channels. Drugs can act at a myriad of sites to influence this process. So can diseases. There are at a minimum ion channel sites, neurotransmitter sites, and allosteric sites as targets of drug (and disease) action. Data are developing so quickly that the details are changing constantly. However, as a general principle, understanding this architecture of receptor-mediated chemical neurotransmission should provide the reader with the basis to understand a vast array of drug actions, and how such actions modify and impact chemical neurotransmission.

Summary

This chapter has introduced the reader to three special properties of receptors. The first of these is the classification of receptors by their subtypes and by their molecular configurations. Several receptor subtypes can bind the exact same neurotransmitter. Also, families of receptors can share common molecular characteristics even if they do not share the same neurotransmitter. Specifically, individual receptors within superfamilies of receptors can all be arranged in a similar configuration with second messengers or with ion channels.

The second of the special properties of receptors discussed here is the action of receptors with neurotransmitters and drugs that bind to them to produce a spectrum of output ranging from full agonists, to partial agonists, to antagonists, to partial inverse agonists, to full inverse agonists.

Finally, the reader has been introduced to the concept of allosteric modulation of one receptor by another. This provides for regulation of neurotransmission through either boosting or blocking one receptor's action by another. The allosterically modulating receptor was shown to act *indirectly* either as a referee or as a coach, but not by participating directly in the action game of neurotransmission.

CHAPTER 4

CHEMICAL NEUROTRANSMISSION AS THE TARGET OF DISEASE ACTIONS

Receptors and Enzymes as Targets of Disease Action in the Central Nervous System

The reader should now know that enzymes and receptors make things happen. Chapter 2 has already discussed that the most powerful way known to change the functioning of a neuron with a *drug* is to interact at one of its key receptors or to inhibit one of its important enzymes. However, this is only one perspective of psychopharmacology, namely that enzymes and receptors are the sites of *drug* action. A second and equally important perspective in psychopharmacology will be developed in this chapter. That perspective is that enzymes and receptors are also the sites of *disease* actions.

If receptors and enzymes are so important for explaining the actions of *drugs* on chemical neurotransmission, it should not be surprising that brain *diseases* that disrupt chemical neurotransmission do so by altering these same enzymes and receptors. The resulting disruption of the normal flow of chemical neurotransmission is thought to lead to the behavioral or motor abnormalities expressed by patients who suffer from psychiatric and neurological disorders. Obviously, different aspects of neurotransmission are hypothetically disrupted in different brain disorders. Given the vast complexity of chemical neurotransmission, there are obviously a lot of possibilities for sites of abnormally acting receptors and/or enzymes.

Psychopharmacology is a science dedicated in part to discovering where these molecular lesions exist in the nervous system in order to learn what is wrong with chemical neurotransmission. Knowing the molecular problem that leads to abnormal neurotransmission can generate a rationale for developing a drug therapy to correct it, thereby removing the psychiatric and neurological symptoms of the brain disorder. Although this concept is complex in its application to specific brain disorders, it will first be discussed in a broad and general manner in this chapter. Later, once the reader is familiar with these general concepts outlined here, these same concepts will be applied to specific psychiatric and neurological disorders in subsequent chapters.

This chapter will discuss how diseases of the central nervous system (CNS) are approached by three disciplines: neuroscience, biological psychiatry, and psychopharmacology. We will then show how these three approaches can be applied to learning how brain disorders modify chemical neurotransmission. Specific concepts that will be explained are the molecular neurobiology of psychiatric disorders, neuronal plasticity, and excitotoxicity. Also, the reader will learn how CNS disorders may be linked either to no neurotransmission, too much neurotransmission, an imbalance among neurotransmitters, or the wrong rate of neurotransmission.

Diseases in the Central Nervous System: A Tale of Three Disciplines

Neuroscience

Neuroscience is the study of brain and neuronal functioning, usually emphasizing normal brain functioning in experimental animals rather than in man (Table 4–1). Obviously, one must first understand normal brain functioning and normal chemical neurotransmission in order to have any chance of detecting – let alone understanding – neurobiological abnormalities that cause psychiatric and neurological disorders. For example, neurobiological investigations have led to the clarification of certain principles of chemical neurotransmission, to the enumeration of specific neurotransmitters, to the discovery of multiple receptor subtypes for each neurotransmitter, to the understanding of the enzymes that synthesize and metabolize the neurotransmitters, and to the unfolding discoveries of how genetic information controls this whole process. The discipline of neurobiology uses drugs as tools to interact selectively with enzymes and receptors – and with the DNA and RNA systems that control the synthesis of enzymes and receptors – in order to elucidate their functions in the

Table 4–1. *Neuroscience*

Limited definition
    The study of brain and neuronal functioning

Approach
    Studies using experimental animals
    The use of drugs to probe neurobiological and molecular regulatory mechanisms

Findings relevant to psychopharmacology
    Discovery of neurotransmitters and their enzymes and receptors
    Principles of neurotransmission
    Genetic and molecular regulation of neuronal functioning
    Neurobiological regulation of animal behaviors

normal brain. Many of the lessons derived from this approach have already been discussed in the preceding chapters.

Biological Psychiatry

Biological psychiatry, on the other hand, is oriented towards discovering the abnormalities in brain biology associated with the causes or consequences of mental disorders (Table 4–2). This discipline uses the results of neurobiological investigations of normal brain functioning as a basis for the search for the substrate of abnormal brain functioning in psychiatric disorders.

Scientists have long suspected that an abnormality in brain enzymes or receptors is the cause of mental illness, and have been searching for an enzyme or receptor deficiency that could be identified as the cause of specific psychiatric disorders. Unfortunately, there has been little progress using this approach. More recently, the focus has shifted to pursuing the discovery of an abnormality in DNA in hereditary psychiatric disorders that could lead to abnormalities in the synthesis of gene products. By understanding how abnormal gene products participate in neuronal functioning and chemical neurotransmission, the hope is that a rationale could be found for reversing these abnormalities with drug therapies. This could be easiest to pursue if the abnormal gene products prove to be enzymes or receptors.

The tools of biological psychiatry are often less elegant than those of basic neurobiology, since practical and ethical considerations limit the manner in which patients and their CNS can be studied, compared to the techniques available for use in laboratories and in animals. The tools available for use in humans include studies of enzymes and receptors in postmortem brain tissues and in peripheral tissues that can be ethically sampled in living patients, such as blood platelets or lymphocytes, whose enzymes and receptors may be similar to those in brain. Metabolites of neurotransmitters can be studied in cerebrospinal fluid, plasma, and urine.

Metabolic rates and cerebral blood flow reflecting neuronal firing patterns – as well as some receptors – can be visualized in living patients by use of positron emission tomography (PET) scans. Receptors for neurotransmitters can also be studied indirectly by using selective drug probes that cause hormones to be released into

Table 4–2. *Biological psychiatry*

Limited definition

The study of abnormalities in brain neurobiology associated with the causes or consequences of mental illnesses

Approach

Studies using patients with psychiatric disorders

Taking direction from psychopharmacological studies that indicate that drugs with known mechanisms of action on receptors or enzymes predictably alter symptoms in a specific psychiatric disorder

Search for abnormalities in receptors, enzymes, neurotransmitters, genes or gene products that correlate with the diagnosis of a particular mental illness

Biochemical measurements using blood, urine, cerebrospinal fluid, peripheral tissues such as platelets or lymphocytes, postmortem brain tissues, or plasma hormones after provoking hormone secretion by drugs

Measurements of structural abnormalities using CT or MRI brain scans

Measurements of functional or physiological abnormalities using PET, EEG, evoked potentials, or magnetoencephalography

Findings relevant to psychopharmacology

Few strong biological findings demonstrating lesions in specific psychiatric disorders

Example: discovery of changes in serotonin receptors and metabolites in depression, schizophrenia, and suicidal behavior

Search for the genetic basis of specific neurological and psychiatric illnesses

---

the blood that can be measured and therefore serve as a reflection of brain receptor stimulation. Structural brain abnormalities can be detected using computed tomography (CT) and magnetic resonance imaging (MRI). Functional abnormalites in brain electrical activity can be detected by measuring it with electroencephalography (EEG), evoked potentials, or magnetoencephalography. Genetic materials can be studied by sampling a wide variety of body tissues, since all cells – including brain cells – contain the same DNA. Abnormalities identified in one cell's DNA therefore implies that the same abnormality exists in the brain's DNA.

Biological psychiatry studies are only beginning to clarify the neuronal dysfunctioning associated with specific psychiatric and neurological disorders. The specific findings in specific disorders are discussed in subsequent chapters. In overview, however, it can be stated in all modesty that very little is yet known to enable biological psychiatry to prove the molecular pathophysiology of CNS disorders.

One successful example of a CNS disorder with a known genetic and molecular basis is the model exemplified by Tay-Sachs disease, in which a specific type of mental retardation is known to be caused by a deficiency of a specific enzyme, namely hexosaminidase A. Unfortunately, no such deficiencies in enzymes or receptors have yet been found for any psychiatric disorder. This frustrating outcome of searching virtually every known enzyme in every known psychiatric condition is only compounded by studies of the substrates and metabolites of the enzymes, which have been similarly lacking in identifying clear disease entities. Many provocative hints exist in such studies, but we currently understand how drugs target enzymes and receptors much better than we understand how diseases do this.

A more promising situation exists with early leads from genetic studies of DNA in certain neurological and muscular disorders including some forms of Alzheimer's disease, ataxia, Huntington's disease, amyotrophic lateral sclerosis (Lou Gehrig's disease), and muscular dystrophy. Certain investigators have identified abnormal genes in such disorders, and there is even some information about how these abnormal genes lead to abnormal gene products.

It is hoped that the rapid pace of such advances will soon generate rational targets for new drugs that could reverse the abnormal genetically driven molecular activities, and thereby also reverse the clinical symptoms of the genetic disorder of the nervous system.

Psychopharmacology

As mentioned previously, the discipline of psychopharmacology is oriented not only towards discovering new drugs and understanding the actions of drugs upon the CNS; it is also oriented towards understanding diseases of the CNS by altering them through the use of drugs whose actions are known (Table 4–3). That is, if a drug with a well-understood mechanism of action on a receptor or enzyme causes reproducible effects upon the symptoms of a patient with a brain disorder, it is likely that that symptom is also linked to the same receptor or enzyme that the drug is targeting. Using drugs as tools in this manner can help map which receptors and enzymes are linked to which psychiatric or neurological disorder. Since drug actions are much better known than disease actions at the present time, the use of drug tools in this manner has so far proved to be the more productive approach to un-

Table 4–3. *Psychopharmacology*

Limited definition
    The use of drugs to treat symptoms of mental illness
    The science of drug discovery, targeting enzymes and receptors

Approach
    Studies in patients with psychiatric disorders
    Serendipitous clinical observations
    In clinical investigations, the use of drugs with known mechanisms of action to provoke biological or behavioral responses that would provide clues where abnormalities in brain functioning may exist in specific psychiatric disorders
    In drug discovery, theory-driven targeting of enzymes and receptors hypothesized to regulate symptoms in a psychiatric disorder

Psychopharmacological results
    In clinical investigations, the first observation is often serendipitous discovery of clinical efficacy, and then the biochemical mechanism of action is discovered
    In drug discovery, specific enzymes or receptors are first targeted for drug action: the earliest experiments use chemistry to synthesize drugs; experimental animals to test the biochemical, behavioral, and toxic actions of the drugs; and human subjects, both normal volunteers and patients, to test the safety and efficacy of the drugs
    Discovery and use of antidepressants, anxiolytics, antipsychotics, and cognitive enhancers as well as drugs of abuse

derstanding diseases compared to the biological psychiatry approach of looking for abnormal receptors, enzymes, or genes. Indeed, much of what is known, hypothesized, or theorized about the neurochemical abnormalities of brain disorders is derived from this approach of using drugs as tools.

Therefore, in general, contemporary knowledge of CNS disorders – as will be discussed for specific entities in subsequent chapters – in fact is largely predicated upon knowing how drugs act on disease symptoms, and then inferring pathophysiology by knowing how the drugs act. Thus, pathophysiology is inferred rather than proven, since we do not yet know the primary enzyme, receptor, or genetic deficiency in any given psychiatric or neurological disorder.

The discipline of psychopharmacology has therefore been useful not only in generating empirically successful treatments for CNS disorders; psychopharmacology has also been useful in generating the leading theories and hypotheses about psychiatric and neurological disorders. These theories in fact direct the biological psychiatry approach where to look for proof of disease abnormalities. Thus, psychopharmacology is bidirectional in the sense that certain drugs (i.e., those that have a known neurochemical mechanism of action and that are also effective in treating a brain disorder) help to generate hypotheses about the causes of those brain disorders. Also, the other direction of psychopharmacology is that in those cases where brain disorders have a known or suspected pathophysiology, drugs can be rationally designed to act on a specific receptor or enzyme predicted to correct the known or suspected pathophysiology in order to treat that disorder.

It would be advantageous for new drug development to proceed from knowledge of pathophysiology to the invention of new therapeutics, but this must await the elucidation of such pathophysiologies, and as emphasized here, this is largely yet unknown. Virtually all drugs that have been discovered to date to be useful in psychopharmacology were found by serendipity (good luck), or by empiricism, that is, by probing disease mechanisms with a drug of known action but no prior proof that such actions would be necessarily therapeutic. It is hoped the other route to drug development will be increasingly available as the molecular causes of such disorders are elucidated in coming years.

How Diseases Modify Synaptic Neurotransmission

Despite a frustrating lack of knowledge of specific pathophysiological mechanisms for various psychiatric disorders, a good deal of progress has been made in our thinking about mechanisms whereby diseases can modify synaptic neurotransmission. Discussed here are several general concepts relating to how psychiatric disorders are thought to be associated with modifications in synaptic neurotransmission.

Molecular Neurobiology and Psychiatric Disorders

A modern formulation of psychiatric disorders involves the integration of at least four key elements: (1) genetic vulnerability to the expression of a disease; (2) life-event stressors that come that individual's way (such as divorce, financial problems, etc.); (3) the individual's personality, coping skills, and social support available from others; and (4) other environmental influences upon the individual and his genome including viruses, toxins, and various diseases.

The first element of this group – inheriting an abnormal gene, which causes the synthesis of an absent or abnormal gene product, causing in turn the expression of overt pathology – is classically seen as a single factor in many medical diseases (Fig. 4–1). This unidimensional genetic mechanism of disease is not yet well established for psychiatric disorders. This model does seem to fit certain psychiatric disorders, such as Huntington's disease, but this model does not seem to fit well for the vast majority of psychiatric disorders.

Better explaining the pathophysiology and genetic basis of many psychiatric disorders may be the "two-hit hypothesis." That is, in order to manifest an overt psychiatric disorder, one must not only sustain the first "hit," namely a genetic vulnerability, but one must also sustain a second "hit" of some type from the environment (see Figs. 4–2 through 4–7). Thus, psychiatric disorders are increased in incidence in first-degree relatives of patients with a wide variety of psychiatric disorders, but not to an extent that allows one to predict which specific individuals will or will not eventually develop a specific psychiatric disorder. This has given rise to the concept that one may not inherit the mental disorder so much as the vulnerability to the mental disorder (the first hit). The chance of actually manifesting this vulnerability apparently depends upon numerous other factors (i.e., second hits). Some mental disorders, such as schizophrenia or bipolar illness, may have a higher chance of being expressed in vulnerable individuals, compared to disorders such as depression, anxiety, or obsessive compulsive disorder, which may more frequently lay dormant in the vulnerable individual (Fig. 4–2). Thus, genetic endowment gives an individual the risk of a certain disorder, and certain disorders may have more of a propensity to become manifest than other disorders, but the vulnerability alone is not enough to express overt psychiatric illness.

What may dictate whether a disorder remains only a latent possibility versus breaking down into overt psychiatric pathology may be the interaction of one's genome with the environment. Several environmental interactions are hypothesized

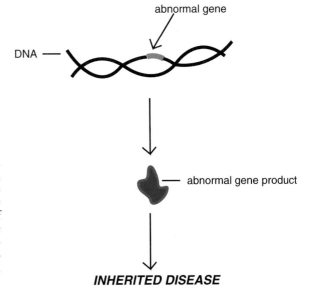

FIGURE 4–1. This figure depicts the **classical view** of an **inherited disease**. In this case, the **abnormal gene** expresses some sort of **abnormal gene product**. The consequences of making this deficient gene product is that cellular functioning is compromised, resulting in the **inherited disease**.

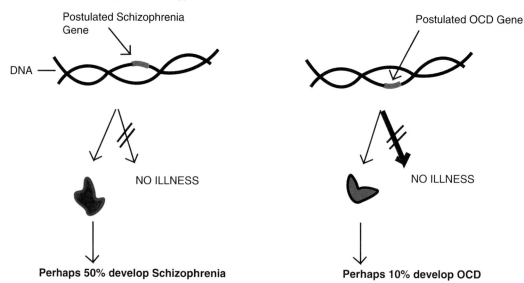

FIGURE 4–2. Depicted here is the more common observations of **how psychiatric disorders are inherited**. That is, a postulated abnormal gene only **sometimes** makes an abnormal gene product, so that only **some** of the owners of abnormal genes ever get the psychiatric illness lying dormant in their genes. On the left is shown a disorder where there is a very high genetic loading, meaning that many of those with the abnormal gene end up getting the disease contained in that gene. Specifically, a **postulated gene for schizophrenia** will cause illness in perhaps up to **50% of those who have that gene**. The remaining 50% have the postulated schizophrenia gene yet **do not develop schizophrenia**. On the right is shown a disorder where there is a relative low genetic loading, meaning that only a fraction of those with the abnormal gene end up getting the disease contained in that gene. Specifically, this may be the case for a variety of disorders such as obsessive compulsive disorder (OCD), panic disorder, social phobia, and depression. In such cases, the **postulated abnormal gene** for the condition (e.g., OCD) will cause illness in perhaps only **10% of those who have that gene**. The remaining 90% have the postulated abnormal gene, yet **do not develop the psychiatric illness**.

to affect the expression of information present in the genome. These include *early life experiences* that cause a person to develop learned patterns of coping that together comprise his or her personality, or in some cases, personality disorder (Figs. 4–3 and 4–4). Also, there are *adult life experiences* that an individual encounters from social interaction with the environment, including events commonly called "stressful" such as divorce, death of a loved one, financial difficulties, and medical problems (Fig. 4–4). Finally, the environment provides biochemical influences on the genome such as exposure to viruses, toxins, or diseases (Fig. 4–4).

Personality traits (Fig. 4–3) may be genetically influenced (e.g., impulsivity, shyness) or environmentally determined by early childhood developmental experiences. Personality traits generate coping skills that can either blunt the impact of adult life events, or can exacerbate the impact of adult life events upon that individual's genome (Fig. 4–3). The ability of an individual to buffer stress or even to grow and prosper when exposed to stressors, versus break down into a mental disorder, may be the product of which life events occur, and how much coping skill and social support exist prior to being layered onto a genome. Also, that genome may be robust or vulnerable, and the particular vulnerability may explain why some people develop

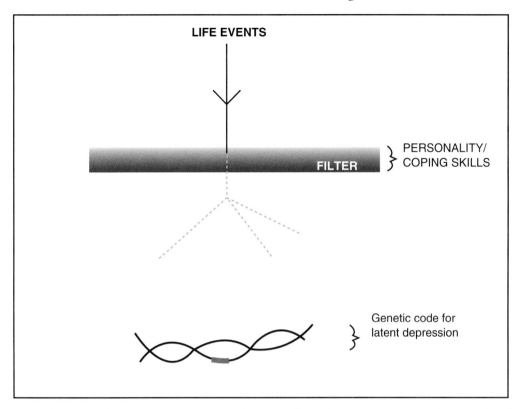

FIGURE 4–3. This figure demonstrates how **life events** from the environment **test the postulated genes** for a psychiatric illness (in this case, a postulated gene capable of triggering **depression**). Life events, sometimes called stressors, challenge the organism, and this manifests itself as a biological demand on the individual's genome. Such stressors are modified by the individual and processed so that the nature of the biological demand may be similarly modified. That is, one who has developed an adaptive **personality** with good **coping skills** and social support may be able to mitigate, blunt, or lessen the biological demand upon his **genetic code for latent depression**. On the other hand, one who has developed an abnormal **personality** with poor **coping skills** may actually worsen, accelerate, or even recruit potentially damaging psychosocial stressors to play on his/her genome. Thus, personality and coping skills are either a **filter** or a **magnifying glass** through which psychosocial stressors pass on their journey to test and challenge the genome where a potential psychiatric disorder may or may not be waiting for a chance to be expressed.

depression, others obsessive compulsive disorder, and others no disorder at all, in the presence of similar life experiences and similar personalities.

The nature of genetic risk may thus be quite different for different psychiatric disorders. Given comparable genetic material and comparable personalities/coping skills, it may be the severity of psychosocial stressors from the environment that determines how often a vulnerable individual in the population develops a mental illness. According to this model, the more biologically determined disorders with the more vulnerable genomes would require only minor stressors to develop that mental illness (e.g., schizophrenia in Fig. 4–5). On the other hand, a less vulnerable disorder such as depression might theoretically require moderate stressors in order to become manifest (Fig. 4–5). Finally, some stressors could be so severe (e.g., rape,

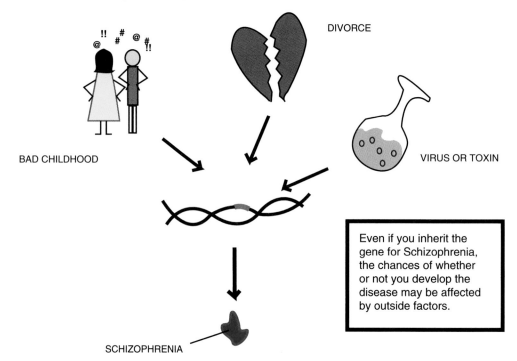

DIVORCE

BAD CHILDHOOD

VIRUS OR TOXIN

Even if you inherit the gene for Schizophrenia, the chances of whether or not you develop the disease may be affected by outside factors.

SCHIZOPHRENIA

FIGURE 4–4. This figure represents the "**two hit**" **hypothesis** for psychiatric illnesses with a genetic component. In this hypothesis, inheriting an abnormal gene (the **first** "**hit**" shown as a red gene on the black strand of DNA) is not sufficient to manifest a psychiatric disorder. One must also sustain just the right **second** "**hit**" from the environment, postulated to be life events such as a **bad childhood** or **divorce**, or insults from the environment such as a **virus** or a **toxin**. Thus, those with just one hit do not develop the disorder, even though they have the gene identical to those who do develop the psychiatric disorder. What distinguishes those who ultimately develop an illness from those who do not is whether the individual at risk and vulnerable for the illness (i.e., the red gene for **schizophrenia**) also is exposed to just the right second hit (shown as inputs onto the gene) necessary to trigger the abnormal gene into making its abnormal gene product and therefore causing the disease in that individual (shown as schizophrenia here).

combat, witnessing atrocities) that even a normal robust genome might break down to a mental disorder (e.g., posttraumatic stress disorder [PTSD] in Fig. 4–5).

Neuronal Plasticity and Psychiatric Disorders

The synapse is a dynamic and constantly changing area of the brain. Synapses are laid down and maintained, and in some cases may be removed. Many things influence this process of adding, maintaining, and removing synapses. Since the synapse is the substrate of chemical neurotransmission, information transfer in the brain is vitally dependent upon the outcomes of these processes of branching, pruning, growing, or dying of neuronal axons and dendrites (see Chapter 1 and Figs. 1–11, 1–12, and 1–13). If they are interrupted early in development, the brain may not reach its full potential, such as in mental retardation and as is now speculated to occur in schizophrenia (Fig. 4–6). If they are interrupted late in life, the brain may regress from the potential it has realized, such as in various dementias (Fig. 4–6).

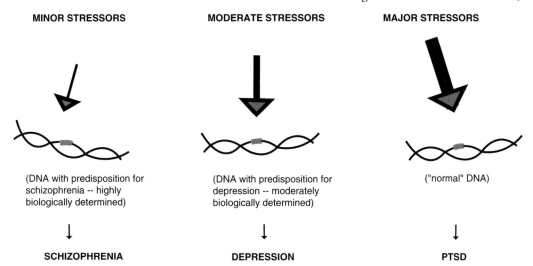

MINOR STRESSORS

MODERATE STRESSORS

MAJOR STRESSORS

(DNA with predisposition for schizophrenia -- highly biologically determined)

(DNA with predisposition for depression -- moderately biologically determined)

("normal" DNA)

SCHIZOPHRENIA

DEPRESSION

PTSD

FIGURE 4–5. Some disorders have a relatively **high predisposition for manifestation** in a vulnerable individual, whereas others have a relatively **low predisposition**, as previously shown in Figure 4–2. Thus, it may take only relatively **minor or usual stressors** for the vulnerable individual to have his/her **schizophrenia gene activated** into producing a disease (*left panel*). On the other hand, since fewer individuals with the postulated genetic potential for depression (or manic depressive illness) may actually manifest this disorder, it may take at least **moderate or more unusual stressors** for the vulnerable individual to have his/her **manic depressive disorder gene activated** into producing a disease (*middle panel*). Finally, even those with "normal" DNA, with no known predisposition to any given psychiatric disorder, may decompensate under **major and overwhelming stressors** such as rape, combat, or natural disasters to produce a breakdown of cellular functioning through the breakdown of "normal" DNA to produce yet other psychiatric disorders (*right panel*). This latter mechanism is one hypothesis for the mechanism of **posttraumatic stress disorder (PTSD)**, for example.

Drug treatments themselves may not only modify neurotransmission acutely, but could potentially interact with neuronal plasticity. Harnessing the neurochemistry of the brain's plasticity is an important goal of several areas of new drug development. For example, certain growth factors may provoke the neuron to sprout new axonal or dendritic branches, and to establish new synaptic connections (see Chapter 1 and Fig. 1–12).

Other factors may be involved in the opposite process of the natural pruning of the branches, destroying and turning over old, useless, or unused arborizations. If a disease renders such pruning processes out of control, it may be involved in the permanent degeneration of certain neurons (Fig. 4–7). Such a disease could be caused by a genetically programmed mechanism that gets out of control and eventually prunes neurons to death. It can also be caused by the ingestion of toxins or toxic drugs of abuse.

The role of plasticity in the action of drugs or diseases upon neurotransmission in the CNS is only beginning to be explored. Drugs are not yet available that can turn on and direct the plasticity process. Theoretically, it should become possible to establish new or to reestablish preexisting neuronal branches and their synapses. Such possible modifications of degenerative nerve diseases are being pursued in two different ways. First, the search is on for abnormal genes or abnormal gene products

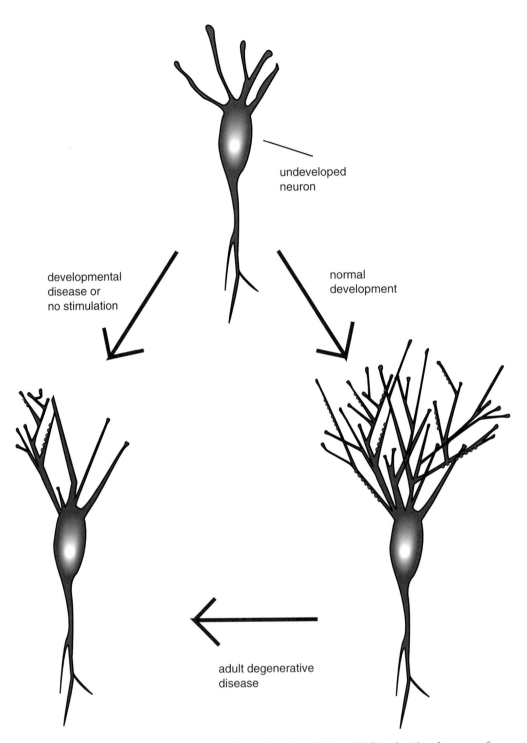

FIGURE 4–6. An **undeveloped neuron** may fail to develop during childhood either because of a **developmental disease** of some sort, or because of the **lack of appropriate neuronal or environmental stimulation** for proper development (*left arrow*). In other cases, the undeveloped neuron does develop normally (*right arrow* showing **normal development**), only to lose these gains when an **adult-onset degenerative disease** strikes it (*bottom arrow*).

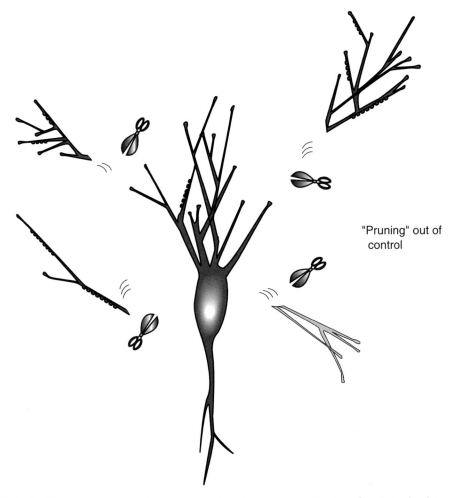

"Pruning" out of control

FIGURE 4–7. Neurons appear to have a normal maintenance mechanism for their dendritic tree where they are able to "prune" or remove old, unused, or useless synapses and dendrites (normal mechanism shown in Fig. 1–13). One postulated mechanism for some degenerative diseases is that this otherwise normal **"pruning" mechanism** may get **out of control,** eventually rendering the neuron useless or even killing it by **"pruning it to death."**

that are mediating the breakdown of neurons. Once identified, it should theoretically be possible to stop the production or block the action of unwanted gene products or to turn on the production or provide a substitute for the desired but absent gene products, depending upon the specific need for the specific disease. Second, transplantation of neurons is being investigated as a manner of substituting new neurons for degenerated neurons. This is not a Frankenstein-style transplant of an entire brain, but rather a selective introduction of specific and highly specialized nerves that produce specialized chemicals and neurotransmitters capable of compensating for and replacing the functions of the degenerated and destroyed neurons that caused disease in the first place. This is already occurring in Parkinson's disease, where dopamine-producing neurons have been successfully transplanted into the brains of

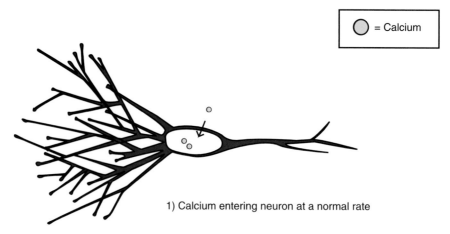

1) Calcium entering neuron at a normal rate

FIGURE 4–8. **Calcium** is an ion that is a key **regulator of neuronal excitability**, and is constantly coming in and out of neurons through ion channels of various sorts that are conducting the normal business functions of the neuron. When this occurs at a **normal rate**, this modifies neuronal excitability but is not damaging to the neuron (but see Figs. 4–9 and 4–10).

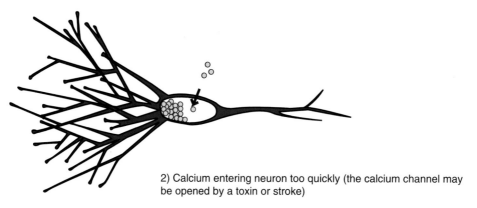

2) Calcium entering neuron too quickly (the calcium channel may be opened by a toxin or stroke)

FIGURE 4–9. **Calcium** may also rush into cells **too quickly** if its ion channels are **opened too much**, such as is postulated to occur by certain **toxins**, by **stroke**, or by **neurodegenerative conditions** (see Fig. 4–10).

animals and patients with this condition. Experimental use of cholinergic neurons holds promise for the treatment of experimental models of Alzheimer's disease.

Excitotoxicity

One current hypothesis for neuronal cell death is that of excitotoxicity. In this scenerio, an excitatory amino acid, like glutamate, does not act at a normal amount of excitation characteristic for excitatory neurotransmission (Fig. 4–8), but instead overexcites a cell (Fig. 4–9), causing too much calcium to enter the cell through

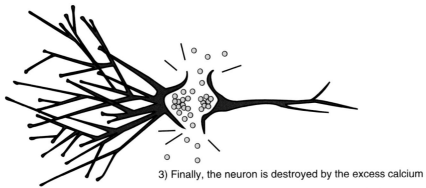

3) Finally, the neuron is destroyed by the excess calcium

FIGURE 4–10. If **too much calcium** gets into the neuron and overwhelms any sinks and buffers there, it can **destroy the neuron** and cause it to degenerate and die. This mechanism of excessive excitation is called **excitotoxicity** and is a major current hypothesis for various psychiatric and neurological disorders. This idea postulates that for such diseases. neurons are literally **"excited to death."**

ion channels, eventually poisoning and killing the neuron (Fig. 4–10). If overexcitation is caused by a malfunction of glutamate itself, it would be as if an endogenous assassin were destroying neurons. This has been theorized to occur in certain hereditary degenerative disorders such as Huntington's disease. It could also occur in certain disorders that release too much glutamate, such as ischemia and stroke. Still other disorders could be related to excitotoxicity from exogenous assassins taken in from the environment. This has been shown for the toxin MPTP, which causes a form of Parkinson's disease, and is speculated to be the case for idiopathic Parkinson's disease itself, as well as perhaps amyotrophic lateral sclerosis, Alzheimer's disease, or other disorders of neuronal cell death.

Discovery of antagonists to excitotoxicity, such as exemplified by the glutamate antagonists, may portend the possibility of developing new drug therapies for neurodegenerative disorders, and other disease processes related to plasticity and neurodevelopmental dysfunction.

No Neurotransmission

There are a myriad of known and suspected mechanisms by which diseases can modify chemical neurotransmission. These can vary from no transmission, such as in the case of a degenerated and absent neuron, to too much neurotransmission from a malfunctioning of the synapse. One of the key consequences of loss of neurons in neurodegenerative disorders such as Parkinson's disease, Huntington's disease, amyotrophic lateral sclerosis (i.e., Lou Gehrig's disease), and Alzheimer's disease, is the fact that no neurotransmission occurs subsequent to neuronal loss (Figs. 4–11 and 4–12). This is a conceptually simple mechanism of disease action with profound consequences. It is also at least in part the mechanism of other disorders such as stroke, multiple sclerosis, and virtually any disorder in which neurons are irreversibly damaged.

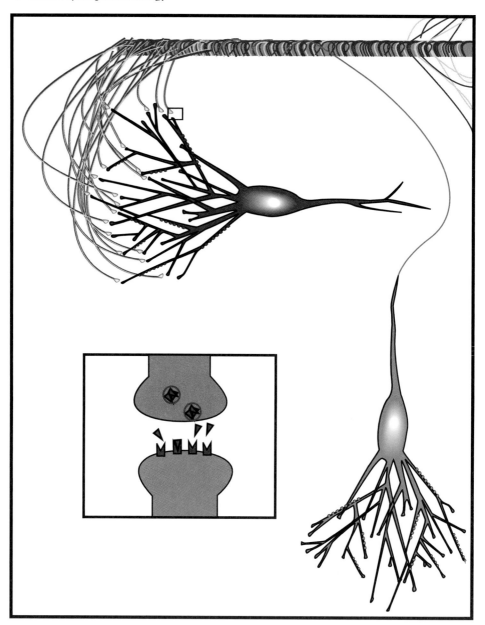

FIGURE 4–11. Shown here is **normal communication between two neurons**, with the synapse between the red and the blue neuron magnified. Normal neurotransmission from the red to the blue neuron is being mediated here by neurotransmitter binding to postsynaptic receptors by the **usual mechanism of synaptic neurotransmission** (but see Figs. 4–12 through 4–21).

One of the earliest attempts to compensate for the dropout of neurons and the consequent loss of neurotransmission (Figs. 4–11 and 4–12) was simply to replace the neurotransmitter (Fig. 4–13). Indeed, this can happen in certain instances such as Parkinson's disease, where the loss of the neurotransmitter dopamine can be replaced.

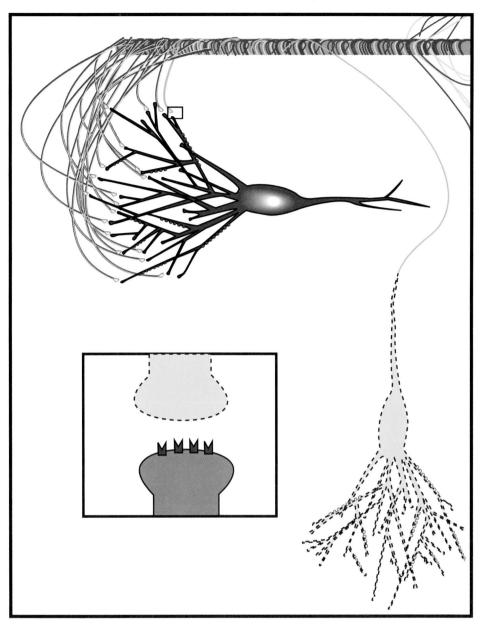

FIGURE 4–12. This figure illustrates what happens in a conceptually simple disease in which a **neuron dies**, leaving behind **no neurotransmission**. The loss of the red neuron means that neuro-transmission at the former site between the red and the blue neuron is now **lost** (but see Figs. 4–13 through 4–16).

Even in this conceptually simple example, however, the therapeutic replacement is in fact not so simple. Dopamine given orally or intravenously cannot get into the brain. The precursor, L-DOPA, can get into the brain, and get converted into dopamine. However, even the precursor needs help in practice, since the coadministration of

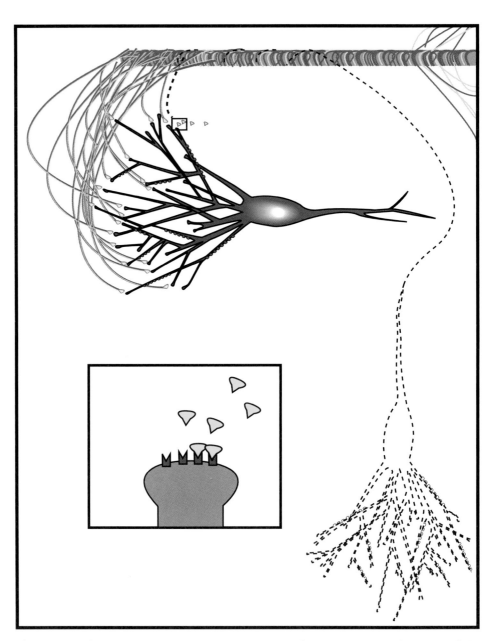

FIGURE 4–13. One of the simplest pharmacological remedies for **replacing the function of the lost neurotransmission from a degenerated neuron** is to replace the neurotransmitter with a drug that mimics the former neuron's neurotransmitter. This is shown here with the yellow drug **replacing the natural neurotransmitter** that was formerly present when the red neuron was present and functioning in Fig. 4–11). This strategy, for example, is used when L-dopa is used to replace the lost neurotransmission in Parkinson's disease when nigrostriatal dopamine neurons degenerate and die.

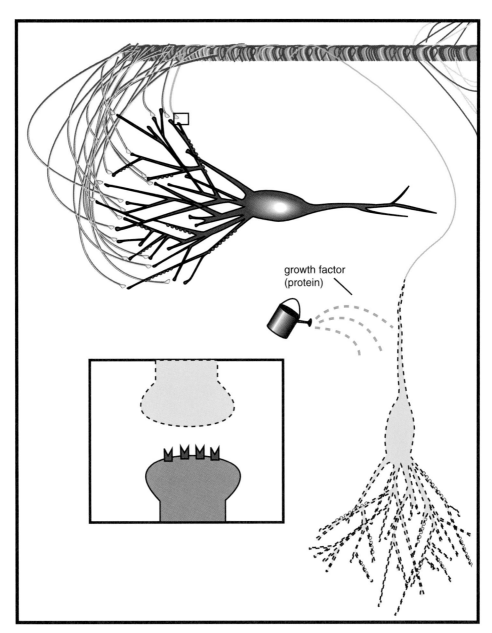

FIGURE 4–14. Shown here and in Fig. 4–15 is a conceptually more complex mechanism of compensating for the loss of a **degenerating neuron**. Indicated here is an ailing but not yet degenerated red neuron. It is no longer functioning to allow normal neurotransmission with the blue neuron (see box) and is about to die. Also indicated is the application of a **growth factor** to the degenerating neuron. This could be conceived as either a natural reparative mechanism that the dying neuron could activate (see Fig. 1–12), or a drug that could mimic this.

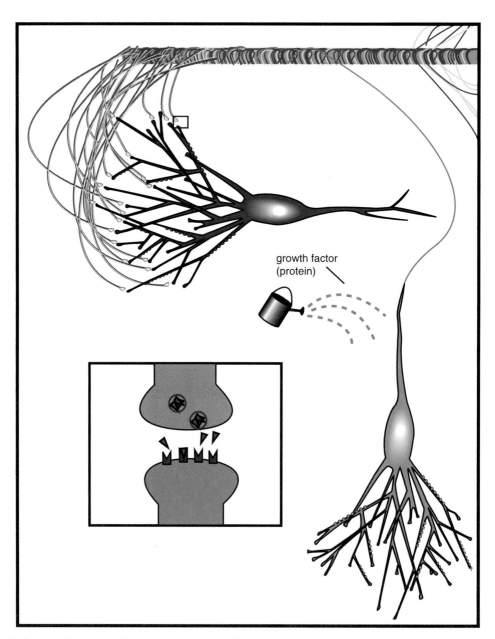

FIGURE 4–15. This figure demonstrates how a **degenerating neuron** might be **rescued by a growth factor**. In this case, the dying neuron of Figure 4–14 is salvaged by a **growth factor**, which restores the function of neurotransmission to **reactivate normal communications** between the red neuron and the blue neuron (see box).

growth factor
(protein)

88

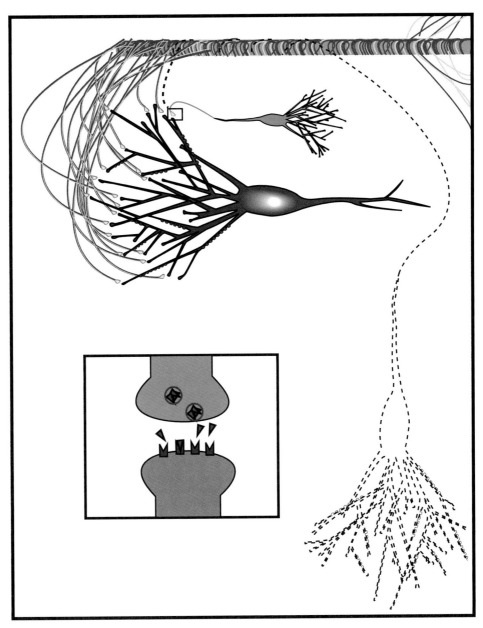

FIGURE 4–16. **Transplantation of a new neuron** by neurosurgical techniques is another potential mechanism for **replacing the function of a degenerated neuron**. In this case, the turquoise transplanted neuron makes the same neurotransmitter as the formerly red neuron made (see Fig. 4–11) prior to degenerating here. Synaptic neurotransmission is restored when the **transplanted neuron takes over the lost function** of the degenerated neuron (see box). This has already been performed for patients with Parkinson's disease, where transplanted fetal substantia nigra neurons can successfully improve functional neurotransmission of degenerated substantia nigra neurons in some patients.

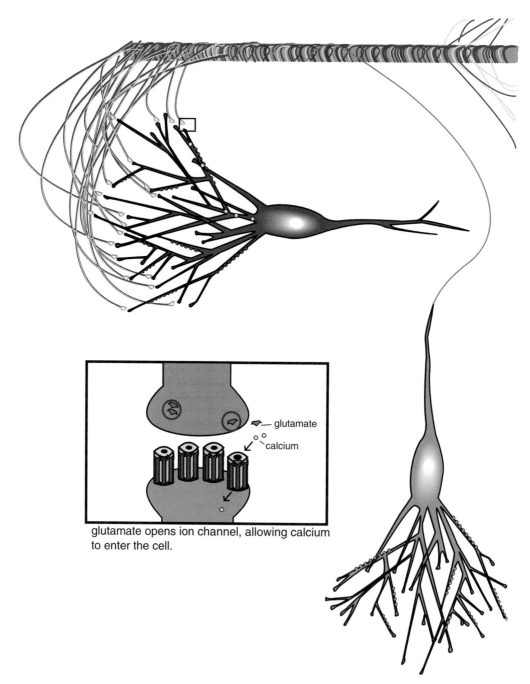

glutamate opens ion channel, allowing calcium
to enter the cell.

FIGURE 4–17. Shown here are details of calcium entering a dendrite of the blue neuron when the red neuron excites it with glutamate during **normal excitatory neurotransmission**. This was previously shown in a more simplistic model in Figure 4–8. Glutamate released from the red neuron travels across the synapse, docks into its agonist slot on its receptor, and as ionic gatekeeper, opens the calcium channel to allow calcium to enter the postsynaptic dendrite of the blue neuron to mediate an excitatory neurotransmission (see box).

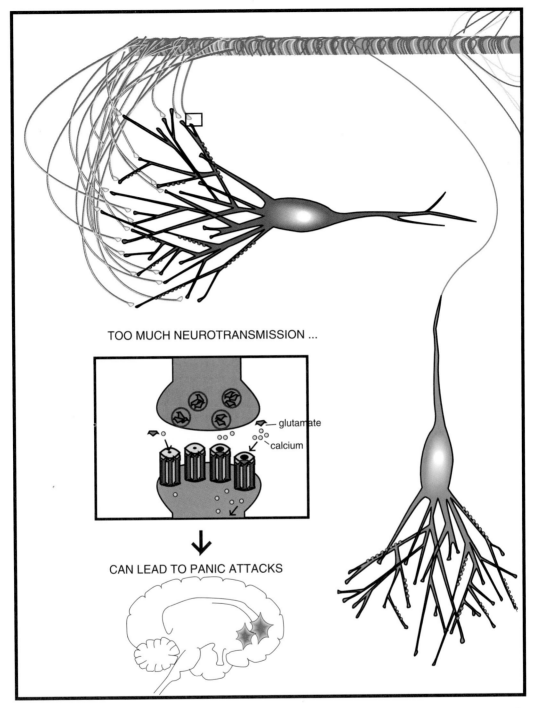

TOO MUCH NEUROTRANSMISSION ...

glutamate

calcium

CAN LEAD TO PANIC ATTACKS

FIGURE 4–18. Shown here is what may happen when excitatory neurotransmission causes **too much neurotransmission**. This may possibly occur during the production of various symptoms mediated by the brain, including **panic attacks**. It could also occur during mania, positive symptoms of psychosis, seizures, and other neuronal-mediated disease symptoms. In this case, **too much glutamate** is being released by the red neuron, causing **too much excitation** of the postsynaptic blue neuron's dendrite. Extra release of glutamate causes additional occupancy of postsynaptic glutamate receptors, opening more calcium channels, allowing more calcium to enter the blue dendrite (see box). Although this degree of excessive neurotransmission may be **associated with psychiatric symptoms**, it does not actually damage the neuron (but see Figs. 4–20 and 4–21).

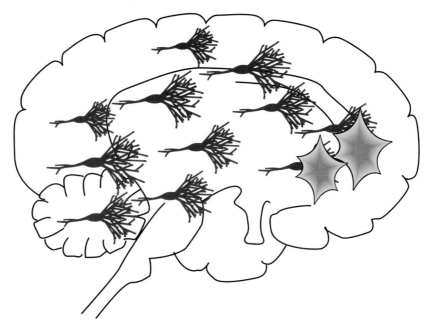

FIGURE 4–19. This figure represents the concept of an **electrical storm** in the brain in which **overexcitation** and **too much neurotransmission** is occurring during the production of various psychiatric symptoms, including those that occur during a **panic attack**. This may also be a model for other disorders of excessive behavioral symptoms that imply too much neurotransmission, including mania, positive symptoms of psychosis, and seizures.

an inhibitor of L-DOPA destruction must be done in order for L-DOPA to work optimally.

We have already discussed the possibility of using drugs to mimic natural growth factors to prevent or halt the process of neurodegeneration (Figs. 4–14 and 4–15), and to use transplants to replace the destroyed neurons (Fig. 4–16).

Too Much Neurotransmission

Another possible disease mechanism is too much neurotransmission (Figs. 4–17 through 4–21). We have already discussed an extreme example of this above, namely excitotoxicity (Figs. 4–9 and 4–10). Other examples of excessive neurotransmission are diseases in which neurotransmission stops short of actually destroying the neuron, but causes the neuron to be overactive (Fig. 4–18). This may be the case for epilepsy, psychosis, and panic (Fig. 4–19). In the case of epilepsy, neurons fire when and where they should not, leading to seizures. It is not yet known why this occurs, but is theorized to be related either to deficient inhibitory neurotransmission or excessive excitatory neurotransmission.

Psychosis possibly shares some analogies with a seizure, in that excessive transmission of dopamine in the mesolimbic areas of brain may lead to symptoms of delusions, hallucinations, and thought disorder in various psychiatric disorders.

Panic disorder may be analogous to a seizure in areas of the brain controlling emotions (such as the parahippocampal gyrus), leading to clinical symptoms char-

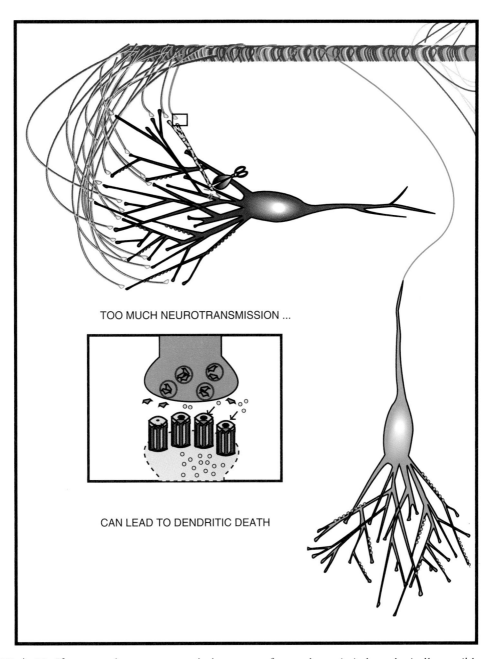

TOO MUCH NEUROTRANSMISSION ...

CAN LEAD TO DENDRITIC DEATH

FIGURE 4–20. If **too much neurotransmission** occurs for too long, it is hypothetically possible that this would **lead to dendritic death**. The mechanism for this may be tantamount to inappropriately activating the normal dendritic pruning process (indicated schematically as scissors snipping off the dendrite; see Fig. 1–13 for a diagram of "normal pruning"). Thus, far too much glutamate release can cause too much opening of the gates of the calcium channel, activating an **excitotoxic demise** of the dendrite (see box).

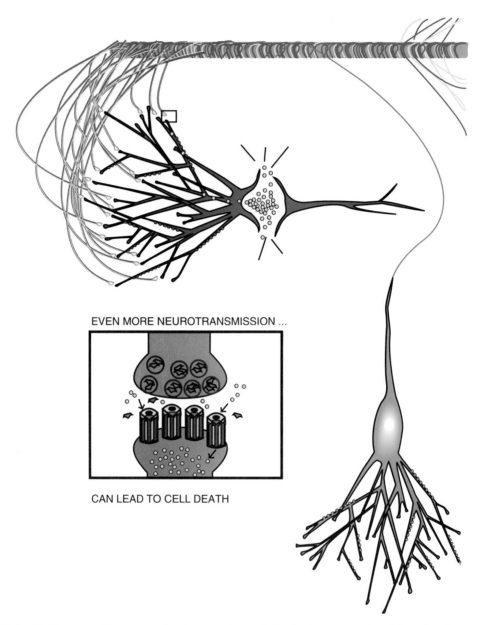

EVEN MORE NEUROTRANSMISSION ...

CAN LEAD TO CELL DEATH

FIGURE 4–21. **Catastrophic overexcitation** can theoretically lead to so much calcium flux into a neuron due to dangerous, wide-ranging opening of calcium channels by glutamate (see box), that not only is the dendrite destroyed but so is the entire neuron. This scenario is one in which the neuron is literally **excited to death**. The same idea was previously represented more simplistically in Figure 4–10. Excitotoxicity is a major current hypothesis to explain the **mechanism of neuronal death in neurodegenerative disorders**, including aspects of schizophrenia, Alzheimer's disease, Parkinson's disease, amyotrophic lateral sclerosis, and ischemic cell damage from stroke.

94

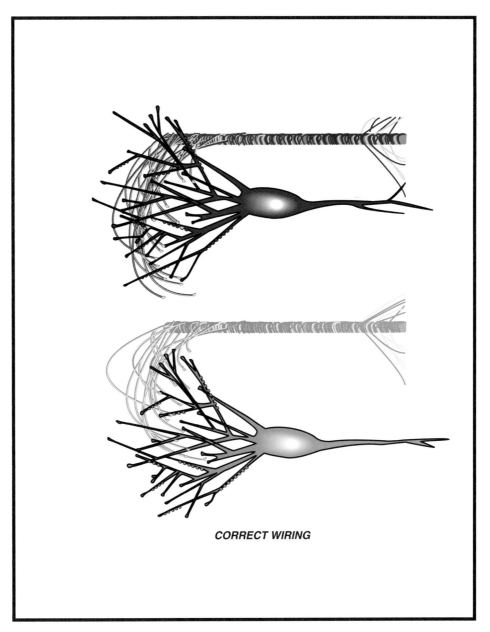

CORRECT WIRING

FIGURE 4–22. This figure represents the **correct wiring** of two neurons. During development, the incoming blue axons from all different parts of the brain are appropriately directed to their appropriate target dendrites on the blue neuron. Similarly, the incoming red axons from various regions of the brain are appropriately paired with their correct dendrites on the red neuron.

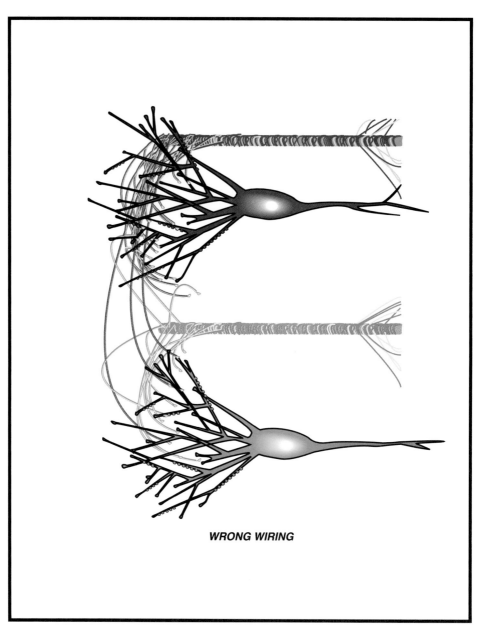

WRONG WIRING

FIGURE 4–23. This figure simplistically represents what might be occurring as a **disease mechanism in neurodevelopmental disorders**. In this case, the neurons do not fail to develop connections; the neurons also do not die or degenerate. What happens here is that the **synapse formation is misdirected**, resulting in the **wrong wiring**. This could lead to abnormal information transfer, confusing neuronal communications, and the inability of neurons to function, such as is postulated to occur in schizophrenia, **mental retardation**, and other neurodevelopmental disorders. This state of chaos is represented here as a **tangle of axons** where red axons inappropriately innervate blue dendrites, and blue axons inappropriately pair up with red dendrites. This is in contrast to the organized state represented in Figure 4–22.

96

acterized by a massive emotional discharge of panic, shortness of breath, chest pain, dizziness, and feelings of impending death or of going crazy.

Thus, disorders such as psychosis, epilepsy, and panic disorder appear to have one level of excessive neurotransmission that may explain their mechanism of producing acute symptoms (Figs. 4–18 and 4–19). Furthermore, these disorders seem to become more resistant to treatment the longer the disorder persists and the poorer the symptoms are uncontrolled, as if there is an underlying mechanism of destruction that accompanies out-of-control symptoms (Figs. 4–20 and 4–21). Thus, excessive neurotransmission itself may be a cause of deficient neurotransmission. As seizures beget seizures, and panic begets panic, psychosis begets psychosis, and mania begets mania, it does not appear that these symptoms are good for the brain. The psychopharmacologist must act to prevent symptoms, not only because symptom control may harness the disruptive influences of excessive neurotransmission upon behavior but because it may ultimately prevent the demise of the neurons mediating these very behaviors (Figs. 4–20 and 4–21). If these disorders of excessive neurotransmission are analogous to the brain "burning" during symptomatic crises such as a seizure, psychosis, panic attack, or mania, treatments might not only "put out the fire" but also salvage the underlying neuronal substrates that are burning as the fuel for the fire.

Other Mechanisms of Abnormal Neurotransmission

Several other mechanisms can be conceptualized. These include the *imbalance* between two neurotransmitters required to regulate a single process. This has been theorized as the mechanism of many of the movement disorders, where balance between the two neurotransmitters dopamine and acetylcholine is not normal. Another possible aberrancy of neurotransmission is that of the *wrong rate* of neurotransmission, possibly disrupting functions such as sleep, or biorhythms. The *wrong neuronal wiring* of the anatomically addressed nervous system could be problematic. This may occur in neurodevelopmental disorders where synapses are laid down in the wrong manner (perhaps in autism, mental retardation, or even schizophrenia) (Figs. 4–22 and 4–23). We have already discussed how degenerative disorders lose neurons and synapses, and the net result of loss of key synapses is an abnormal remaining wiring system of the brain.

Summary

In summary, this chapter has reviewed how enzymes and receptors are not only the targets of drug actions but also the sites of disease actions. We have discussed how diseases of the CNS are approached by three disciplines: neuroscience, biological psychiatry, and psychopharmacology. We have also discussed how disease actions in the brain modify neurotransmission by at least eight mechanisms: (1) modifications of molecular neurobiology; (2) loss of neuronal plasticity; (3) the process of excitotoxicity; (4) no neurotransmission; (5) too much neurotransmission; (6) an imbalance among neurotransmitters; (7) the wrong rate of neurotransmission; and (8) the wrong neuronal wiring.

CHAPTER 5

Depression

In this chapter, the reader will develop a foundation of knowledge about depression and the affective disorders. This chapter will describe the disorders of mood and also the major hypotheses on the biological basis for depression. In doing so, this chapter will formulate some of the key pharmacological principles that apply to neurons using norepinephrine (NE), dopamine (DA), and serotonin (5-hydroxytryptamine [5-HT]) as neurotransmitters. This will set the stage for understanding the pharmacological concepts underlying the use of antidepressant and mood-stabilizing drugs that will be reviewed in Chapter 6.

Clinical descriptions and criteria for how to diagnose affective disorders will only be mentioned in passing. The reader should consult standard reference sources for this material. Here, this chapter will discuss how discoveries of various antidepressants have impacted the diagnostic criteria for depression and modified the natural

Table 5–1. *Public perceptions of mental illness*

71%	Due to emotional weakness
65%	Caused by bad parenting
45%	Victim's fault; can will it away
43%	Incurable
35%	Consequence of sinful behavior
10%	Has a biological basis; involves the brain

history and course of this illness. The goal of this chapter is to acquaint the reader with current ideas about the clinical and biological aspects of depression in order to be prepared to understand how the various antidepressants work.

Clinical Description

Depression is an emotion that is universally experienced by virtually everyone at some time in their lives. Distinguishing the "normal" emotion of depression from an illness requiring medical treatment is often problematic for those who are not trained in the mental health sciences. Stigma and misinformation in our culture create the widespread popular misconception that mental illness such as depression is not a disease, but a deficiency of character that can be overcome with effort.

A recent survey of the general population revealed that 71% thought that mental illnesses were due to emotional weakness; 65% thought it was caused by bad parenting; 45% thought it was the victim's fault and that they could will it away; 43% thought that mental illness was uncurable; 35% thought it was the consequence of sinful behavior; and only 10% thought it had a biological basis or involved the brain (Table 5–1).

Stigma and misinformation can also extend into primary care, where many depressed as well as nondepressed patients present with medically unexplained symptoms. "Somatization" is the term used for such use of physical symptoms to express emotional distress, and may be a major reason for misdiagnosis of mental illness by primary care physicians. Many depressed patients with somatic complaints are considered to have no real or treatable illness, and are not treated for a psychiatric disorder once medical illnesses are evaluated and ruled out. In reality, however, most patients with diffuse unexplained somatic symptoms in primary care settings either have a treatable psychiatric illness (i.e., anxiety or depressive disorder) or are responding to stressful life events. Such patients do not generally have a genuine somatization disorder where "their symptoms are really all in their mind."

Given how frequent and treatable the depressive illnesses are, if there are a few most important points to make in this textbook, one of them is the need for the reader to know how to recognize and treat depression.

Diagnostic Criteria

Accepted, standardized diagnostic criteria are used to separate "normal" depression caused by disappointment or "having a bad day" from the disorders of mood, called

Table 5–2. *DSM IV diagnostic criteria for a major depressive episode*

A.   Five (or more) of the following symptoms have been present during the same 2-week period and represent a change from previous functioning; at least one of the symptoms is either (1) depressed mood or (2) loss of interest or pleasure. *Note*: Do not include symptoms that are clearly due to a general medical condition, or mood-incongruent delusions or hallucinations.

   1.   Depressed mood most of the day, nearly every day, as indicated by either subjective report (e.g., feels sad or empty) or observation made by others (e.g., appears tearful). *Note*: In children and adolescents, can be irritable mood.
   2.   Markedly diminished interest or pleasure in all, or almost all, activities most of the day, nearly every day (as indicated by either subjective account or observation made by others).
   3.   Significant weight loss when not dieting or weight gain (e.g., a change of more than 5% of body weight in a month), or decrease or increase in appetite nearly every day. *Note*: In children, consider failure to make expected weight gains.
   4.   Insomnia or hypersomnia nearly every day.
   5.   Psychomotor agitation or retardation nearly every day (observable by others, not merely subjective feelings of restlessness or being slowed down).
   6.   Fatigue or loss of energy nearly every day.
   7.   Feelings of worthlessness or excessive or inappropriate guilt (which may be delusional) nearly every day (not merely self-reproach or guilt about being sick).
   8.   Diminished ability to think or concentrate, or indecisiveness, nearly every day (either by subjective account or as observed by others).
   9.   Recurrent thoughts of death (not just fear of dying), recurrent suicidal ideation without a specific plan, or a suicide attempt or a specific plan for committing suicide.

B.   The symptoms do not meet criteria for a Mixed Episode.
C.   The symptoms cause clinically significant distress or impairment in social, occupational, or other important areas of functioning.
D.   The symptoms are not due to the direct physiological effects of a substance (e.g., a drug of abuse, a medication, or other treatment) or a general medical condition (e.g., hyperthyroidism).
E.   The symptoms are not better accounted for by Bereavement (i.e., after the loss of a loved one), the symptoms persist for longer than 2 months or are characterized by marked functional impairment, morbid preoccupation with worthlessness, suicidal ideation, psychotic symptoms, or psychomotor retardation.

affective disorders. Such criteria are in constant evolution, with current nosologies being set by the *Diagnostic and Statistical Manual of Mental Disorders* (DSM-IV) (Tables 5–2 and 5–3) in the United States and the *International Classification of Diseases* (ICD-10) in other countries. The reader is referred to these references for the specifics of currently accepted diagnostic criteria.

For our purposes, it is sufficient to recognize that the affective disorders are actually *syndromes*. That is, they are *clusters of symptoms*, only one of which is an abnormality of mood. Certainly the quality of mood, the degree of mood change from the normal (up, mania; or down, depression), and the duration of the abnormal mood are all important features of an affective disorder. In addition, however, clinicians must assess *vegetative features* such as sleep, appetite, weight, and sex drive;

Table 5–3. *DSM IV diagnostic criteria for a manic episode*

A. A distinct period of abnormally and persistently elevated, expansive, or irritable mood, lasting at least 1 week (or any duration if hospitalization is necessary).
B. During the period of mood disturbance, three (or more) of the following symptoms have persisted (four if the mood is only irritable) and have been present to a significant degree:
    1. Inflated self-esteem or grandiosity.
    2. Decreased need for sleep (e.g., feels rested after only 3 hours of sleep).
    3. More talkative than usual or pressure to keep talking.
    4. Flight of ideas or subjective experience that thoughts are racing.
    5. Distractability (i.e., attention too easily drawn to unimportant or irrelevant external stimuli).
    6. Increase in goal-directed activity (either socially, at work or school, or sexually) or psychomotor agitation.
    7. Excessive involvement in pleasurable activities that have a high potential for painful consequences (e.g., engaging in unrestrained buying sprees, sexual indiscretions, or foolish business investments).
C. The symptoms do not meet criteria for a Mixed Episode.
D. The mood disturbance is sufficiently severe to cause marked impairment in occupational functioning or in usual social activities or relationships with others, or to necessitate hospitalization to prevent harm to self or others, or there are psychotic features.
E. The symptoms are not due to the direct physiological effects of a substance (e.g., a drug of abuse, a medication, or other treatment) or a general medical condition (e.g., hyperthyroidism). *Note:* Manic-like episodes that are clearly caused by somatic antidepressant treatment (e.g., medication, electroconvulsive therapy, light therapy) should not count towards a diagnosis of Bipolar I Disorder.

Table 5–4. *Depression is a syndrome*

Clusters of symptoms in depression:
    Vegetative
    Cognitive
    Impulse Control
    Behavioral
    Physical (somatic)

cognitive features such as attention span, frustration tolerance, memory, and negative distortions; *impulse control* such as suicide and homicide; *behavioral features* such as motivation, pleasure, interests, and fatigability; and *physical (or somatic) features* such as headaches, stomachaches, and muscle tension (Table 5–4).

Discovery of Antidepressants

The introduction of antidepressants profoundly impacted the evolution of diagnostic criteria for affective disorders. Prior to the 1950s no effective antidepressants existed.

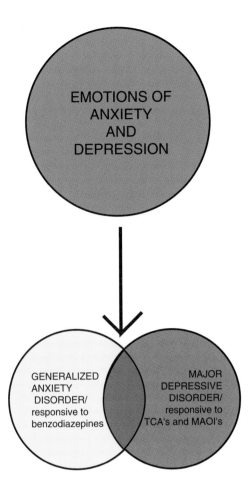

FIGURE 5–1. Prior to the discovery of antidepressants and anxiolytics, there were no widely accepted diagnostic criteria for major depressive disorder or for generalized anxiety disorder. Diagnostic criteria to separate the **emotions of anxiety and depression** into better defined psychiatric diagnoses were assisted by the introduction of therapeutic agents that effectively treated these symptoms. Thus, **generalized anxiety disorder** became increasingly recognized as a syndrome **responsive to benzodiazepine** anxiolytic agents, and **major depressive disorder** a syndrome **responsive to tricyclic antidepressants (TCAs) and monoamine oxidase inhibitors (MAOIs)**.

When the first antidepressants were serendipitously discovered in the 1950s and 1960s, it became important to identify those patients likely to benefit from these drugs. The diagnostic criteria for depression at that time were aimed in part at distinguishing those patients who would respond to the new antidepressants (the tricyclic antidepressants and the monoamine oxidase inhibitors [MAOIs]), versus those patients who would respond to the new anxiolytics also being introduced at the same time (the benzodiazepines). Thus, the concept evolved that major depressive disorder could be clinically distinguished from generalized anxiety disorder (called anxiety neurosis at that time), and that each condition had unique pharmacological treatments. In part, the early diagnostic criteria were used to attempt to identify a "benzodiazepine responsive syndrome" that differed from a "tricyclic antidepressant responsive syndrome" (Fig. 5–1).

Search for Subtypes of Depression

Although effective for depression in general, the early antidepressants did not help everyone with depression. This observation applies as well today, as only two out of three patients with depression will respond to any given antidepressant. In the 1970s and 1980s, the diagnostic criteria for depression began to focus in part on identifying which depressed patients were the best candidates for the various antidepressant treatments that had become available. For example, lithium was found to be effective for the diagnostic subtype of manic depressive disorder and was also introduced into clinical practice at this time.

During this era, the idea evolved that there might be one subgroup of unipolar depressives that was especially responsive to antidepressants, and another that was not. The first group was hypothesized to be a serious, even melancholic clinical form of depression that had a biological basis, a high degree of familial occurrence, was episodic in nature, and was likely to respond to tricyclic antidepressants and MAOIs. Opposed to this was a second form of depression hypothesized to be neurotic and characterological in origin, less severe but more chronic, not especially responsive to antidepressants, and possibly amenable to treatment with psychotherapy.

As discussed in Chapter 4, the search for biological markers (such as the dexamethasone suppression test) for some type of depression that is biologically based and predictive of antidepressant treatment responsiveness has been disappointing up to now. Various theories and hypotheses are still tenable and will be discussed in the following section. However, it is not yet possible to predict who will and who will not respond to a given antidepressant drug. What is now known is that several clinical features of depression are not particularly helpful in making this distinction, and these have fallen out of diagnostic utility in the 1990s. These include biological versus nonbiological; endogenous versus reactive; melancholic versus neurotic; acute versus chronic; familial versus nonfamilial; and others as well.

Epidemiology and Natural History

In the 1990s, diagnostic criteria for depression began to be applied increasingly to describing the epidemiology and natural history of depression so that the effects of treatments could be better measured. Key questions are, What is the incidence of major depressive disorder? How many people have the condition at the present time, and how many in their lifetimes? Are individuals with depression being identified and treated and, if so, how? Also, what is the outcome of their treatment? What is the natural history of their depression without treatment and how is this impacted by treatment?

Answers to these questions are just beginning to evolve (see Tables 5–5 through 5–10). For example, the incidence of affective disorders is approximately 5 to 6% of the population (more than 12 million individuals in the United States), but only about one third of these individuals are in treatment. Depression is just as socially debilitating as coronary artery disease, and more debilitating than diabetes mellitus or arthritis. Up to 15% of severely ill depressed patients will ultimately commit suicide. Suicide attempts are up to 10/100 subjects depressed for a year, with 1 successful suicide per 100 subjects depressed for a year. In the United States, for example, there are approximately 300,000 suicide attempts and 30,000 completed suicides per year, most but not all associated with depression.

The conclusions are impressive: depression is a common, debilitating, life-threatening illness that can be successfully treated, but which commonly is not treated. Public education efforts are ongoing to identify cases and get them effective treatment.

Table 5–5. *Patient education*

The effectiveness of any treatment rests on a cooperative effort by patient and practitioner. The patient should be told of the diagnosis, prognosis, and treatment options, including costs, duration, and potential side effects. In presenting patient and family education about the clinical management of depression, it is useful to emphasize the following information:

Depression is a medical illness, not a character defect or weakness.

Recovery is the rule, not the exception.

Treatments are effective, and there are many options for treatment. An effective treatment can be found for nearly all patients.

The aim of treatment is complete symptom remission, not just getting better, but getting and staying well.

The risk of recurrence is significant: 50% after one episode, 70% after two episodes, 90% after three episodes.

Patient and family should be alert to early signs and symptoms of recurrence and seek treatment early if depression returns.

Table 5–6. *Risk factors for major depression*

Risk Factor	Association
Gender	Major depression is twice as likely in women
Age	Peak age on onset is 20–40 years of age
Family history	1.5 to 3 times higher risk with positive history
Marital status	Separated and divorced persons report higher rates
	Married males lower rates than unmarried males
	Married females higher rates than unmarried females
Postpartum	An increased risk for the 6-month period following childbirth
Negative life events	Possible association
Early parental death	Possible association

Table 5–7. *Depression in the United States*

High rate of occurrence
    5–11% lifetime prevalence
    10–14 million in United States depressed in any year
Episodes can be of long duration (years)
Over 50% rate of recurrence following a single episode; higher if patient has had multiple episodes
Morbidity comparable to angina and advanced coronary artery disease
High mortality from suicide if untreated

Longitudinal Course of Depression

Until recently very little was known about what happens to depression if it is not treated. It is now thought that most untreated episodes of depression last 6 to 24 months (Fig. 5–2). Perhaps only 5 to 10% of untreated cases have their episodes continue for more than 2 years.

Table 5–8. *Facts about suicide and depression*

20–40% of patients with an affective disorder exhibit nonfatal suicidal behaviors, including thoughts of suicide
Estimates associate 16,000 suicides in the United States annually with depressive disorder
15% of those hospitalized for major depressive disorder attempt suicide
15% of patients with severe primary major depressive disorder of at least 1 month's duration eventually commit suicide

Table 5–9. *Suicide and major depression: the rules of sevens*

One out of seven with recurrent depressive illness commit suicide
70% of suicides have depressive illness
70% of suicides see their primary care physician within 6 weeks of suicide
Suicide is the seventh leading cause of death in the United States

Table 5–10. *The hidden cost of not treating major depression*

Mortality
    30,000 to 35,000 suicides per year
    Fatal accidents due to impaired concentration and attention
    Death due to illnesses which an be a sequelae (e.g., alcohol abuse)
Patient morbidity
    Suicide attempts
    Accidents
    Resultant illnesses
    Lost jobs
    Failure to advance in career and school
    Substance abuse
Societal costs
    Dysfunctional families
    Absenteeism
    Decreased productivity
    Job-related injuries
    Adverse effect on quality control in the workplace

Four terms are used to describe the clinical status of depressed patients over time. These are the four Rs: remission, recovery, relapse, and recurrence. They are often confused. The terms "remission" and "recovery" both mean that a depressed patient has experienced at least a 50% reduction in symptoms as assessed on a standard psychiatric rating scale (the Hamilton Depression Scale). This also generally corresponds to a global clinical rating that the patient is much improved or very much improved (not merely minimally improved) (see Fig. 5–2). Sometimes the term "remission" is used interchangeably with "recovery." However, remission properly

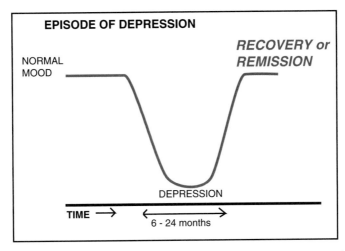

FIGURE 5–2. Depression is episodic, with **untreated episodes** commonly lasting from **6 to 24 months**, followed by **recovery or remission**.

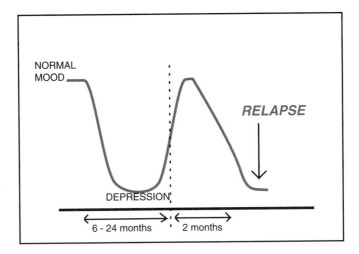

FIGURE 5–3. When depression returns within 2 months of recovery, it is called a **relapse**.

refers to improvement that has lasted less than 2 months, and recovery to improvement that has lasted longer than 2 months.

The term "relapse" means return of a depressive episode within 2 months of improvement (Fig. 5–3). Thus, "relapse" occurs during "remission" and prior to "recovery." On the other hand, if an episode of depression occurs *after* 2 months of improvement, it is called a "recurrence" (Fig. 5–4). Thus "recurrence" occurs after "recovery."

Follow-up studies of depressed patients after 1 year show that approximately 40% still have the same diagnosis, 40% have no diagnosis, and the rest either recover partially or develop the diagnosis of dysthymia (Fig. 5–5). Dysthymia is a low-grade but very chronic form of depression that lasts for more than 2 years (Fig. 5–6). It may represent a relatively stable and unremitting illness of low-grade depression, or it may indicate a state of partial recovery from an episode of major depressive dis-

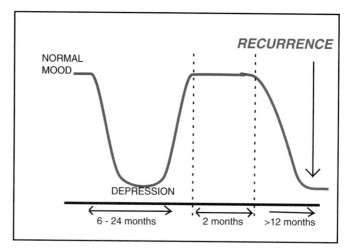

FIGURE 5–4. When depression returns greater than 2 months following recovery, it is called a **recurrence**.

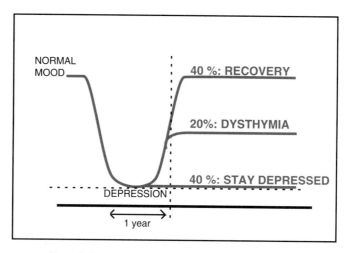

FIGURE 5–5. Follow-up studies of depressed patients show that after 1 year, approximately 40% **stay depressed**, 40% have **recovered**, and the rest either recover partially or develop **dysthymia**.

order. When major depressive episodes are superimposed upon dysthymia, the resulting condition is sometimes called "double depression" (Fig. 5–7) and may account for many of those with poor interepisode recovery.

Longitudinal Treatment of Depression

Guidelines for long-term treatment of patients with antidepressants are just evolving, since early studies with antidepressants only targeted short-term treatment of single depressive episodes, and only recently has there been widespread appreciation of the chronicity and high recurrence rate of major depressive disorder. Thus, modern treatment is now emphasizing that antidepressants should be used not only to treat acute episodes of depression but also to try to prevent future episodes of illness.

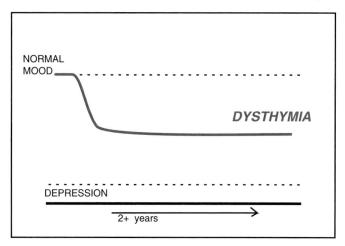

FIGURE 5–6. **Dysthymia** is a low-grade but very chronic form of depression that lasts for more than 2 years.

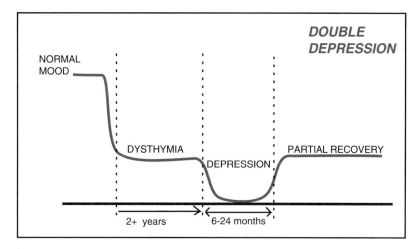

FIGURE 5–7. **Double depression** is a syndrome characterized by oscillating between episodes of major depression and periods of partial recovery or dysthymia.

Treatments are increasingly attempting to gain full remission of symptoms as well, for studies of those with only a partial recovery suggest that the likelihood of a subsequent episode is increased, and that there will be continuing poor or partial recovery between future episodes of major depression. Studies also suggest that treatment for major depressive disorder is more effective earlier in the episode before it becomes chronic or recurrent. This is an emerging theme for many psychiatric disorders today: namely, that uncontrolled symptoms may indicate that some pathophysiological mechanism is ongoing in the brain which, if allowed to persist untreated, may cause the ultimate outcome of illness to be worse (see Figs. 4–19 and 4–20). Depression may beget depression. Depression may thus have a long-lasting or even irreversible neuropathological effect upon the brain, rendering treatment less

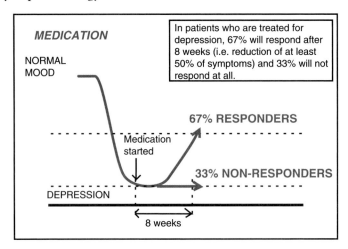

FIGURE 5–8. Virtually every known antidepressant has the same **response rate,** namely that 67% of depressed patients respond to a given medication, and 33% fail to respond.

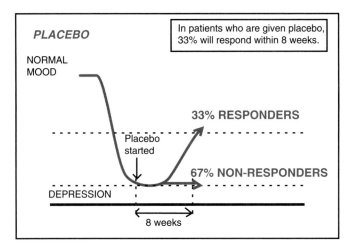

FIGURE 5–9. In controlled clinical trials, 33% of patients respond to **placebo** treatment, and 67% fail to respond.

effective if allowed to progress than if symptoms are removed by appropriate treatment early in the course of the illness.

Studies of antidepressants have traditionally been 4- to 8-week studies. The onset of action of all known antidepressants is delayed for at least 2 to 4 weeks, whereas the onset of therapeutic actions for the benzodiazepines in treating anxiety is often much sooner. Beyond this notion of delayed onset for antidepressants, however, there has been little emphasis until recently on what happens to a depressed patient after the first month or two of treatment. It has long been known that two out of three subjects with depression have a "response" (50% or greater improvement) after a month or two of treatment with any given antidepressant agent (Fig. 5–8). Interestingly, it is also well recognized that one out of three subjects with depression respond to placebo (Fig. 5–9).

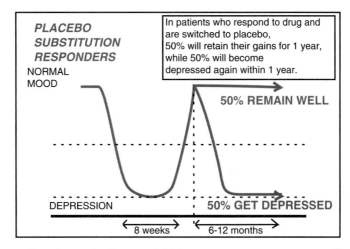

FIGURE 5–10. Depressed patients who have an initial treatment response to an antidepressant will **experience a recurrence at the rate of 50%** within 6 to 12 months if their medication is withdrawn and a **placebo substituted**.

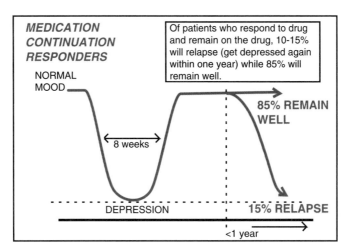

FIGURE 5–11. Depressed patients who have an initial treatment response to an antidepressant will **experience a recurrence only at the rate of 10 to 15%** if their **medication is continued for a year** following recovery.

If antidepressant treatment is withdrawn within the first year after remission, there is roughly a 50% chance of the patient experiencing another episode of major depressive disorder (Fig. 5–10). However, if antidepressant treatment is continued for a year after remission, there is only a 10 to 15% chance of another episode of major depression recurring (Fig. 5–11). Current treatment guidelines are therefore to treat patients having their first-ever major depressive episode with an antidepressant until remission, and then to continue the medication for another 6 to 12 months. For patients who have had multiple prior episodes of major depressive disorder, or inadequate treatment responses, there are not yet clear guidelines for duration of treatment. However, recurrence rates may be even higher in such individuals and treatment duration may need to be longer than a year in selected cases, or even indefinitely until clearer guidelines emerge from future research.

Although a number of antidepressants have been shown to reduce *relapse* from the index episode of depression within the first 6 to 12 months, it is not yet certain whether antidepressants can continue to function as prophylaxis against *recurrence* for longer than 1 year of treatment. Such investigations are currently in progress, but it already appears to be prudent to consider long-term continuation of antidepressants in those who have had several episodes of depression and also a good response to antidepressant drugs when under treatment.

In terms of dose of medication to use for longitudinal treatment to prevent relapse and recurrence in depression, one clinical nostrum has been that the dose of antidepressant used for initial treatment as an inpatient could be cut in half for outpatient maintenance of an indeterminate period of time. This practice was never validated by controlled clinical trials and is outdated today by the results of new studies with antidepressants that show that the dose used to induce a remission is also required to maintain the remission.

Chronic treatment guidelines are therefore beginning to evolve for those who respond well to acute treatment with antidepressants. How about those who fail to respond to antidepressants at all (so-called "treatment-refractory" patients) or those who are "nonresponders" (i.e., they do not experience a full remission, or have less than a 50% reduction in symptoms or are only minimally and unsatisfactorily improved)? Unfortunately, refractory and nonresponding patients are not adequately studied, resulting in unclear treatment guidelines and often inadequate outcomes for them. In practice, treatments for refractory and for nonresponding depressed patients are usually organized by various and sundry algorithms involving in the first instance a sequence of antidepressants, and then combinations of antidepressants. Various algorithms for the use of antidepressants in treatment-refractory patients and in nonresponding patients have evolved more by anecdote than by systematic study over the years and are discussed in the following chapter. However, no U.S. Food and Drug Administration (FDA) – approved guidelines exist in the United States for use of antidepressants in either of these groups.

In summary, the natural history of depression indicates that this is a lifelong illness, likely to relapse within several months of an index episode, especially if antidepressants are discontinued, and prone to multiple recurrences possibly preventable by long-term antidepressant treatment.

Biological Basis of Depression

Monoamine Hypothesis

The first major theory about the biological etiology of depression hypothesized that depression was due to a deficiency of monoamine neurotransmitters, notably NE and 5HT (see Figs. 5–12 through 5–15). Evidence for this was rather simplistic. Certain drugs that depleted these neurotransmitters could induce depression, and the known antidepressants at that time (the tricyclic antidepressants and the MAOIs) both had pharmacological actions that boosted these neurotransmitters. Thus, the idea was that the "normal" amount of monoamine neurotransmitters (Fig. 5–12) became

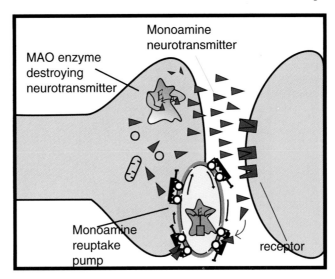

FIGURE 5–12. This figure represents the **normal state** of a monoaminergic neuron. This particular neuron is releasing the neurotransmitter **norepinephrine (NE)** at the normal rate. All the regulatory elements of the neuron are also normal, including the functioning of the enzyme **MAO, which destroys NE**; the **NE reuptake pump**, which terminates the action of NE; and the **NE receptors**, which react to the release of NE.

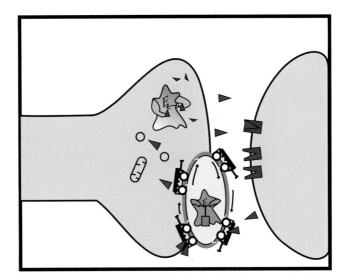

FIGURE 5–13. In the case of **depression**, the neurotransmitter is depleted, causing **neurotransmitter deficiency**.

somehow depleted, perhaps by an unknown disease process, by stress, or by drugs (Fig. 5–13), leading to the symptoms of depression. MAOIs increased the neurotransmitters, causing relief of depression due to inhibition of MAO (Fig. 5–14). Tricyclic antidepressants also increased the neurotransmitters, resulting in relief from depression due to blockade of the monoamine transport pumps (Fig. 5–15).

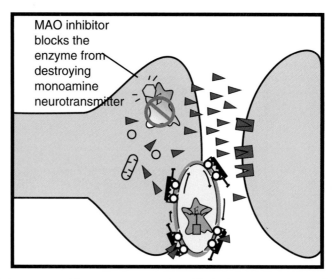

FIGURE 5–14. **MAOIs** act as antidepressants, since they block the enzyme MAO from destroying monoamine neurotransmitters, thus allowing them to accumulate. This accumulation theoretically reverses the prior neurotransmitter deficiency (see Fig. 5–13) and relieves depression by returning the monoamine neuron to the normal state.

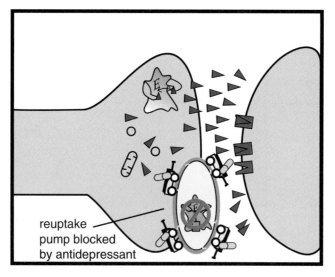

FIGURE 5–15. **Tricyclic antidepressants** act as antidepressants, since they block the neurotransmitter reuptake pump, thus causing neurotransmitter to accumulate. This accumulation theoretically reverses the prior neurotransmitter deficiency (see Fig. 5–13) and relieves depression by returning the monoamine neuron to the normal state.

Monoaminergic Neurons

In order to understand this hypothesis, it is necessary first to understand the normal pharmacological functioning of monoaminergic neurons. The principal monoamine

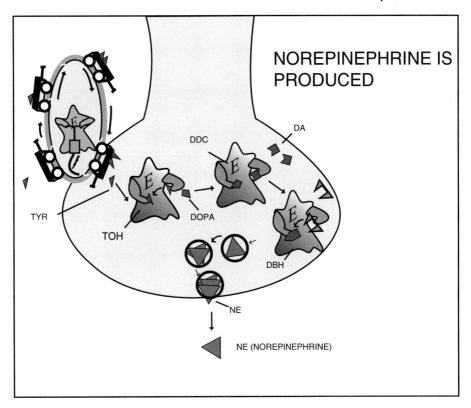

FIGURE 5–16. This figure shows how the neurotransmitter **norepinephrine (NE) is produced** in noradrenergic neurons. This process starts with the amino acid precursor of NE, **tyrosine (tyr)**, being transported into the nervous system from the blood by means of an active transport pump. This active transport pump for tyrosine is separate and distinct from the active transport pump for NE itself (see Fig. 5–17). Once pumped inside the neuron, the tyrosine is acted upon by three enzymes in sequence: first, tyrosine hydroxylase (**TOH**), the rate-limiting and most important enzyme in the regulation of NE synthesis. Tyrosine hydroxylase converts the amino acid tyrosine into **DOPA**. The second enzyme then acts, namely DOPA decarboxylase (**DDC**), which converts DOPA into dopamine (**DA**). The third and final NE synthetic enzyme, dopamine beta hydroxylase (**DBH**), converts DA into NE. NE is then stored in synaptic packages called vesicles until released by a nerve impulse.

neurotransmitters in the brain are the catecholamines NE and DA, and the indolamine 5HT.

Noradrenergic neurons. The noradrenergic neuron utilizes norepinephrine, also known as noradrenaline, for its neurotransmitter. It has already been discussed in Chapter 2 that neurotransmitters are synthesized by means of enzymes that assemble neurotransmitters in the nerve terminal. For the noradrenergic neuron, this process starts with the amino acid precursor of NE, tyrosine, being transported into the nervous system from the blood by means of an active transport pump (Fig. 5–16). Once inside the neuron, the tyrosine is acted upon by three enzymes in sequence: first, tyrosine hydroxylase (TOH), the rate-limiting and most important enzyme in the regulation of NE synthesis. Tyrosine hydroxylase converts the amino acid tyrosine

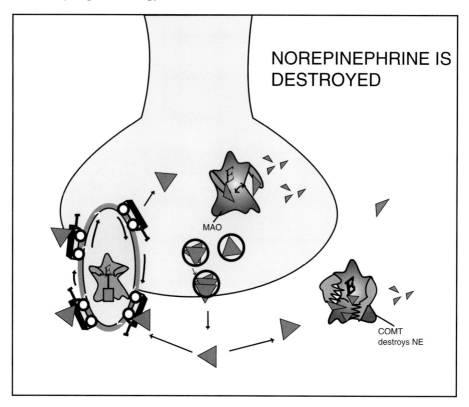

FIGURE 5–17. **Norepinephrine** (NE) can also be **destroyed** by enzymes in the NE neuron. The principal destructive enzymes are monoamine oxidase (**MAO**) and catechol-0-methyltransferase (**COMT**). The action of NE can be terminated not only by enzymes that destroy NE but also by a **transport pump for NE**, which removes it from acting in the synapse without destroying it. This transport pump is separate and distinct from the transport pump for tyrosine used in carrying tyrosine into the NE neuron for NE synthesis (see Fig. 5–16). The transport pump that terminates the synaptic action of NE is sometimes called the "NE transporter" or the "NE reuptake pump." It is selective for NE and not for any other neurotransmitter (see also the dopamine transporter in Fig. 5–20 and the serotonin transporter in Fig. 5–23). The NE transporter is part of the presynaptic machinery, where it acts as a vacuum cleaner whisking NE out of the synapse, off the synaptic receptors, and stopping its synaptic actions. Once inside the presynaptic nerve terminal, NE can either be stored again for subsequent reuse when another nerve impulse arrives, or it can be destroyed by NE-destroying enzymes.

into DOPA. The second enzyme then acts, namely DOPA decarboxylase (DDC), which converts DOPA into DA. DA itself is a neurotransmitter in some neurons. However, for NE neurons, DA is just a precursor of NE. In fact, the third and final NE synthetic enzyme, dopamine beta hydroxylase (DBH), converts DA into NE. NE is then stored in synaptic packages called vesicles until released by a nerve impulse (Fig. 5–16).

NE is not only created by enzymes but can also be destroyed by enzymes (Fig. 5–17). Two principal destructive enzymes act on NE to turn it into inactive metabolites. The first is MAO, which is located in mitochondria in the presynaptic neuron and elsewhere. The second is catechol-0-methyltransferase (COMT), which is thought to be located largely outside of the presynaptic nerve terminal (Fig. 5–17).

The action of NE can be terminated not only by enzymes that destroy NE but also cleverly by a transport pump for NE that removes it from acting in the synapse without destroying it (Fig. 5–17). In fact, such inactivated NE can be restored for reuse in a later neurotransmitting nerve impulse. The transport pump that terminates the synaptic action of NE is sometimes called the "NE transporter" and sometimes the "NE reuptake pump." It is selective for NE and not for any other neurotransmitter. This NE reuptake pump is located as part of the presynaptic machinery, where it acts a vacuum cleaner whisking NE out of the synapse, off the synaptic receptors, and stopping its synaptic actions. Once inside the presynaptic nerve terminal, NE can either be stored again for subsequent reuse when another nerve impulse arrives, or it can be destroyed by NE-destroying enzymes (Fig. 5–17).

The noradrenergic neuron is regulated by a multiplicity of receptors for NE (Fig. 5–18). In the classical subtyping of NE receptors, they were classified as either alpha or beta, depending upon their preference for a series of agonists and antagonists. Next, the NE receptors were subclassified into alpha 1 and alpha 2 as well as beta 1 and beta 2. More recently, adrenergic receptors have been even further subclassified both on pharmacological and molecular differences.

For a general understanding of NE receptors, the reader should begin with an awareness of two key receptors: the postsynaptic beta 1 receptor, and the presynaptic alpha 2 receptor (Fig. 5–18). There are also postsynaptic beta 2 receptors and postsynaptic alpha 1 and alpha 2 receptors, as well as further subtypes of adrenergic receptors, but these will not be emphasized for now.

The presynaptic alpha 2 receptor is important because it is an *autoreceptor*. That is, when the presynaptic alpha 2 receptor recognizes synaptic NE, it turns off further release of NE. Since this alpha 2 receptor is located on the axon nerve terminal, it is sometimes called a *terminal autoreceptor*. Thus the presynaptic alpha 2 terminal autoreceptor acts as a brake for the NE neuron, also known as a negative feedback regulatory signal. Stimulating this receptor (i.e., stepping on the brake) stops the neuron from firing. This probably occurs physiologically to prevent overfiring of the NE neuron, since it can shut itself off once the firing rate gets too high and the autoreceptor becomes stimulated. It is worthy of note that drugs can not only mimic the natural functioning of the NE neuron by stimulating the presynaptic alpha 2 neuron, but drugs that antagonize this same receptor will have the effect of cutting the brake cable and enhancing the release of NE.

The postsynaptic beta 1 receptor recognizes NE released into the synapse and acts to set up a molecular cascade in the postsynaptic neuron, thereby causing neurotransmission to pass from the presynaptic neuron to the postsynaptic neuron (Fig. 5–18).

Dopaminergic neurons. Dopaminergic neurons utilize the neurotransmitter DA, which is synthesized in dopaminergic nerve terminals by two out of three of the same enzymes that also synthesize NE (Fig. 5–19). However, DA neurons lack the third enzyme, namely dopamine beta-hydroxylase, and thus cannot convert DA to NE. Therefore, it is DA that is stored and used for neurotransmitting purposes.

The DA neuron has a presynaptic transporter (reuptake pump) that is unique for DA (Fig. 5–20), but works analogously to the NE transporter (Fig. 5–17). On the other hand, the same enzymes that destroy NE (Fig. 5–17) also destroy DA (MAO and COMT) (Fig. 5–20).

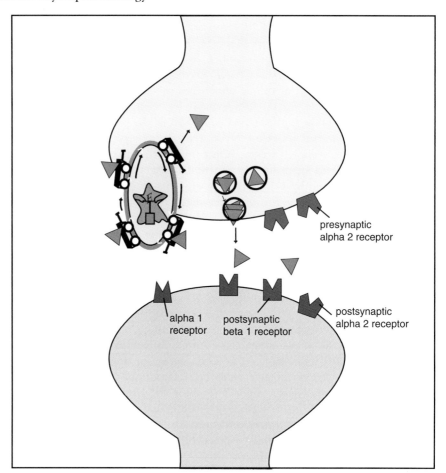

FIGURE 5–18. The noradrenergic neuron is regulated by a multiplicity of **receptors for NE**. Pictured here are the **NE transporter**, and several NE receptors, including alpha 1, alpha 2, and beta 1 adrenergic receptors. Three of these receptors are located on the postsynaptic neuron, including the **beta 1 receptor** and both the **alpha 1** and the **alpha 2** adrenergic receptors. Postsynaptic NE receptors generally act by recognizing when NE is released from the presynaptic neuron, and reacting by setting up a molecular cascade in the postsynaptic neuron, thereby causing neurotransmission to pass from the presynaptic neuron to the postsynaptic neuron. The **presynaptic alpha 2 receptor** is important because it is an autoreceptor. That is, when the presynaptic alpha 2 receptor recognizes synaptic NE, it turns off further release of NE. Thus the presynaptic alpha 2 terminal autoreceptor acts as a brake for the NE neuron. Stimulating this receptor (i.e., stepping on the brake) stops the neuron from firing. This probably occurs physiologically to prevent overfiring of the NE neuron, since it can shut itself off once the firing rate gets too high and the autoreceptor becomes stimulated.

Receptors for dopamine also regulate dopaminergic neurotransmission (Fig. 5–21). A plethora of dopamine receptors exist, including at least five pharmacological subtypes and several more molecular isoforms. Perhaps the most extensively investigated dopamine receptor is the dopamine-2 receptor, as it is stimulated by dopaminergic agonists for the treatment of Parkinson's disease, and blocked by dopamine antagonist neuroleptics for the treatment of schizophrenia. Dopamine receptors can

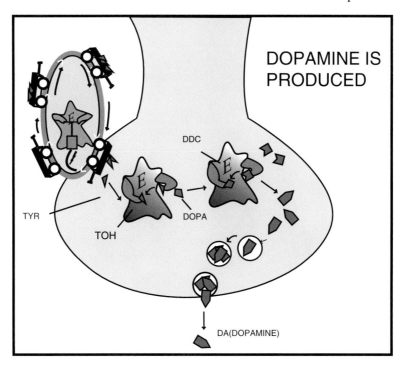

FIGURE 5–19. **Dopamine (DA)** is produced in dopaminergic neurons from the precursor **tyrosine (tyr)**, which is tranported into the neuron by an active transport pump, and then converted into DA by two out of three of the same enzymes that also synthesize norepinephrine (Fig. 5–16). The DA synthesizing enzymes are tyrosine hydroxylase (**TOH**), which produces **DOPA**, followed by DOPA decarboxylase (**DDC**), which produces DA.

be presynaptic, where they function as negative feedback regulatory, or postsynaptic, where they are involved in neurotransmission from the presynaptic neuron to the postsynaptic neuron (Fig. 5–21).

Serotonergic neurons. Analogous enzymes, transport pumps, and receptors exist in the 5HT neuron (Figs. 5–22 through 5–24). For synthesis of serotonin in serotonergic neurons, however, a different amino acid, tryptophan, is transported into the brain from the plasma to serve as the 5HT precursor (Fig. 5–22). Two synthetic enzymes then convert tryptophan into serotonin: first tryptophan hydroxylase converts tryptophan into 5-hydroxytryptophan (5HTP), and then aromatic amino acid decarboxylase converts 5HTP into 5HT (Fig. 5–22). Like NE and DA, 5HT is also destroyed by MAO, and converted into an inactive metabolite (Fig. 5–23). Also, the 5HT neuron has a presynaptic transport pump selective for serotonin called the serotonin transporter (Fig. 5–23), analogous to the NE transporter in NE neurons (Fig. 5–17) and to the DA transporter in DA neurons (Fig. 5–20).

Receptor subtyping for the serotonergic neuron has proceeded at a very rapid pace, with at least four major categories of 5HT receptors, each further subtyped depending upon pharmacological or molecular properties (Fig. 5–24). 5HT receptors are a good example of how the description of neurotransmitter receptors is in constant flux, and is constantly being revised. For a general understanding of the 5HT

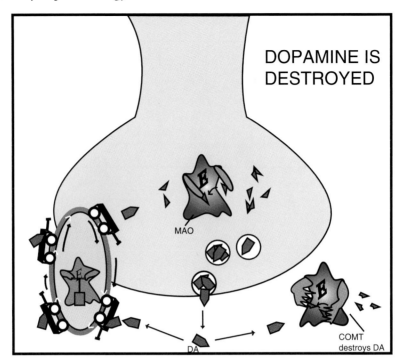

FIGURE 5–20. **Dopamine (DA)** is destroyed by the same enzymes that destroy norepinephrine (see Fig. 5–17), namely monoamine oxidase (**MAO**) and catechol-0-methyltransferase (**COMT**). The DA neuron has a presynaptic transporter (**reuptake pump**) that is unique for DA, but works analogously to the NE transporter (Fig. 5–17).

neuron, the reader can begin with an understanding that there are two key receptors that are presynaptic (5HT1A and 5HT1D) and several that are postsynaptic (5HT1A, 5HT1D, 5HT2A, 5HT2C, 5HT3, and 5HT4) (Figs. 5–24 through 5–32), the most important of these perhaps being the 5HT2A, sometimes also called the 5HT2 receptor (Figs. 5–31 and 5–32).

Presynaptic 5HT receptors are autoreceptors, and detect the presence of 5HT, causing a shutdown of further 5HT release and 5HT neuronal impulse flow. When 5HT is detected in the cell dendrites and cell body, it occurs via a 5HT1A receptor that is also called a *somatodendritic* autoreceptor (Figs. 5–24 and 5–25). This causes a slowing of neuronal impulse flow through the serotonin neuron (Fig. 5–26). When 5HT is detected in the synapse by presynaptic 5HT receptors, it occurs via a 5HT1D receptor that is also called a *terminal autoreceptor* (Fig. 5–27) – analogous to the alpha 2 adrenergic terminal autoreceptor in the noradrenergic neuron explained above (Fig. 5–18). In the case of the 5HT1D terminal autoreceptor, 5HT occupancy of this receptor causes a blockade of 5HT release (Figs. 5–28 and 5–30). On the other hand, drugs that block the 5HT1D autoreceptor can promote 5HT release (Fig. 5–29).

Postsynaptic 5HT receptors such as 5HT2A receptors (Fig. 5–31) regulate the translation of 5HT release from the presynaptic nerve into a neurotransmission in the postsynaptic nerve (Fig. 5–32). The 5HT2 (5HT2A) receptor is especially emphasized as an important postsynaptic 5HT receptor subtype because it is implicated in the mechanism of action of antidepressants, as will be developed next in Chapter

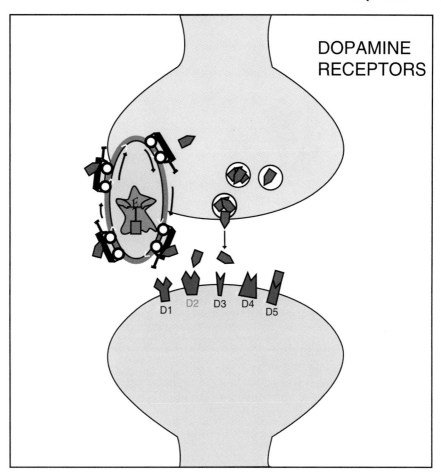

FIGURE 5–21. **Receptors for dopamine** (DA) regulate dopaminergic neurotransmission. A plethora of dopamine receptors exist, including at least five pharmacological subtypes and several more molecular isoforms. Perhaps the most extensively investigated dopamine receptor is the dopamine-2 receptor, as it is stimulated by dopaminergic agonists for the treatment of Parkinson's disease and blocked by dopamine antagonist neuroleptics for the treatment of schizophrenia.

6. However, more is being learned about the importance of postsynaptic 5HT1A and 5HT2C receptors, especially for the mechanism of various pharmacological agents that act on 5HT neurons. These will also be discussed in greater detail later.

Classical Antidepressants and the Monoamine Hypothesis

The first antidepressants to be discovered came from two classes of agents: first, the tricyclic antidepressants (so named because their chemical structure has three rings) and the MAOIs (so named because they inhibit the neurotransmitter destroying enzyme MAO). When tricyclic antidepressants block the NE transporter, they increase the availability of NE in the synapse, since the vacuum cleaner pump can no longer sweep NE out of the synapse (Figs. 5–15 and 5–17). When tricyclic antidepressants block the DA pump (Fig. 5–20) or the 5HT pump (Fig. 5–23), they

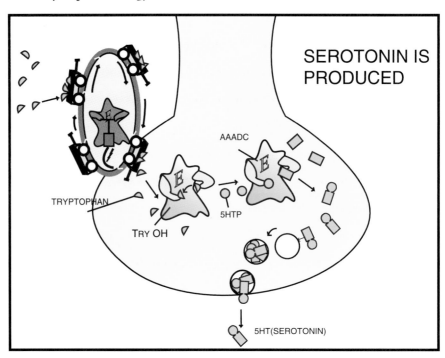

FIGURE 5–22. **Serotonin** (5-hydroxytryptamine [5HT]) is **produced** from enzymes after the amino acid precursor tryptophan is transported into the serotonin neuron. The **tryptophan transport pump** is distinct from the serotonin transporter (see Fig. 5–23). Once transported into the serotonin neuron, tryptophan is converted into 5-hydroxytryptophan (**5HTP**) by the enzyme tryptophan hydroxylase (**Try OH**). 5HTP is then converted into 5HT by the enzyme aromatic amino acid decarboxylase (**AAADC**). Serotonin is then stored in synaptic vesicles, where it stays until released by a neuronal impulse.

similarly enhance the synaptic availability of DA or 5HT, respectively, and by the same mechanism (Fig. 5–15). When MAOIs block NE, DA, and 5HT breakdown, they boost the levels of these neurotransmitters (Fig. 5–14).

Since it was recognized by the 1960s that all the classical antidepressants thus boost NE, DA, and 5HT by one manner or another (Figs. 5–14 and 5–15), the original idea was that one or another of these neurotransmitters, also chemically known as monoamines, might be deficient in the first place in depression (Fig. 5–13). Thus, the "monoamine hypothesis" was born. A good deal of effort was expended especially in the 1960s and 1970s to identify the theoretically predicted deficiencies of the monoamine neurotransmitters. This effort to date has unfortunately yielded mixed and sometimes confusing results.

Some studies suggest that NE metabolites are deficient in some patients with depression, but this has not been uniformly observed. Other studies suggest that the 5HT metabolite 5HIAA is reduced in the cerebrospinal fluid (CSF) of depressed patients. On closer examination, however, it has been found that only some of the depressed patients had low CSF 5HIAA, and these tended to be those with suicide attempts of a violent nature. Subsequently, it was also reported that CSF 5HIAA is decreased in other populations subject to violent outbursts of poor impulse control,

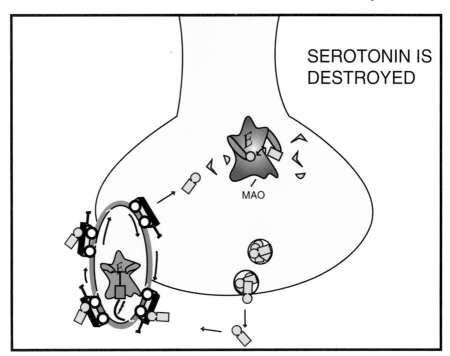

FIGURE 5–23. **Serotonin is destroyed** by the enzyme monoamine oxidase (**MAO**) and converted into an inactive metabolite. The 5HT neuron has a presynaptic transport pump selective for serotonin called the **serotonin transporter**, analogous to the norepinephrine (NE) transporter in NE neurons (Fig. 5–17) and to the DA transporter in DA neurons (Fig. 5–20).

but who were not depressed, namely patients with antisocial personality disorder who were arsonists, and patients with borderline personality disorder with self-destructive acts. Thus, low CSF 5HIAA may be linked more closely with impulse control problems, rather than with depression.

Another problem with the monoamine hypothesis is that certain drugs that boost monoamines are not antidepressants (e.g., cocaine), and others that fail to boost monoamines are antidepressants (e.g., iprindole, mianserin). Perhaps the key difficulty with the monoamine hypothesis is that the timing of antidepressant effects on neurotransmitters is far different from the timing of the antidepressant effects on mood. That is, antidepressants boost monoamines *immediately*, but as mentioned earlier, have a significant *delay* in the onset of their therapeutic actions, which is in fact many days to weeks *after* they have already boosted the monoamines. Because of these and other difficulties, the focus of hypotheses for the etiology of depression began to shift from the monoamine neurotransmitters themselves to their receptors.

Neurotransmitter Receptor Hypothesis of Depression

This theory posits that something is wrong with the receptors for the key monoamine neurotransmitters (Figs. 5–33 through 5–35). According to this theory, an abnormality in the functioning of receptors for monoamine neurotransmitters thus

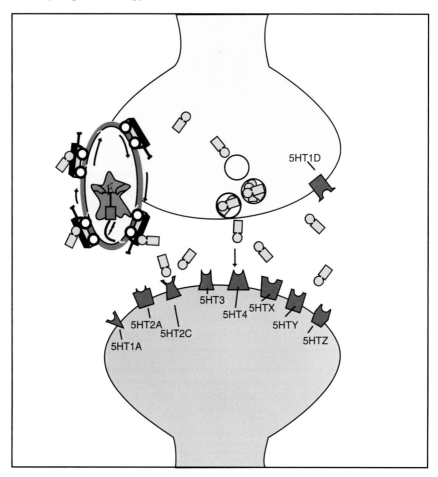

FIGURE 5–24. **Receptor subtyping for the serotonergic neuron** has proceeded at a very rapid pace, with at least four major categories of 5HT receptors, each further subtyped depending upon pharmacological or molecular properties. In addition to the serotonin transporter, there is a key presynaptic serotonin receptor (the 5HT1D receptor) and several postsynaptic serotonin receptors (5HT1A, 5HT1D, 5HT2A, 5HT2C, 5HT3, 5HT4, and many others denoted by 5HT X, Y, and Z).

leads to depression (Fig. 5–35). Such a disturbance in neurotransmitter receptors may be itself caused by depletion of monoamine neurotransmitters (Fig. 5–34).

Depletion of monoamine neurotransmitters (compare Figs. 5–33 with 5–34) has already been discussed as the central theme of the monoamine hypothesis of depression (see Figs. 5–12 and 5–13). The neurotransmitter receptor hypothesis of depression takes this theme one step further, namely that the depletion of neurotransmitter causes compensatory up-regulation of postsynaptic neurotransmitter receptors (Fig. 5–35).

Direct evidence of this is generally lacking, but postmortem studies do consistently show increased numbers of serotonin-2 receptors in the frontal cortex of patients who commit suicide. Indirect studies of neurotransmitter receptor functioning in patients with major depressive disorder suggest abnormalities in various neurotransmitter receptors when using neuroendocrine probes or peripheral tissues such

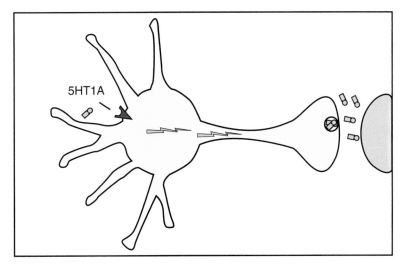

FIGURE 5–25. Presynaptic **5HT1A receptors** are autoreceptors, are located on the cell body and dendrites, and are therefore called somatodendritic autoreceptors.

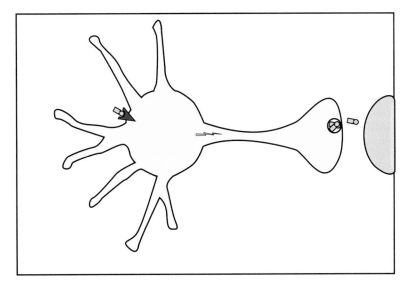

FIGURE 5–26. The **5HT1A somatodendritic autoreceptors** depicted in the previous figure (Fig. 5–25) act by detecting the presence of 5HT, and causing a **shutdown of 5HT neuronal impulse flow**, depicted here as decreased electrical activity.

as platelets or lymphocytes. Modern molecular techniques are exploring for abnormalities in gene expression of neurotransmitter receptors and enzymes in families with depression, but have not yet been successful in identifying molecular lesions.

Summary

In this chapter, we have introduced two major psychopharmacological themes, namely the affective disorders and the monoamine neurotransmitters. We have de-

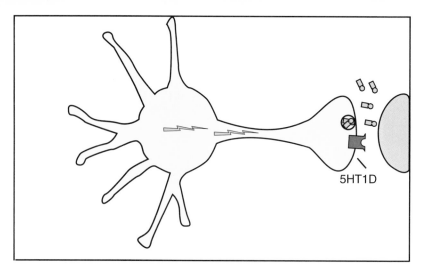

FIGURE 5–27. Presynaptic **5HT1D receptors** are also a type of autoreceptor, but are located on the presynaptic axon terminal, and are therefore called terminal autoreceptors.

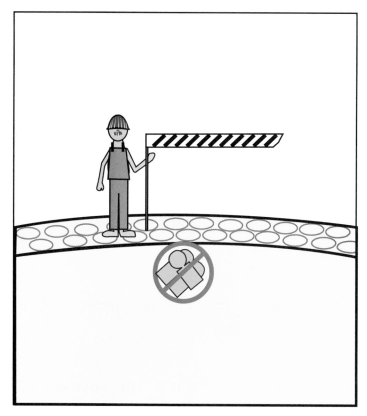

FIGURE 5–28. Presynaptic **5HT1D** terminal autoreceptors act as regulators of 5HT release. If the **5HT1D receptor is stimulated**, it **blocks the release of 5HT**.

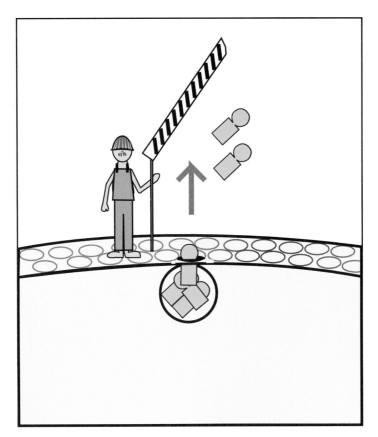

FIGURE 5–29. When presynaptic **5HT1D terminal autoreceptors are blocked**, this promotes the release of 5HT.

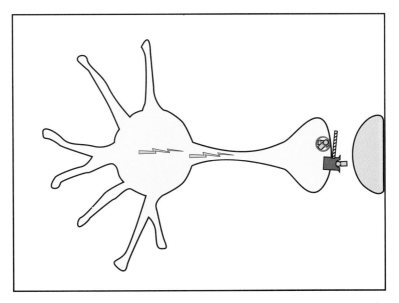

FIGURE 5–30. Depicted here is the consequence of the 5HT1D terminal autoreceptor being stimulated. The terminal autoreceptor of Figure 5–27 is occupied here by **5HT, causing the blockade of 5HT release**, just as shown in Figure 5–28.

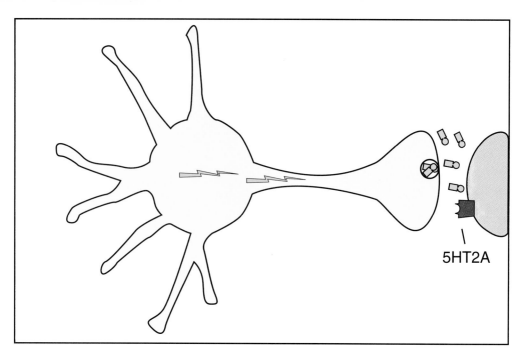

FIGURE 5–31. A key postsynaptic regulatory receptor is the **5HT2A receptor**.

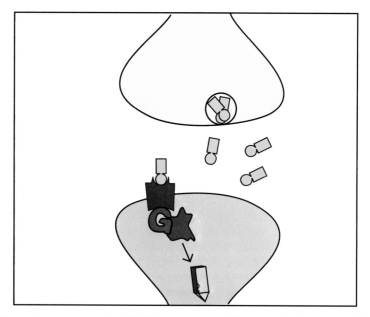

FIGURE 5–32. When the **postsynaptic 5HT2A receptor** of Figure 5–31 is occupied by 5HT, it causes neuronal impulses in the postsynaptic neuron to be altered via the production of **second messengers**.

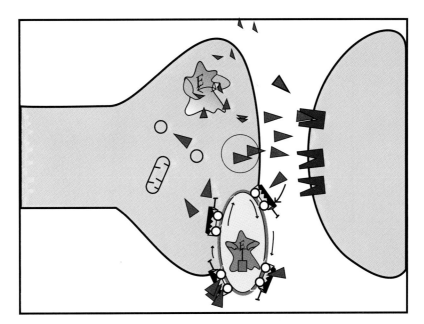

FIGURE 5–33. Monoamine receptor hypothesis of depression. This theory posits that something is wrong with the receptors for the key monoamine neurotransmitters. According to this theory, an abnormality in the receptors for monoamine neurotransmitters thus leads to depression. Such a disturbance in neurotransmitter receptors may be itself caused by depletion of monoamine neurotransmitters. Depicted here is the **normal monoamine neuron** with the normal amount of monoamine neurotransmitter and the normal amount of correctly functioning monoamine receptors.

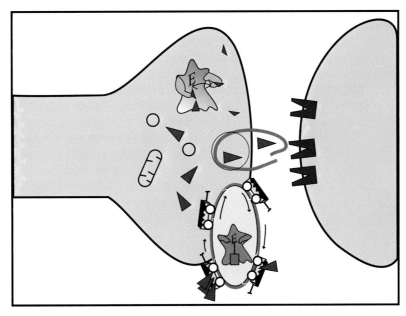

FIGURE 5–34. In this figure, **monoamine neurotransmitter is depleted** (see red circle), just as shown in Figure 5–13.

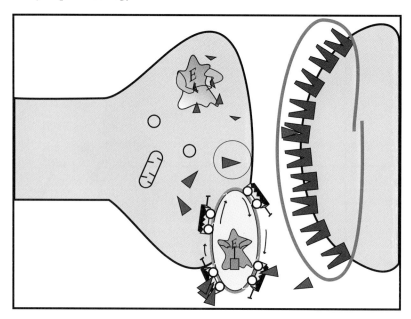

FIGURE 5–35. The consequences of monoamine neurotransmitter depletion of Figure 5–34 is that the **postsynaptic receptors abnormally up-regulate** (indicated in red circle). This up-regulation correlates with the production of the depressive illness, and is hypothetically linked to the cause of depression.

scribed the clinical features, epidemiology, and longitudinal course of various types of depression. We have also described the three monoamine neurotransmitter systems: noradrenergic, dopaminergic, and serotonergic. Specifically, the synthesis, metabolism, transport systems, and receptors for each monoaminergic system were outlined and then applied to the leading theories for the biological basis of depression. These theories are the monoamine hypothesis and the neurotransmitter hypothesis of depression.

The material in this chapter should provide the reader with the basis for understanding the pharmacological basis of the treatment of depression discussed in the following chapter. It should also provide useful background information about the monoamine neurotransmitter systems that serve as the pharmacological basis for several other classes of psychotropic drugs discussed throughout this book.

ANTIDEPRESSANTS AND MOOD STABILIZERS

This chapter will review pharmacological concepts underlying the use of antidepressant and mood stabilizing drugs. The goal of this chapter is to acquaint the reader with current ideas about how the various antidepressants and mood stabilizers work. This chapter will explain mechanisms of action of these drugs by building upon general pharmacological concepts introduced in earlier chapters.

Discussion of antidepressants in this chapter is at the conceptual level, and not at the pragmatic level. The reader should consult standard drug handbooks for details of doses, side effects, drug interactions, and other issues relevant to the prescribing of these drugs in clinical practice.

Discussion of antidepressants and mood stabilizers will begin with the classical monoamine oxidase inhibitors (MAOIs) and tricyclic antidepressants (TCAs), and then move into those agents introduced into clinical practice more recently. This chapter will also explore several antidepressants under development but not yet introduced into clinical practice. Finally, this chapter will mention the use of combinations of drugs, of electroconvulsive therapy (ECT), and of psychotherapy for treatment of mood disorders.

Antidepressant drugs

Overview of the Neurotransmitter Receptor Hypothesis of Antidepressant Action

In fairness, it must be stated that we really do not have a complete and adequate explanation of how antidepressant drugs work. What we do know with considerable confidence is that antidepressants are effective in relieving depression significantly more frequently than placebo. We also know that all effective antidepressants have identifiable immediate interactions with one or more neurotransmitter receptor or enzyme.

As discussed in the preceding chapter, this immediate pharmacological action often has the effect of boosting the levels of neurotransmitter (Figs. 5–14 and 5–15; see also Fig. 6–1). The following sections will review those specific receptors and enzymes that each of the various antidepressants influence virtually immediately after administration to a depressed patient. Just how all these different immediate pharmacological actions result ultimately in an antidepressant response a few weeks after administering an antidepressant agent (i.e., the final common pathway of antidepressant treatment response) is the subject of intense research interest and debate (Fig. 6–1).

The leading theory to explain the ultimate mechanism of delayed therapeutic action of the class of antidepressant drugs as a group is the "neurotransmitter receptor down-regulation hypothesis of antidepressant action" (Figs. 6–1 through 6–6). This is a hypothesis related to the "neurotransmitter receptor hypothesis of depression" discussed in the preceding chapter (Fig. 5–35). As previously discussed, this latter hypothesis proposes that depression itself is linked to abnormal functioning of neurotransmitter receptors, particularly up-regulation of serotonin-2 receptors.

Whether or not neurotransmitter receptors are abnormal in depression, the neurotransmitter receptor hypothesis of antidepressant action proposes that antidepressants, no matter what their initial actions on receptors and enzymes, eventually cause a down-regulation of key neurotransmitter receptors in a time course consistent with the delayed onset of antidepressant action of these drugs (Figs. 6–1 through 6–6).

Thus, the normal state becomes one of depression as neurotransmitter is depleted and then postsynaptic receptors up-regulate (Fig. 6–2). Boosting neurotransmitters by MAO inhibition (Figs. 6–3 and 6–4) or by blocking reuptake pumps for monoamine neurotransmitters (Figs. 6–5 and 6–6) eventually result in the down-regulation of postsynaptic neurotransmitter receptors in a delayed time course more

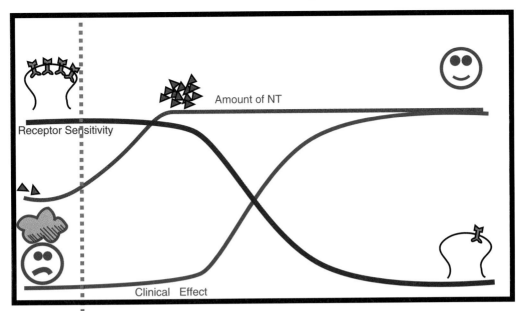

FIGURE 6−1. This figure depicts the different time courses for three effects of antidepressant drugs, namely changes in mood, changes in neurotransmitters (NT), and changes in receptor sensitivity. Specifically, the **amount of NT** changes relatively rapidly after the **antidepressant is introduced**. However, the **clinical effect** is delayed, as is the down-regulation of neurotransmitter **receptor sensitivity**. This temporal correlation of clinical effects with changes in receptor sensitivity has given rise to the hypothesis that changes in neurotransmitter receptor sensitivity may actually mediate the clinical effects of antidepressant drugs.

closely related to the timing of recovery from depression (Figs. 6−1, 6−4, and 6−6).

The evidence for this hypothesis will be summarized as the immediate pharmacological actions of each of the individual drugs are explained in the sections that follow. It may be useful to keep this overview hypothesis for the entire class of antidepressants in mind as one reads about individual antidepressant agents. Although we shall see that there are problems and inconsistencies in the neurotransmitter receptor hypothesis as an overall explanation for how all antidepressants work, it remains a leading theory of antidepressant action. Thus, neurotransmitter receptors are implicated not only in theories about the *cause of depression* (e.g., Figs. 5−33 through 5−35) but also about the actions of *antidepressants* (e.g., Figs. 6−1 through 6−6).

In summary, it appears that most known antidepressants have a common action on certain neurotransmitter receptors of down-regulating (i.e., decreasing or desensitizing) them in a delayed time course more typical of the time of onset of their therapeutic effects (Figs. 6−1 and 6−6). Although the actions of antidepressants on some neurotransmitter receptors and enzymes are immediate, the actions of antidepressants on other neurotransmitter receptors are delayed (Fig. 6−1). Since the therapeutic actions of antidepressants are also delayed, attention is increasingly being

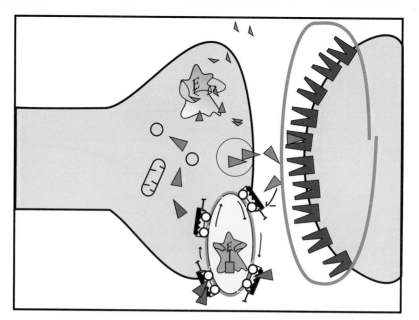

FIGURE 6–2. *The down-regulation hypothesis of antidepressant action* – **part** 1. Shown here is the monoaminergic neuron in the **depressed state**, with **up-regulation of receptors** (indicated in the red circle).

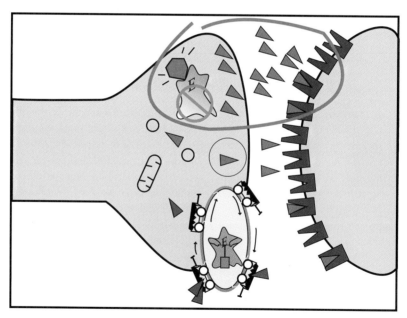

FIGURE 6–3. *The down-regulation hypothesis of antidepressant action* – **part** 2. Here, a **mono-amine oxidase (MAO) inhibitor** is blocking the enzyme and therefore stopping the destruction of neurotransmitter. This causes **more neurotransmitter to be available** in the synapse (indicated in the red circle).

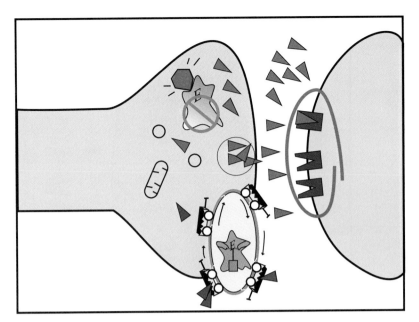

FIGURE 6–4. *The down-regulation hypothesis of antidepressant action* – **part 3**. The consequence of **long-lasting blockade of monoamine oxidase (MAO)** by an MAOI is for the neurotransmitter **receptors to down-regulate** (indicated in the red circle).

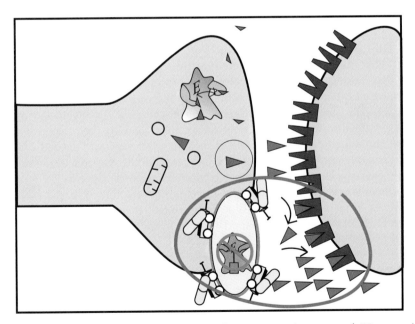

FIGURE 6–5. *The down-regulation hypothesis of antidepressant action* – **part 4**. Here, a **tricyclic antidepressant** blocks the reuptake pump, causing **more neurotransmitter** to be available in the synapse (indicated in the red circle). This is very similar to what happens after MAO is inhibited (see Fig. 6–3).

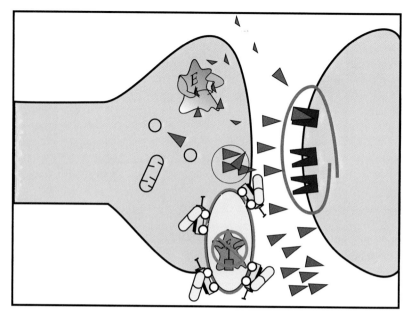

FIGURE 6–6. *The down-regulation hypothesis of antidepressant action* – **part 5**. The consequence of **long-lasting blockade** of the reuptake pump by a **tricyclic antidepressant** is for the neurotransmitter **receptors to down-regulate** (indicated in the red circle). This is the same outcome as with long-lasting blockade of MAO (see Fig. 6–4).

paid to how the initial and immediate actions at receptors and enzymes translate into delayed actions at other receptors.

This change in emphasis from the immediate pharmacological mechanisms of the drugs to their delayed pharmacological actions is of interest for a number of reasons. First, understanding how initial actions lead to delayed actions can give insight into the normal regulatory processes of neurotransmission. Second, such an understanding may explain why some patients fail to respond to antidepressants, since it is possible that in such patients the initial pharmacological actions are not translated into the required delayed pharmacological actions. Knowing the biological basis for treatment nonresponse may lead to the development of a greatly needed advance in the pharmacotherapy of depression, namely an effective treatment for refractory or nonresponding depressed patients (see discussion in the Chapter 5). Finally, if one understands the key pharmacological events that are linked to the therapeutic actions of the drugs, it may be possible to accelerate them with future drugs. If so, it could lead to another highly desired advance in the pharmacotherapy of depression, namely a rapid-onset antidepressant.

In any event, the state of the art today is that the neurotransmitter receptors most consistently known to be down-regulated by the greatest number of known antidepressants are the beta 1 receptor in the norepinephrine (NE) synapse and the serotonin-2 receptor in the 5-hydroxytryptamine (5HT) synapse. Much of the evidence for this comes from preclinical studies in experimental animals, but evidence is beginning to accrue that down-regulation of serotonin receptors does occur in depressed patients undergoing treatment with antidepressants, and may be linked to therapeutic outcomes in these patients.

Table 6–1. *Monoamine oxidase inhibitors (MAOIs)*

Classical MAOIs – irreversible and nonselective
  Phenelzine (Nardil)
  Tranylcypromine (Parnate)
  Isocarboxazid (Marplan)
RIMAs – Reversible inhibitors of MAO A
  Moclobemide (Aurorix)
Selective inhibitors of MAO B
  Deprenyl (selegiline; Eldepryl)

Monoamine Oxidase Inhibitors

The first clinically effective antidepressants to be discovered were immediate inhibitors of the enzyme MAO (see Table 6–1 and Figs. 5–14, 6–3, and 6–4). They were discovered by accident when an antituberculosis drug was observed to help depression, which coexisted in some of the patients who had tuberculosis. This antituberculosis drug, which was also an antidepressant, was soon discovered to inhibit the enzyme MAO. It was soon thereafter shown that inhibition of MAO was unrelated to its antitubercular actions, but was the immediate biochemical event that led to its ultimate antidepressant actions. This discovery soon led to the synthesis of more drugs in the 1950s and 1960s that inhibited MAO, but lacked unwanted additional properties (such as antituberculosis properties). Although best known as powerful antidepressants, the MAOIs are also therapeutic agents for certain anxiety disorders such as panic disorder and social phobia (discussed later in Chapter 8).

The original MAOIs are all irreversible enzyme inhibitors, which bind to MAO irreversibly and destroy its function forever, with enzyme activity returning only after new enzyme is synthesized (see Figs. 2–29, 2–33, 5–14, 6–3, and 6–4). Sometimes such inhibitors are called "suicide inhibitors" because once the enzyme binds the inhibitor (Fig. 2–33), it essentially commits suicide in that it can never function again until a new enzyme protein is synthesized by the neuron's DNA in the cell nucleus (see Fig. 1–8).

MAO exists in two subtypes, A and B. Both forms are inhibited by the original MAOIs, which are therefore nonselective. The A form metabolizes the neurotransmitter monoamines most closely linked to depression (i.e., serotonin and norepinephrine). It therefore also metabolizes the amine most closely linked to control of blood pressure (norepinephrine). Because of these observations, MAO A inhibition is linked both to antidepressant actions and to the troublesome hypertensive side effects of the MAOIs. The B form is thought to convert some amine substrates, called protoxins, into toxins that may cause damage to neurons. MAO B inhibition is linked to prevention of neurodegenerative processes, such as in Parkinson's disease.

Two developments have occurred with MAOIs in recent years. One is the production of selective inhibitors of MAO A or of MAO B. The other advance is to make selective MAO A inhibitors that are reversible. The implications of these advances are multiple. One of the most troublesome properties of the original nonselective irreversible MAOIs is the fact that after they inhibit MAO, amines taken in from the diet can cause dangerous elevations in blood pressure. Normally, such

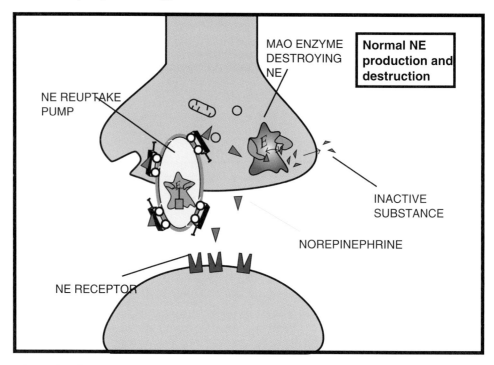

FIGURE 6–7. This figure shows the normal process of **norepinephrine** (NE) being both produced and **destroyed**. **MAO (monoamine oxidase)** is the enzyme that normally acts to destroy NE to keep it in balance.

dietary amines are safely metabolized by MAO prior to their causing blood pressure elevations (Figs. 6–7 and 6–8). However, when MAO A is inhibited, blood pressure can rise suddenly and dramatically, and can even cause intracerebral hemorrhage and death after eating certain tyramine-containing foods or beverages (Fig. 6–9). This risk can be controlled by restricting the diet so that dangerous foods are eliminated, and also restricting the simultaneous use of certain dangerous medications (i.e., the pain killer Demerol [meperidine], the serotonin selective reuptake inhibitors, and sympathomimetic agents). The risk of hypertensive crisis and the hassle of restricting diet and medications have generally been the price a patient has had to pay in order to get the therapeutic benefits of the MAOIs.

In the case of MAO B inhibitors, no significant amount of MAO A is inhibited, and there is essentially no risk of hypertension from dietary amines. Patients taking MAO B inhibitors to prevent progression of Parkinson's disease, for example, do not require any special diet. On the other hand, MAO B inhibitors are also not effective antidepressants at doses that are selective for MAO B.

A new class of MAOIs is just coming into clinical practice for the treatment of depression, known as reversible inhibitors of MAO A (RIMAs). This is a nifty development in new drug therapeutics for depression, because it has the potential of making the MAO A inhibition for the treatment of depression much safer. That is, the "suicide inhibitors" are associated with the dangerous hypertensive episodes mentioned above and which are caused when patients eat food rich in tyramine (such

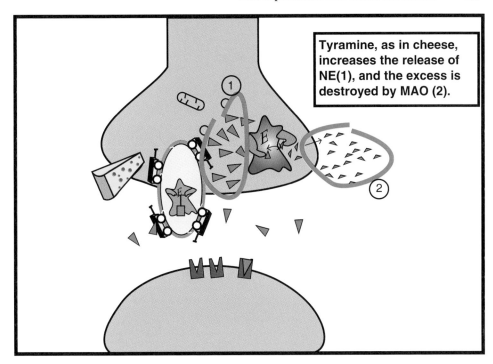

Tyramine, as in cheese, increases the release of NE(1), and the excess is destroyed by MAO (2).

FIGURE 6–8. **Tyramine** is an amine present in food such as **cheese**. Indicated in this figure is how tyramine (depicted as cheese) acts to **increase the release of norepinephrine (NE)** (see red circle 1). However, in normal circumstances, the enzyme **MAO (monoamine oxidase) readily destroys the excess NE** that is released by tyramine, and no harm is done (see red circle 2).

as cheese). This so-called cheese reaction is caused when the tyramine in the diet releases norepinephrine and other sympathomimetic amines (Fig. 6–9). When MAO is inhibited irreversibly, the levels of these amines rise to a dangerous level because they are not destroyed by MAO. Blood pressure soars, even causing blood vessels to rupture in the brain.

Enter the reversible MAO inhibitors. If someone eats cheese, tyramine will still release sympathomimetic amines, but these amines will chase the reversible inhibitor off the MAO enzyme, allowing the dangerous amines to be destroyed (Fig. 6–10). This is sort of like having your cake – or cheese – and eating it, too. The reversible MAOIs have the same therapeutic effects of the suicide inhibitors, without the danger of a cheese reaction if a patient inadvertently takes in otherwise dangerous dietary tyramine.

As MAOIs are finding increasing applications in anxiety disorders such as panic disorder and social phobia in addition to depression, the RIMAs have the potential of making the treatment of these additional disorders by MAO A inhibition much safer as well.

Tricyclic Antidepressants

The tricyclic antidepressants (Table 6–2) were so-named because their organic chemical structure contains three rings (Fig. 6–11). The tricyclic antidepressants were

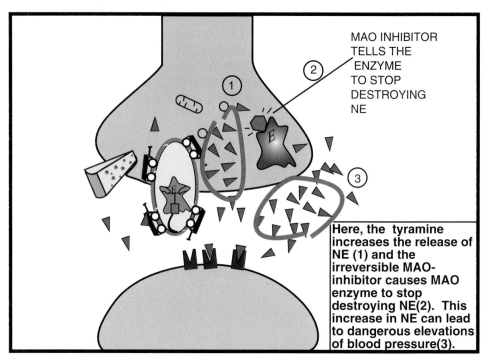

FIGURE 6–9. Here, tyramine is releasing norepinephrine (NE) (see red circle 1) just as previously shown in Figure 6–8. However, this time **MAO (monoamine oxidase)** is also being **inhibited** by a typical, irreversible MAOI. This results in MAO **stopping its destruction of norepinephrine (NE)** (see arrow 2). As already indicated earlier in Figure 6–3, such MAO inhibition in itself causes the **accumulation of NE.** However, when MAO inhibition is taking place in the presence of tyramine, the combination can lead to a very large accumulation of NE (see red circle 3). Such a great degree of NE accumulation can cause dangerous elevations of blood pressure.

synthesized about the same time as other three-ringed molecules that were shown to be effective tranquilizers for schizophrenia (i.e., the early antipsychotic neuroleptic drugs such as chlorpromazine) (Fig. 6–12). The tricyclic antidepressants were a disappointment when tested as antipsychotics. Even though they had a three-ringed structure, they were not effective in the treatment of schizophrenia and were almost discarded. However, during testing for schizophrenia, they were discovered to be antidepressants. That is, careful clinicians detected antidepressant properties in the schizophrenic patients, although not antipsychotic properties in these patients. Thus, the antidepressant properties of the tricyclic antidepressants were serendipitously observed in the 1950s and 1960s, and eventually the TCAs were marketed for the treatment of depression.

Long after their antidepressant properties were observed, the tricyclic antidepressants were discovered to block the reuptake pumps for both serotonin and norepinephrine (and to a lesser extent, dopamine) (Figs. 5–15, 6–5, and 6–6). In addition, essentially all the tricyclic antidepressants have at least three other actions: blockade of muscarinic cholinergic receptors, blockade of H1 histamine receptors, and blockade of alpha 1 adrenergic receptors (Fig. 6–13). Whereas blockade of the serotonin and norepinephrine reuptake pumps is thought to account for the *therapeutic actions*

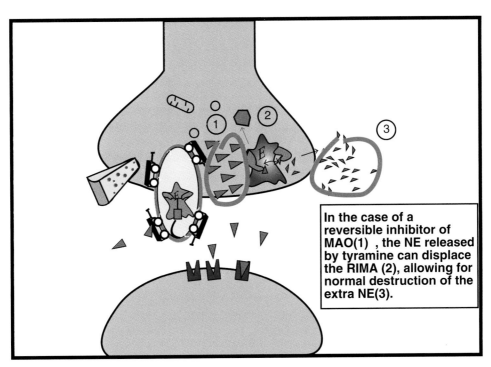

In the case of a reversible inhibitor of MAO(1) , the NE released by tyramine can displace the RIMA (2), allowing for normal destruction of the extra NE(3).

FIGURE 6–10. Shown in this figure is also the **combination of an MAO (monoamine oxidase) inhibitor and tyramine**. However, in this case the MAOI is of the **reversible** type (reversible inhibitor of MAO A or **RIMA**). In contrast to the situation shown in the previous figure (Fig. 6–9), the accumulation of norepinephrine (NE) caused by tyramine (indicated in red circle 1) can actually strip the RIMA off MAO (arrow 2). MAO – now devoid of its inhibitor – can merrily do its job, which is to destroy the NE (red circle 3) and thus prevent the dangerous accumulation of NE. Such a reversal of MAO by NE is only possible with a RIMA, and not with the classical MAOIs, which are completely irreversible.

Table 6–2. *Tricyclic antidepressants*

Clomipramine (Anafranil)
Imipramine (Tofranil)
Amitriptyline (Elavil; Endep; Tryptanol)
Nortriptyline (Pamelor)
Protriptyline (Vivactil)
Maprotiline (Ludiomil)
Amoxapine (Asendin)
Doxepin (Sinequan; Adapin)
Desipramine (Norpramin)
Trimipramine (Surmontil)

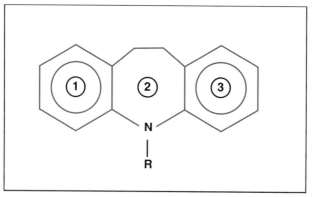

FIGURE 6–11. This is the chemical structure of a tricyclic antidepressant (TCA). The three rings show how this group of drugs got their name.

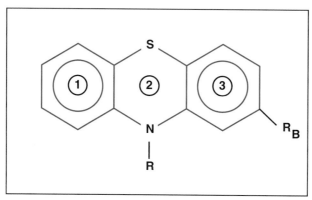

FIGURE 6–12. This is a general chemical formula for the phenothiazine type of antipsychotic drugs. These drugs also have three rings, and the first antidepressants were modeled after such drugs.

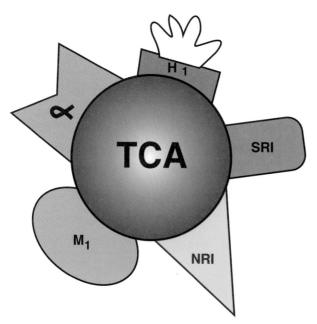

FIGURE 6–13. Shown here is an icon of a tricyclic antidepressant (TCA). These drugs are actually five drugs in one: (1) a serotonin reuptake inhibitor (SRI); (2) a norepinephrine reuptake inhibitor (NRI); (3) an anticholinergic/antimuscarinic drug (M1); (4) an alpha adrenergic antagonist (alpha); and (5) an antihistamine (H1).

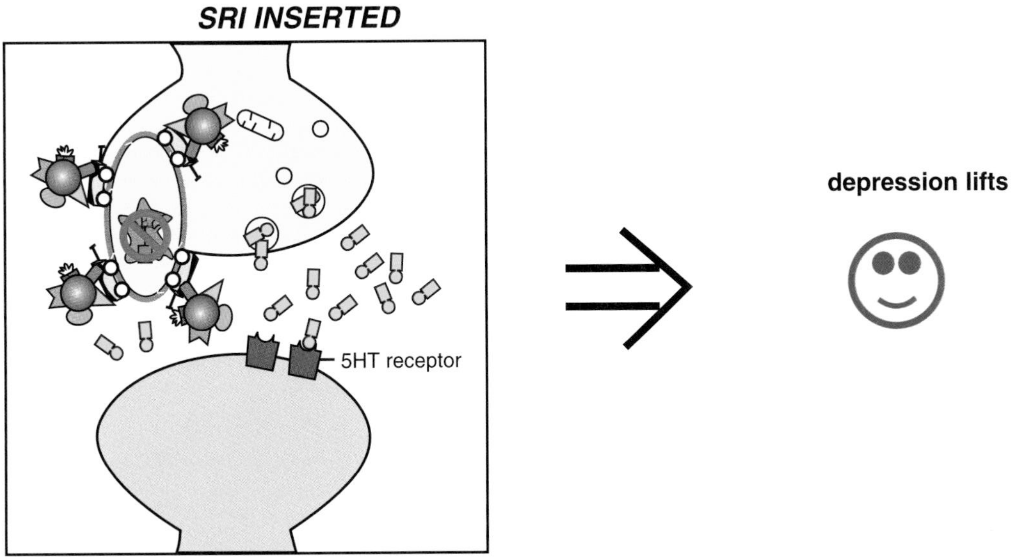

SRI INSERTED

FIGURE 6–14. *Therapeutic actions of the tricyclic antidepressants (TCAs)* – **part** 1. In this diagram, the icon of the **TCA** is shown with its serotonin reuptake inhibitor (**SRI**) portion inserted into the serotonin reuptake pump, blocking it, and causing an **antidepressant effect**.

of these drugs (Figs. 6–14 and 6–15), the other three pharmacological properties are thought to account for the *side effects* of the TCAs (Figs. 6–16, 6–17, and 6–18). Some of the tricyclic antidepressants also have the ability to block serotonin-2 receptors, which may contribute to the therapeutic actions of those agents with this property. Blockade of serotonin-2 receptors is discussed further in the section below on serotonin antagonist/reuptake inhibitors (SARIs).

In terms of the *therapeutic actions* of tricyclic antidepressants, they essentially work as allosteric modulators of the neurotransmitter reuptake process. Specifically, the TCAs are negative allosteric modulators. When the neurotransmitters norepinephrine or serotonin bind to their own selective receptor transporter sites, they are normally transported back into the presynaptic neuron as discussed in Chapters 2 (see Fig. 2–14), 3 (Fig. 3–18), and 5 (Fig. 5–15). However, when certain antidepressants bind to an allosteric site close to the neurotransmitter transporter, this causes the neurotransmitter to no longer be able to bind there, thus blocking synaptic reuptake transport of the neurotransmitter (Figs. 6–14 and 6–15). Therefore, norepinephrine and serotonin cannot be shuttled back into the presynaptic neuron.

In terms of side effects of the tricyclic antidepressants, blockade of alpha 1 adrenergic receptors causes orthostatic hypotension and dizziness (Fig. 6–16). Anticholinergic actions at muscarinic cholinergic receptors cause dry mouth, blurred vision, urinary retention, and constipation (Fig. 6–17). Blockade of H1 histamine receptors causes sedation and weight gain (Fig. 6–18).

The term "tricyclic antidepressant" is archaic by today's pharmacology. First, the antidepressants that block biogenic amine reuptake are not all tricyclic anymore: the new agents can have one, two, three, or four rings in their structures. Second, the tricyclic antidepressants are not merely antidepressant, since some of them

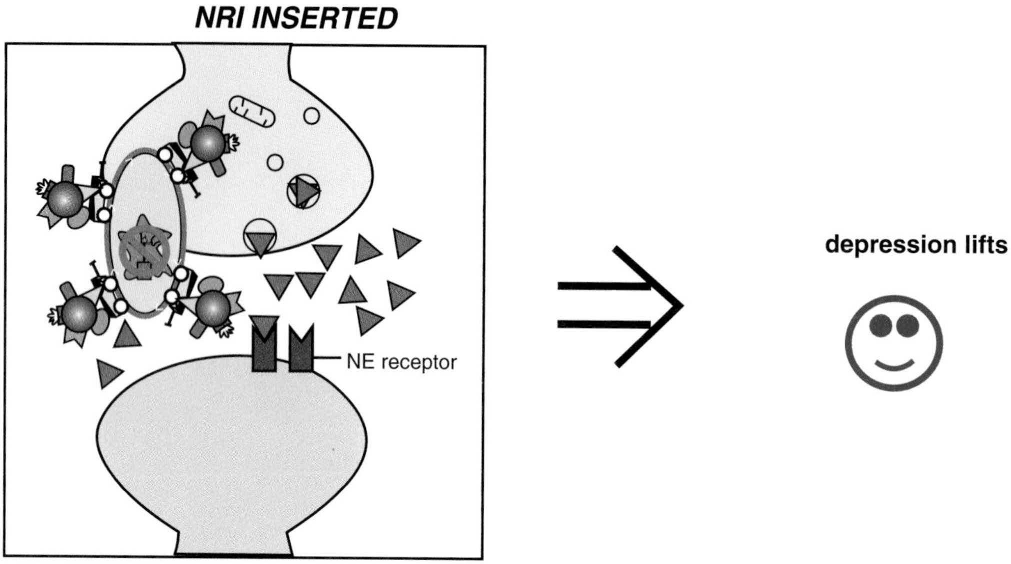

NRI INSERTED

depression lifts

FIGURE 6–15. *Therapeutic actions of the tricyclic antidepressants (TCAs) – part 2.* In this diagram, the icon of the **TCA** is shown with its norepinephrine reuptake inhibitor (**NRI**) portion inserted into the norepinephrine reuptake pump, blocking and causing an **antidepressant effect**. Thus, both the serotonin reuptake portion (see Fig. 6–14) and the NRI portion of the TCAs act pharmacologically to cause an antidepressant effect.

have anti–obsessive compulsive disorder effects, others have antipanic effects (see chapter 8).

Serotonin Selective Reuptake Inhibitors

The troublesome side effects of the tricyclic antidepressants sparked the search for reuptake-blocking drugs that lacked the side effects of the TCAs. Also, the TCAs are dangerous in overdose, which depressed patients are prone to take. In fact, a 15-day supply of most TCAs is a lethal dose in many patients. The logical manner to eliminate the side effects of the TCAs would be to eliminate blockade of the three receptors muscarinic cholinergic, H1 histaminergic, and alpha 1 adrenergic. This was accomplished by a group of agents called the serotonin selective reuptake inhibitors (SSRIs) (Table 6–3 and Fig. 6–19). The SSRIs retained the ability to block the 5HT transporter (Fig. 6–20).

However, the SSRIs went one step further: they also removed the norepinephrine reuptake blocking properties (Fig. 6–13 versus Fig. 6–19). This caused a great deal of debate and consternation prior to clinical testing, as many clinicians and pharmacologists feared that elimination of the NE blockade would weaken the therapeutic effects normally associated with the TCAs.

Imagine the thrill and surprise when the SSRIs were shown not only to be as effective in depression as the older TCAs but without the troublesome or dangerous side effects of the TCAs; paradoxically, the SSRIs have proven to be even more useful than most of the TCAs, with additional efficacy for obsessive compulsive disorder, which most of the TCAs lack (see Chapter 8). Also, the acceptability of the SSRIs

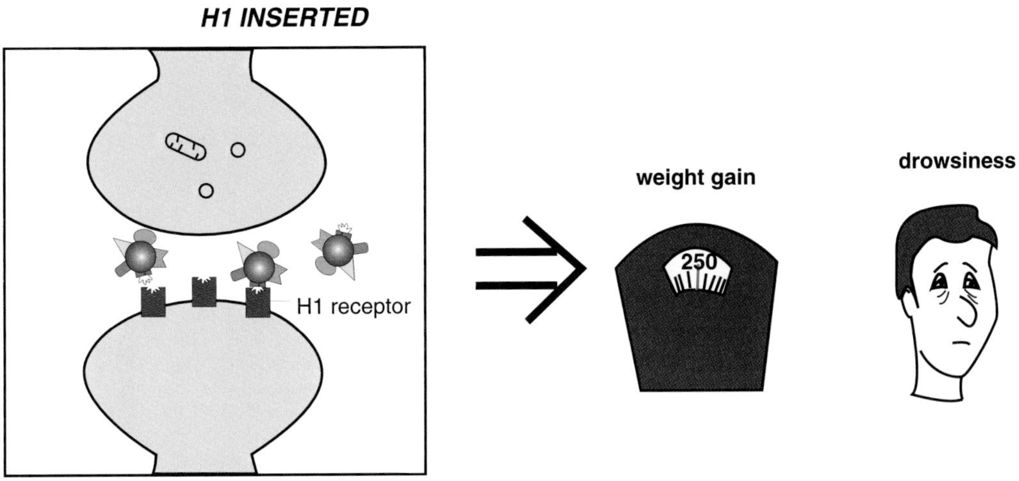

H1 INSERTED

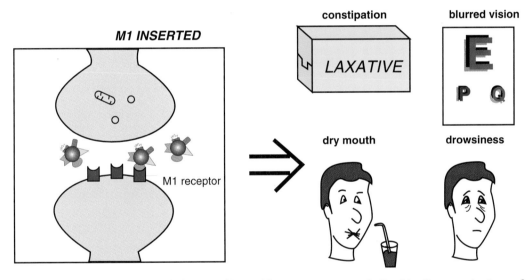

FIGURE 6–16. *Side effects of the tricyclic antidepressants* – part 1. In this diagram, the icon of the **TCA** is shown with its **H1** (antihistamine) portion inserted into histamine receptors, causing the side effects of **weight gain and drowsiness**.

FIGURE 6–17. *Side effects of the tricyclic antidepressants* – part 2. In this diagram, the icon of the **TCA** is shown with its **M1** (anticholinergic/antimuscarinic) portion inserted into acetylcholine receptors, causing the side effects of **constipation, blurred vision, dry mouth, and drowsiness**.

has made them much easier to administer, has enhanced patient compliance, and has made them especially appropriate for long-term administration just as the data are evolving that long-term treatment of depression is indicated to maintain remission, prevent relapse, and prevent recurrence (see Chapter 5).

On the other hand, some new problems emerged. Agitation and akathisia (a type of motor restlessness) were observed, especially with fluoxetine. Sexual dysfunction, especially anorgasmia in women and delayed ejaculation in men, is caused in a

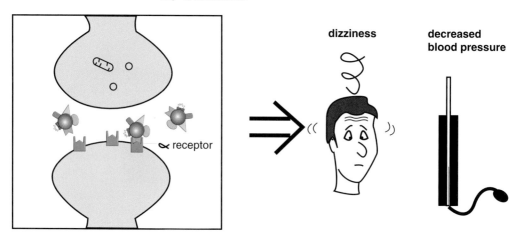

∝ INSERTED

dizziness

decreased
blood pressure

∝ receptor

FIGURE 6–18. *Side effects of the tricyclic antidepressants* – **part** 3. In this diagram, the icon of the **TCA** is shown with its **alpha** (alpha adrenergic antagonist) portion inserted into alpha adrenergic receptors, causing the side effects of **dizziness, decreased blood pressure, and drowsiness**.

Table 6–3. *Serotonin selective reuptake inhibitors (SSRIs)*

Fluoxetine (Prozac)
Sertraline (Zoloft)
Paroxetine (Paxil)
Fluvoxamine (Luvox)
Citalopram

significant number of patients by all members of the SSRI class. In the United States, a furor broke out in the lay press after some cases of suicide were reported following the administration of fluoxetine. Careful analysis of the database for fluoxetine administration throughout the world, however, has so far failed to establish that fluoxetine increases suicide rate. In a disorder like depression that is associated with suicide and also associated with antidepressant treatment, it is inevitable that suicide will frequently be associated with antidepressant treatment.

There is an old clinical adage that depressed patients who are starting to recover after the initiation of antidepressant treatment may finally get up the energy to make and execute a suicide plan, so that clinicians must keep alert to the possibility of suicide even as the patient is improving. Thus, all of the antidepressants have a certain general risk of being associated with suicide, if not in a directly causative relationship. On the other hand, most of the data support the proposition that antidepressants reduce the suicide rate, not increase it, including fluoxetine.

Additional uses of SSRIs in panic disorder, obsessive compulsive disorder, social phobia, and other novel indications are discussed in Chapter 8.

Recent studies of SSRIs in experimental animals suggest how the neurotransmitter hypothesis of antidepressant action can be amplified. That is, emphasis has moved

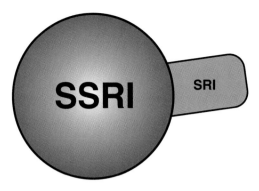

FIGURE 6–19. Shown here is the icon of a selective **serotonin** reuptake inhibitor (**SSRI**). In this case, four out of the five pharmacological properties of the TCAs (tricyclic antidepressants; Fig. 6–13) were removed. Only the serotonin reuptake inhibitor (**SRI**) portion remains; thus the SRI action is selective, which is why these agents are called **selective SRIs**.

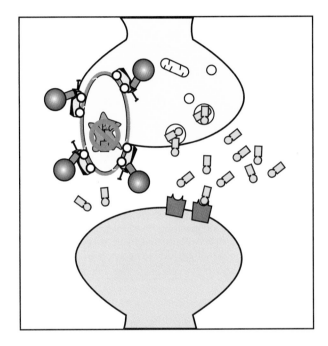

FIGURE 6–20. In this diagram, the **SRI** (serotonin reuptake inhibitor) portion of the **SSRI** molecule is shown inserted in the serotonin reuptake pump, blocking it and causing an **antidepressant effect**. This is analogous to one of the dimensions of the tricyclic antidepressants (TCAs), already shown in Figure 6–14.

from events occurring at the axon terminal (Figs. 6–1 through 6–6) to the somatodendritic autoreceptors near the cell body (Figs. 6–21 through 6–25). In the depressed state (Fig. 6–21), postsynaptic receptors may be up-regulated, and serotonin may be deficient not only at the axon terminal area but also at somatodendritic autoreceptors. When an SSRI is given acutely, 5HT rises due to blockade of the 5HT transport pump. However, this occurs at first only at the cell body area in the midbrain raphe, and not in the areas of the brain where the axons terminate (Fig. 6–22). The effect of maintaining this increased 5HT at somatodendritic autoreceptors is to down-regulate and desensitize them (Fig. 6–23).

Once the autoreceptors are down-regulated, 5HT no longer polices its own release, resulting in a flurry of 5HT release from its axons and an increase in neuronal

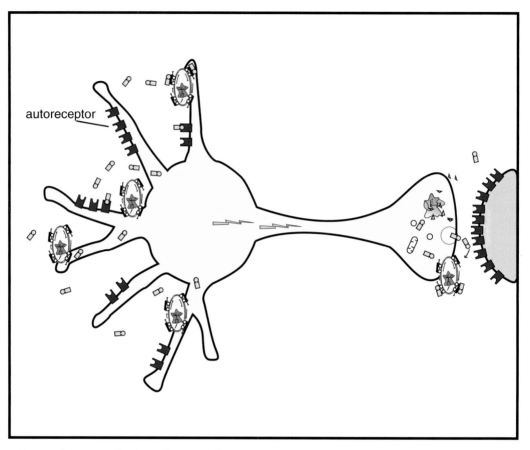

autoreceptor

FIGURE 6–21. *Mechanism of action of serotonin selective reuptake inhibitors (SSRIs)* – **part 1.**
Depicted here is a **serotonin neuron in a depressed patient.** In depression, the serotonin neuron is
conceptualized as having a relative **deficiency of the neurotransmitter serotonin.** Also, the number
of **serotonin receptors** is **up-regulated,** or increased, including both presynaptic **autoreceptors** as
well as **postsynaptic receptors.**

impulse flow (Fig. 6–24). There is a delay in how soon the increased somatodendritic
5HT due to blockade of the 5HT transport pump can down-regulate the somatodendritic autoreceptors in order to allow the neuron to be able to increase its 5HT
in axonal terminals and to increase its neuronal impulses. The delay in 5HT arriving
at the axon terminals may account not only for a delay in the down regulation of
postsynaptic 5HT2 receptors but also for a delay in the therapeutic consequences of
SSRIs (Fig. 6–25). This theory thus suggests the pharmacological cascading mechanism whereby the SSRIs exert their therapeutic actions: it is hypothetically due to
the restoration of neuronal impulse traffic in the 5HT neurons causing an increase
in 5HT release in axon terminal synapses with perhaps consequential postsynaptic
5HT2 receptor down regulation.

There are potentially exciting corollaries to this hypothesis. First, if the ultimate
increase in 5HT at axonal synapses is critical, then its failure to occur may explain
why some patients respond to an SSRI and some do not. Also, if new drugs could

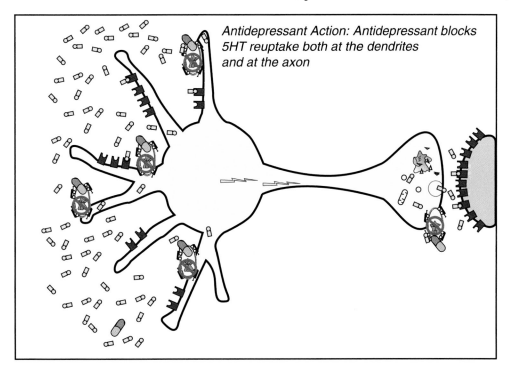

Antidepressant Action: Antidepressant blocks 5HT reuptake both at the dendrites and at the axon

FIGURE 6–22. *Mechanism of action of serotonin selective reuptake inhibitors (SSRIs)* – **part 2.** When an SSRI is administered, it immediately blocks the serotonin reuptake pump (see icon of a capsule blocking the reuptake pump). However, this causes **serotonin to increase initially only in the somatodendritic area**, and not in the axon terminals.

be designed to increase 5HT at the right place at a faster rate, it could result in a much needed rapid acting antidepressant. Such ideas are mere research hypotheses at this time, but could lead to additional studies clarifying the molecular events that are key mediators of depressive illness as well as of antidepressant treatment responses.

Norepinephrine and Dopamine Reuptake Blockers (Adrenergic Modulators)

Bupropion is the prototypical agent of the norepinephrine and dopamine reuptake blocker (NDRI) group (Fig. 6–26), with other drugs in clinical testing at the present time. For many years, the mechanism of action of bupropion was unclear. Bupropion itself has weak reuptake properties for dopamine, and weaker yet for norepinephrine. The action of the drug, however, has always appeared to be more powerful than these weak properties could explain, leading to explanations that bupropion acted rather vaguely as a dopamine or adrenergic modulator of some type. Recently, it has been discovered that bupropion is metabolized to an active metabolite, which is not only a more powerful norepinephrine and dopamine reuptake blocker than bupropion itself, but is also concentrated in the brain. In some ways, therefore,

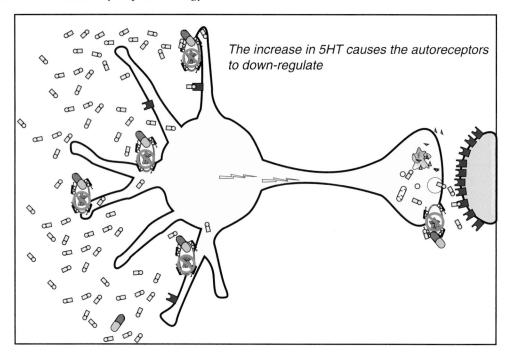

The increase in 5HT causes the autoreceptors to down-regulate

FIGURE 6–23. *Mechanism of action of serotonin selective reuptake inhibitors (SSRIs)* – part 3. The consequence of serotonin increasing in the somatodendritic area of the serotonin neuron as depicted in the previous figure (Fig. 6–22) is for the **somatodendritic serotonin 1A autoreceptors to down-regulate**.

bupropion is more of a prodrug (i.e., precursor) than a drug itself. That is, it gives rise to the real drug, namely its hydroxylated active metabolite, and it is this metabolite that is the actual mediator of antidepressant efficacy, primarily via norepinephrine and dopamine reuptake blockade blockade (Fig. 6–27). Numerous investigational agents are being tested as antidepressants that are dual norepinephrine and dopamine reuptake inhibitors, norepinephrine-selective reuptake inhibitors, or dopamine-selective reuptake inhibitors.

Bupropion is an effective antidepressant, is generally activating or even stimulating, and has an increased incidence of grand mal seizures compared to other antidepressants, which also cause seizures, but in lesser frequency. A new controlled-release formulation of bupropion is a promising improvement that may reduce both the frequency of dosing to only once or twice a day as well as the side effects associated with peak plasma blood levels of the drug. Interestingly, bupropion does not appear to be associated with production of bothersome sexual dysfunction that can occur with the SSRIs, probably because bupropion lacks a significant serotonergic component to its mechanism of action. Thus, it may be a useful antidepressant not only for patients who cannot tolerate the serotonergic side effects of SSRIs but also for patients whose depression does not respond to serotonergic boosting by SSRIs.

Bupropion is prescribed predominantly in the United States and mostly by psychiatrists, whereas most other antidepressants are prescribed throughout the world and predominantly by nonpsychiatric practitioners who treat depression.

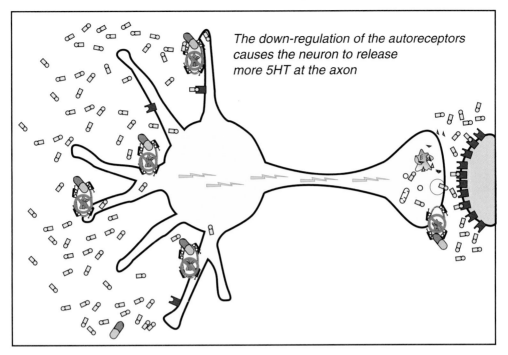

The down-regulation of the autoreceptors causes the neuron to release more 5HT at the axon

FIGURE 6–24. *Mechanism of action of serotonin selective reuptake inhibitors (SSRIs) – part 4.* Once the somatodendritic autoreceptors down-regulate as depicted in Figure 6–23, there is no longer inhibition of impulse flow in the serotonin neuron. Thus, **neuronal impulse flow is turned on.** The consequence of this is for **serotonin to be released in the axon terminal.** However, **this increase is delayed** compared to the increase of serotonin in the somatodendritic areas of the serotonin neuron depicted in Figure 6–22. This delay is the result of the time it takes for somatodendritic serotonin to down-regulate the serotonin 1A autoreceptors, and turn on neuronal impulse flow in the serotonin neuron. This delay may account for why antidepressants do not relieve depression immediately. It is also the reason why the mechanism of action of antidepressants may be linked to increasing neuronal impulse flow in serotonin neurons with serotonin levels increasing in axon terminals before an SSRI can exert its antidepressant effects.

Serotonin-Norepinephrine Reuptake Inhibitors (Dual Reuptake Inhibitors)

A new class of therapeutic agent is being introduced, called dual reuptake inhibitors, or sometimes serotonin-norepinephrine reuptake inhibitors (SNRIs) (Fig. 6–28). The designation "dual reuptake inhibitors" can be confusing because many agents have dual pharmacological actions including the inhibition of both NE and 5HT reuptake. What is unique about venlafaxine, the prototype agent of this group of SNRIs, is that it shares the NE and 5HT (and to a lesser extent DA) reuptake inhibitory properties of the classical TCAs, but without alpha 1, cholinergic, or histamine receptor blocking properties (Figs. 6–28 and 6–29). Depending upon the dose, venlafaxine has different degrees of inhibition of 5HT reuptake (most potent and present at low doses), NE reuptake (moderate potency and present at higher doses), and DA reuptake (least potent and present at highest doses).

Although well documented as effective antidepressants, it is not yet clear if they have advantages over the SSRIs in terms either of efficacy or side effects. Theoreti-

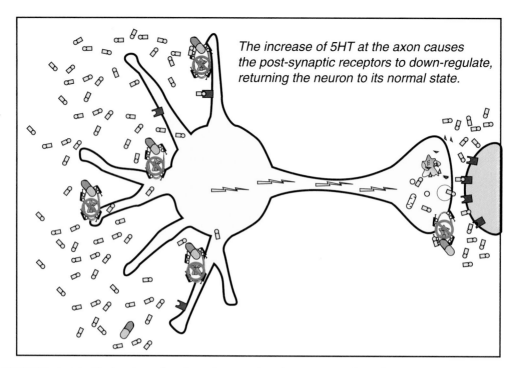

The increase of 5HT at the axon causes the post-synaptic receptors to down-regulate, returning the neuron to its normal state.

FIGURE 6–25. *Mechanism of action of serotonin selective reuptake inhibitors – part 5.* Finally, once the SSRIs have blocked the reuptake pump (Fig. 6–22), increased somatodendritic serotonin (Fig. 6–22), down-regulated somatodendritic serotonin 1A autoreceptors (Fig. 6–23), turned on neuronal impulse flow (Fig. 6–24) and increased release of serotonin from axon terminals (Figure 6–24), the final step shown here may be the down-regulation of postsynaptic serotonin receptors. This has also been shown in previous figures demonstrating the actions of monoamine oxidase inhibitors (MAOIs) (Fig. 6–4) and the actions of tricyclic antidepressants (Fig. 6–6).

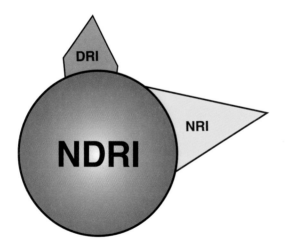

FIGURE 6–26. Shown here is the icon of a **norepinephrine and dopamine** reuptake inhibitor (**NDRI**). In this case, four out of the five pharmacological properties of the tricyclic antidepressants (TCAs; Fig. 6–13) were removed. Only the norepinephrine reuptake inhibitor (**NRI**) portion remains; to this is added a dopamine reuptake inhibitor (**DRI**) action.

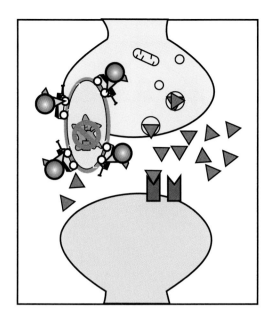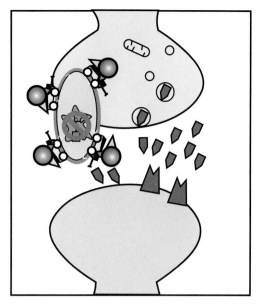

FIGURE 6–27. In this diagram, the norepinephrine reuptake inhibitor (**NRI**) and the dopamine reuptake inhibitor (**DRI**) portions of the **NDRI** molecule are shown inserted in the norepinephrine and the dopamine reuptake pumps, respectively, blocking them and causing an **antidepressant effect**.

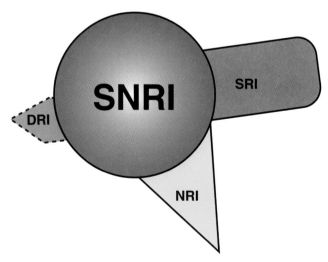

FIGURE 6–28. Shown here is the icon of a dual reuptake inhibitor that combines the actions of both a **serotonin** reuptake inhibitor (**SRI**) and a **norepinephrine** reuptake inhibitor (**NRI**). In this case, three out of the five pharmacological properties of the tricyclic antidepressants (TCAs; Fig. 6–13) were removed. Both the SRI portion and the NRI portion of the TCA remain; however, the alpha, antihistamine, and anticholinergic portions are removed. These **serotonin/norepinephrine reuptake inhibitors** are called **SNRIs** or **dual inhibitors**. A small amount of dopamine reuptake inhibition (DRI) is also present in some of these agents, especially at high doses.

153

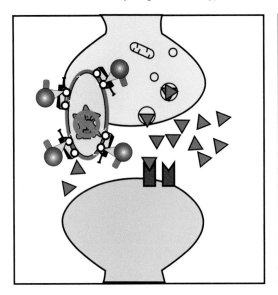 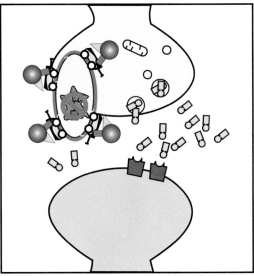

FIGURE 6–29. In this diagram, the dual actions of the serotonin/norepinephrine reuptake inhibitors (**SNRIs**) are shown. Both the norepinephrine reuptake inhibitor (NRI) portion of the SNRI molecule (left panel) and the serotonin reuptake inhibitor (SRI) portion of the SNRI molecule are inserted into their respective reuptake pumps. Consequently, both reuptake pumps are blocked, and the drug mediates an **antidepressant effect**. This is analogous to two of the dimensions of the tricyclic antidepressants (TCAs), already shown in Figures 6–14 and 6–15. It is also analogous to the single action of SSRIs (Fig. 6–20) added to the single action of the NSRIs (Fig. 6–27).

cally, the addition of NE (and to a lesser extent, DA) reuptake blockade to 5HT reuptake blockade (Fig. 6–29) might lead to an enhanced efficacy profile compared to the SSRIs. Would a dual reuptake blocker be tantamount to giving an SSRI and bupropion simultaneously?

Studies are in progress to determine whether onset of action is faster with serotonin and norepinephrine dual reuptake blockade (SNRI) when compared to a selective single reuptake blocker like the SSRIs or an adrenergic modulator (NDRI) such as bupropion. Other studies are also in progress to find out whether the dual 5HT/NE reuptake inhibitors have a greater degree of efficacy compared to other pharmacological classes of antidepressants. Finally, novel therapeutic uses for dual 5HT/NE reuptake inhibitors, such as chronic pain, are being investigated. The first such agent to be introduced into clinical practice is venlafaxine. Another similar agent in clinical testing is duloxetine.

Serotonin-2 Antagonist/Reuptake Inhibitors: Dual Actions as Antagonists of Serotonin-2 Receptors and as Serotonin Reuptake Inhibitors

Several antidepressants share the ability to block both serotonin-2 receptors as well as serotonin reuptake. In fact, some of the tricyclic antidepressants discussed above (such as amitriptyline, nortriptyline, doxepin, and others) have this combination of actions at the serotonin synapse. Since the potency of blockade of serotonin-2 receptors varies considerably among the tricyclics, it is not clear how important this action is to the therapeutic actions of tricyclic antidepressants in general.

However, there is another chemical class of antidepressants known as phenylpiperazines, the most powerful pharmacological action of which is to block serotonin-2 receptors. This class includes the agents trazodone and nefazodone. Both of these agents also block serotonin reuptake, but do so in a less potent manner than either the tricyclic antidepressants or the SSRIs. Since the pharmacological mechanism of action of these agents is thought to derive predominantly from a combination of powerful antagonism of serotonin-2 receptors combined with weaker blockade of serotonin reuptake, these agents are classified separately as SARIs.

Trazodone is the first member of this SARI group of antidepressants. It also blocks alpha 1 receptors and histamine receptors (Fig. 6–30). Perhaps due to its histamine receptor blocking properties, trazodone is extremely sedating, and in fact is an excellent non–dependence forming hypnotic, but was never actually formally approved or marketed for this indication. It is also an antidepressant, and pharmacologically is distinguished from the tricyclic antidepressants by lacking not only potent norepinephrine reuptake blocking properties but also potent blockade of cholinergic receptors. A rare but troublesome side effect is priapism (prolonged erections in men, usually painful), which can be treated by injecting alpha adrenergic agonists into the penis to reverse the priapism and prevent vascular damage to the penis.

Nefazodone is a new member of the SARI class of antidepressant. Like trazodone, it is a powerful 5HT2 antagonist with secondary actions as a serotonin reuptake inhibitor (Fig. 6–30). It is far less sedating than trazodone, perhaps because it is less potent as a blocker of histamine receptors. Nefazodone also blocks alpha receptors. In contrast to trazodone, nefazodone is a weak blocker not only of serotonin reuptake but also of norepinephrine reuptake.

The major distinction between the SARIs and other classes of antidepressants is that SARIs are predominantly 5HT2 antagonists, yet combine a lesser amount of 5HT reuptake inhibition. When 5HT reuptake is inhibited selectively, as with the SSRIs, it causes essentially all serotonin receptors to be stimulated by the increased levels of 5HT that result. Although this has proven to be quite useful for treating depression and other disorders, this also has its cost. For example, stimulation of 5HT1A receptors in the raphe may help depression, but stimulating 5HT2 receptors in the forebrain may cause agitation or anxiety, and stimulating 5HT2 receptors in the spinal cord may lead to sexual dysfunction. Thus, an agent that combines 5HT reuptake blockade with stronger 5HT2 antagonism would theoretically reduce the undesired actions of 5HT stimulating 5HT2 receptors (see Fig. 6–31). In this case, competition between weak reuptake blockade and strong 5HT2 antagonism results in net antagonism at the 5HT2 receptor.

The SARIs in fact appear to lack the activating properties of some of the SSRIs, such as agitation, anxiety, and akathisia, and also lack the sexual dysfunction associated with the SSRIs. Nefazodone appears to lack the strong sedating, antihistaminic, and in vivo alpha 1 antagonist properties of trazodone, to which it is chemically related. The elimination of unwanted antihistamine activity could explain the enhanced tolerability (especially improved sedation) of nefazodone over trazodone.

Another difference between trazodone and nefazodone is that there are only very weak alpha antagonist properties of nefazodone in vivo, even though it antagonizes binding at alpha 1 receptors in vitro. The difference may be that nefazodone also

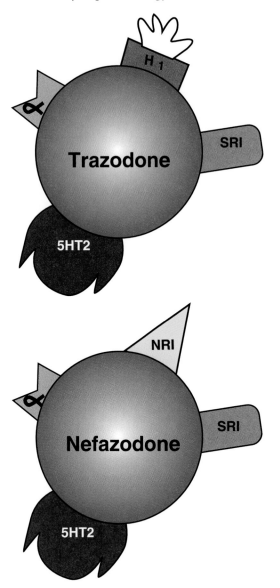

FIGURE 6–30. Shown here are icons for two of the serotonin-2 antagonist/reuptake inhibitors (**SARIs**). These agents also have a **dual action**, but the two mechanisms are different from the dual actions of the SNRIs (serotonin norepinephrine reuptake inhibitors). The SARIs act by potent **blockade both of serotonin-2 (5HT2) receptors, combined with SRI (serotonin reuptake inhibitor) actions**. Nefazodone also has weak norepinephrine reuptake inhibition (NRI) as well as weak alpha adrenergic blocking properties. Trazodone also contains antihistamine properties and alpha antagonist properties, but lacks NRI properties.

has the ability to inhibit norepinephrine uptake, which trazodone lacks (see Fig. 6–30). Thus, at the norepinephrine synapse, relatively equal amounts of alpha blockade and norepinephrine reuptake blockade may be offsetting for nefazodone (Fig. 6–32). That is, norepinephrine reuptake blockade causes increased synaptic norepinephrine that competes with nefazodone for the alpha receptor, and offsets its actions there. However, with trazodone, there is no norepinephrine reuptake blockade to offset alpha receptor antagonism (Fig. 6–30), and thus alpha antagonist properties predominate for trazodone (Fig. 6–33). This difference may account for the reduced

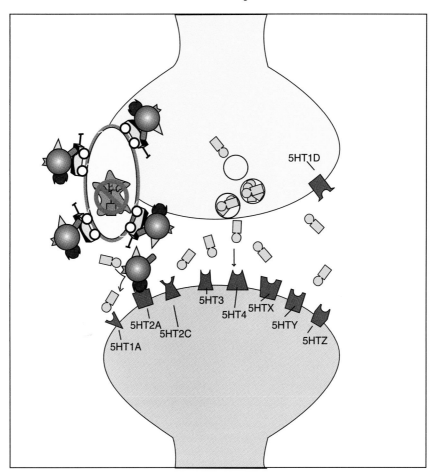

FIGURE 6–31. In this diagram, the dual actions of a **serotonin-2 antagonist/reuptake inhibitor (SARI)** are shown. These agents act both presynaptically and postsynaptically. Presynaptic actions are indicated by the serotonin reuptake inhibitor (**SRI**) portion of the icon inserted into the serotonin reuptake pump, blocking it. Postsynaptic actions are indicated by the **serotonin-2 receptor antagonist** portion of the icon (5HT2) inserted into the serotonin 2 receptor, blocking it. It is believed that both actions contribute to the therapeutic actions of SARIs as antidepressants. Blocking serotonin actions at 5HT2 receptors may also diminish side effects mediated by stimulation of 5HT2 receptors when the SRI acts to increase 5HT at all receptors subtypes. The serotonin-2 antagonist properties are stronger than the serotonin reuptake properties, so serotonin antagonism predominates at the 5HT2 receptor.

incidence of orthostatic hypotension and so far as of this writing, no cases of priapism with nefazodone compared to trazodone.

Improving the side-effect profile of trazodone by eliminating unwanted receptor blocking properties is a strategy comparable to enhancing the tolerability of the SSRIs over the TCAs once the histamine, muscarinic, and alpha properties of the TCAs were removed. Whether nefazodone will prove to have novel efficacy due to its novel predominant 5HT2 antagonist properties is yet to be shown.

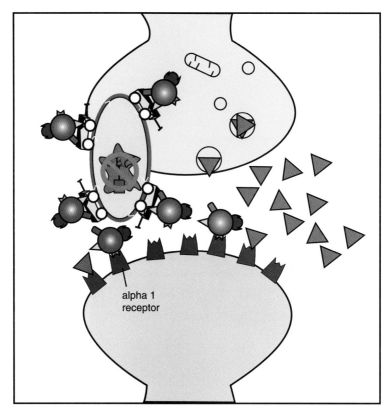

FIGURE 6–32. Actions of the serotonin-2 antagonist/reuptake inhibitor (SARI) nefazodone at the norepinephrine synapse. Nefazodone has two weak but opposite actions at noradrenergic synapses that may tend to cancel themselves. Postsynaptically, alpha receptors are blocked. Simultaneously, norepinephrine reuptake is also blocked presynaptically, raising norepinephrine levels. The increased norepinephrine is free to compete with nefazodone for the postsynaptic alpha receptor, and to offset its actions there.

Antidepressants in Clinical Trials and Future Antidepressants

This section is intended for the advanced reader with considerable knowledge of psychopharmacology. The novice may wish to skip ahead to the section on mood-stabilizing drugs.

Although no antidepressant has improved the efficacy of the TCAs or the MAOIs, the SSRIs, the SNRIs, and the new SARIs all have improved the side-effect profiles. Currently, what is needed is an antidepressant that works faster and that works for more than two out of three patients. Several theoretical candidates are in development. A sampling of these are given below, and all are variations on the theme of modulating either adrenergic neurons or serotonergic neurons with novel pharmacological mechanisms.

Adrenergic Modulators

NOREPINEPHRINE SELECTIVE REUPTAKE INHIBITORS   Several agents in clinical development block NE reuptake, but not 5HT reuptake. Preliminary evidence in-

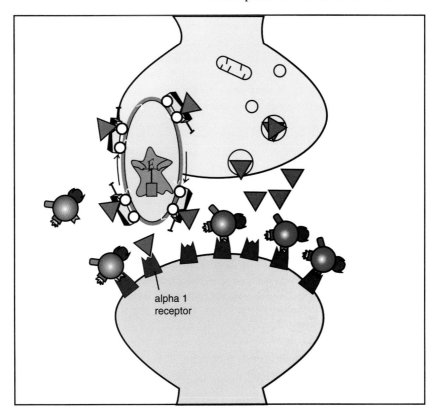

FIGURE 6–33. Actions of the serotonin-2 antagonist/reuptake inhibitor **(SARI)** trazodone at the **norepinephrine synapse**. In contrast to nefazodone, trazodone has only one action at the noradrenergic synapse. Postsynaptically, alpha receptors are blocked. Simultaneously, there is no norepinephrine reuptake blockade to offset this, so **alpha blockade predominates** for trazodone.

dicates antidepressant properties, but a different side effect profile than the SSRIs, as discussed above with bupropion. Special efficacy in depression or expanded use outside of depression is not yet established.

ALPHA 2 ANTAGONISTS   Although no selective alpha 2 antagonists are currently marketed, the nonselective agents, mianserin (also has some serotonin 2 antagonism) and mirtazepine (also has some alpha 1 antagonism) are available in Europe, and these and others are in testing worldwide. The locus coeruleus noradrenergic cell bodies as well as their presynaptic nerve terminals throughout the brain are populated with alpha 2 adrenergic receptors. As discussed in Chapter 5, the alpha 2 receptors are negative feedback receptors that brake the flow of norepinephrine out of these neurons, and turn off the release of this neurotransmitter. Blocking alpha 2 receptors has the effect of cutting the brake cable, and the release of norepinephrine continues unfettered. Theoretically, blocking presynaptic alpha 2 receptors should stop the negative feedback of norepinephrine blocking its own release. This should enhance NE action in the synapse. This could cause a robust down-regulation of beta 1 adrenergic receptors, as this has been shown in preclinical models. It might even be faster in down-regulating these receptors than by blocking NE reuptake. Although promising in terms of efficacy as antidepressants in some studies, various selective alpha 2 antagonists have had unacceptable side effects, including priapism in men, and dangerous drug interactions causing hypertension, as well as anxiety. Since the discovery of numerous alpha adrenergic receptor subtypes, it may be possible to design drugs that are safer.

BETA AGONISTS   Beta adrenergic receptors can be rapidly down-regulated by agonists, and if this is desired for an antidepressant action, beta agonists may be useful. To date, it has not been possible to identify beta agonists that successfully penetrate the brain yet are not cardiotoxic. Pursuing safer beta agonists, perhaps as partial agonists, may optimize the pharmacological properties.

SECOND-MESSENGER SYSTEMS   Enhancing adrenergic functioning distal to the receptor occupancy site can theoretically be accomplished by targeting either the G proteins or the adenylate cyclase enzyme. Both types of agents are under development. Rolipram has shown promise as an antidepressant that blocks the destruction of cyclic adenosine monophosphate (AMP) second messenger.

Modulating Serotonin Systems

SEROTONIN REUPTAKE ENHANCERS   Tianeptine is an example of an agent that allosterically modifies serotonin reuptake in a manner that is almost the opposite to that of the SSRIs. Although this might theoretically seem to have the potential to cause depression rather than treat it, tianeptine in fact appears to be antidepressant.

PURE 5HT2 ANTAGONISTS   Mianserin, mirtazepine (Remeron; Org 3770), trazodone, nefazodone, and others all have 5HT2 antagonist properties, although each is associated with additional pharmacological actions. Whereas it might be predicted that a pure 5HT2 antagonist might be a cleaner and safer antidepressant, those that have been tested to date actually look less impressive than standard antidepressants. Perhaps some other novel use of pure 5HT2 antagonists will be found. Examples include amesergide and ritanserin.

5HT1A AGONISTS   Although these compounds have been used predominantly as anxiolytics, clinical testing suggests that they may also be antidepressants (see detailed discussion of 5HT1A agonists as anxiolytics in Chapter 7). Modern drug delivery technology may well enhance the utility of such agents, as they allow once-a-day drug administration, with higher doses and lower side effects than the regimen currently employed to treat anxiety.

SINGLE-MOLECULE POLYPHARMACY   Although conventional pharmacological wisdom has always been to target a single action of a drug in order to eliminate unwanted actions that usually account for the side effects of agents, there is a countermovement afoot. Based upon observations that treatment-refractory cases are treated empirically with drug combinations, it seems possible that a multiplicity of pharmacological actions may lead to a rapid onset of antidepressant action, or to an antidepressant effect in a higher proportion of patients. In fact, several of the newer

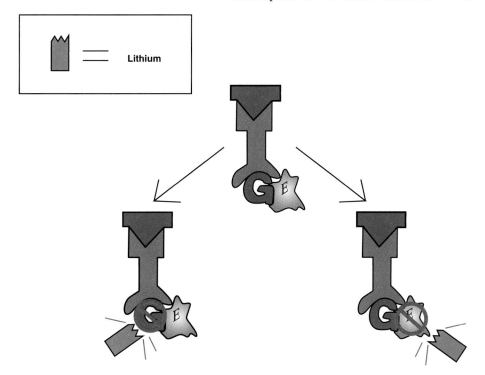

FIGURE 6–34. The **mechanism of action of lithium** is not well understood, but is hypothesized to act by **modifying second-messenger systems**. One possibility is that lithium alters **G-proteins** and their ability to transduce signals inside the cell once the neurotransmitter receptor is occupied by the neurotransmitter. Another theory is that lithium alters **enzymes** that interact with the second-messenger system, such as inositol monophosphatase, or others.

antidepressants exhibit "intramolecular polypharmacy." That is, the SNRI venlafaxine inhibits both 5HT and NE reuptake; the SARI nefazodone blocks both 5HT2 receptors and 5HT reuptake. Several combinations of two sites of targeted and presumed therapeutic actions for a single drug are currently in clinical testing.

Mood-Stabilizing Drugs

Lithium

Mood disorders characterized by elevations of mood above normal as well as depressions below normal are classically treated with lithium. Lithium is an ion whose mechanism of action is not certain. Candidates for its mechanism of action are sites beyond the receptor, in the second-messenger system, perhaps either as an inhibitor of an enzyme involved in the phosphatidyl inositol system, called inositol monophosphatase, or as a modulator of G proteins (Fig. 6–34). Lithium not only treats acute episodes of mania and hypomania, but was the first demonstrated psychotropic agent shown to prevent recurrent episodes of illness. Lithium may also be effective in treating and preventing episodes of depression in patients with manic depressive disorder. Unfortunately, lithium has many side effects that can severely limit its utility and acceptability in clinical practice.

Carbamazepine and Valproic Acid

Based upon theories that mania may "kindle" further episodes of mania, a logical parallel with seizure disorders was drawn. Thus, trials of certain anticonvulsants including carbamazepine and valproic acid were conducted, eventually demonstrating the efficacy of these agents both in manic depressive disorder in general as well as in such patients refractory to lithium. The mechanism of action of carbamazepine and valproic acid are uncertain, but some leading theories link these drugs to modulation of the gamma-amino-butyric acid (GABA) system.

Experimental Lithium-Mimetics and the Future Mood Stabilizers

Given the limitations of current treatments for mania, the search for an improved lithium-mimetic continues. One such target is to produce an inhibitor of inositol monophosphatase. Another is to target G proteins. Such agents may avoid the considerable side effects of lithium, including neurological, renal, and others. Some evidence exists that calcium channel blockers may also help to treat mania in some patients.

Drug Combinations for Treatment-Refractory Patients – Rational Polypharmacy

So far, we have discussed many individual members of the "depression pharmacy" (Fig. 6–35). More than a dozen different single interventions may thus be useful for treating the typical case of depression. However, psychopharmacologists are increasingly being called upon to provide treatment for patients who do not respond to their initial treatment with one or another of the various antidepressant treatments available from the depression pharmacy (Fig. 6–35).

Such treatment-refractory cases have classically been approached with an algorithm, trying at first single agents from different pharmacological classes, and then boosting single agents with a second drug, making for a variety of possible drug combinations (Fig. 6–36). Classically, one combination to try was to boost a TCA with lithium (the classic combo). One can even combine with great caution a TCA and an MAOI (the cautious combo). More recently, standard TCAs have been boosted with thyroid hormones, even in patients with normal thyroid functioning, and especially if their mood disorders are bipolar (manic depressive) and rapid cycling (hormone combo). Another hormone combination therapy is to combine a first line antidepressant, especially an SSRI, with estrogen replacement therapy in perimenopausal or postmenopausal women refractory to treatment with monotherapies.

Most recently, there has been a tendency to enhance serotonin agents with various boosting agents such as buspirone, fenfluramine, and trazodone or nefazodone (serotonin combo; Fig. 6–37). This may be especially desirable for "serotonin spectrum disorders" such as depression combined with symptoms of obsessive compulsive disorder, panic disorder, social phobia, or bulimia. Another pharmacological boosting strategy is to enhance adrenergic activity by boosting one of the noradrenergic/

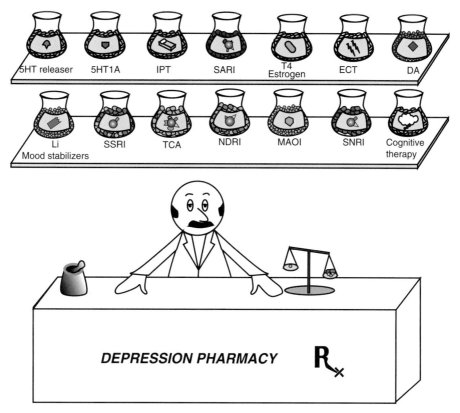

FIGURE 6–35. There are many treatments for depression, indicated here as therapies on the shelf of the depression pharmacy. Many of these treatments are used as single interventions in the treatment of depression. However, if the single agents fail, some of these agents may be used in various combinations (see Fig. 6–34). The therapies include serotonin releasers (**5HT releasers**); serotonin 1A receptor agonists (**5HT1A agents**); interpersonal psychotherapy (**IPT**); serotonin antagonists/reuptake inhibitors (**SARIs**); thyroid hormone (**T4**) or estrogen; electroconvulsive therapy (**ECT**); dopaminergic agents (**DA**); lithium (**Li**) or mood stabilizers; serotonin selective reuptake inhibitors (**SSRIs**); tricyclic antidepressants (**TCAs**); norepinephrine dopamine reuptake inhibitors (**NDRI**); monoamine oxidase inhibitors (**MAOIs**); serotonin norepinephrine reuptake inhibitors (**SNRIs**); and **cognitive therapy** (psychotherapy).

dopaminergic agents, such as the TCA desipramine, or bupropion, or moderate to high doses of venlafaxine, with additional adrenergic agents such as amphetamine, methylphenidate, pemoline, bromocriptine, phenteramine, or mazindol (the adrenergic combo; Fig. 6–37). This may be especially useful for patients with retarded or melancholic depression, or those who require concomitant mood stabilizers for bipolar disorders. In the most refractory of all patients, it may be necessary to use both serotonin and adrenergic combination strategies (heroic combo; Fig. 6–37). Failure to respond to a variety of antidepressants, singly or in combination, is the key factor indicating consideration of ECT. Unfortunately, there are not very good clinical guidelines for using antidepressants in combination, and this strategy is best left to psychopharmacology subspecialists familiar with this approach and their application to the most resistant patients unable to respond to simpler and possibly safer approaches.

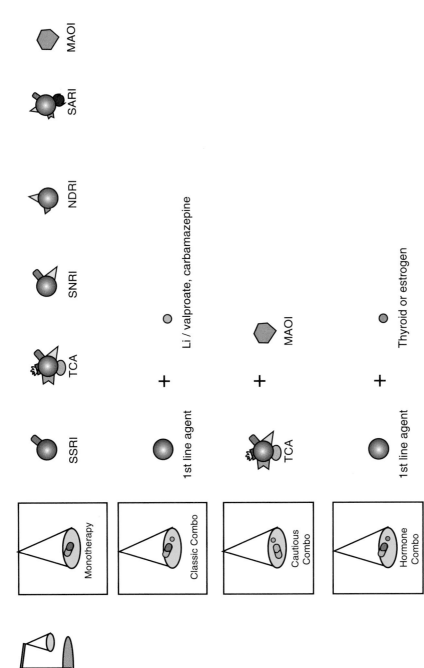

FIGURE 6–36. The treatment of depression generally begins with a single agent, called a **first-line agent**, as **monotherapy**. If the single agents fail, then drugs are often used in **combination**. For example, the classical combination of agents is a first-line agent with lithium or a mood stabilizer as augmentation (**classic combo**). A powerful if potentially dangerous combination is to use a tricyclic antidepressant and a monoamine oxidase inhibitor simultaneously (**cautious combo**). Another strategy is to augment a first-line agent with a hormone such as thyroid hormone or estrogen (**hormone combo**).

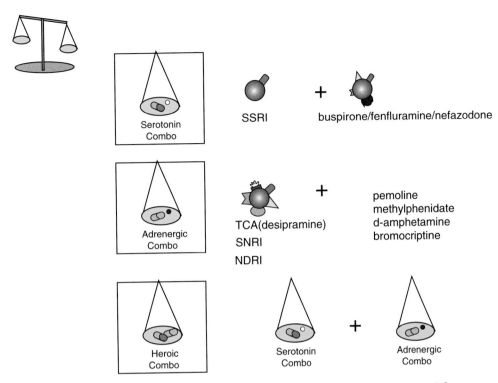

FIGURE 6–37. Other strategies for combining antidepressants involve attempts to amplify seroto-nergic action with a serotonin selective reuptake inhibitor (SSRI) plus another serotonin augmenting agent such as a serotonin 1A receptor agonist (buspirone); a serotonin releaser (fenfluramine) or a serotonin antagonist/reuptake inhibitor (SARI) (serotonin combos). Similarly, a related augmentation strategy is to amplify adrenergic actions with a TCA, SNRI, or NSRI combined with agents such as pemoline, methylphenidate, *d*-amphetamine or bromocriptine (adrenergic combos). In very difficult cases unable to respond to virtually any of the above combos, one might even combine serotonin and adrenergic combos (heroic combo).

Various combinations of antidepressants are discussed in further detail in Chapter 8, where the use of such agents to treat anxiety disorders is reviewed. The same combinations discussed there are also sometimes useful in treatment refractory and treatment-resistant nonresponding patients with depression.

Electroconvulsive Therapy

This is the only therapeutic agent for the treatment of depression that is rapid in onset, and can start after even a single treatment, and typically within a few days. The mechanism is unknown, but is thought to be related to the probable mobilization of neurotransmitters caused by the seizure. In experimental animals, ECT down-regulates beta receptors (analogous to antidepressants), but up-regulates 5HT2 receptors (opposite of antidepressants). Memory losses and social stigma are the primary problems associated with ECT and which limit its use.

ECT is thus especially useful as a therapy when rapid onset of clinical effect is desired, and when patients are refractory to a number of antidepressant drugs. If the mechanism of therapeutic action of ECT could be unraveled, it might be possible to find a new antidepressant drug capable of rapid onset of antidepressant effects or of special value for treatment-refractory patients. Until then, ECT will remain a valuable member of the therapeutic armamentarium for depression.

Psychotherapy

In recent years, modern psychotherapy research has begun to standardize and test selected psychotherapies in a manner analogous to how antidepressants are tested in clinical trials. Thus, psychotherapies are now being tested by being administered according to standard protocols by therapists receiving standardized training and using standardized manuals, also in standard "doses" for fixed durations. Such use of psychotherapies is being compared in clinical trials to placebo or antidepressants. The results have shown that brief interpersonal therapy (IPT) and cognitive therapy for depression may be as effective as antidepressants themselves in certain patients. Research is only beginning in how to combine psychotherapy with drugs. Proof of efficacy of certain psychotherapies is thus beginning to evolve.

Summary

This chapter has discussed the mechanisms of action of the major antidepressant drugs. The acute pharmacological actions of these agents on receptors and enzymes have been described, as well as the major hypothesis that attempts to explain how all current antidepressants ultimately work. That hypothesis is known as the neurotransmitter receptor hypothesis of antidepressant action. Specific agents that the reader should now understand include the MAOIs, tricyclic antidepressants, serotonin selective reuptake inhibitors, adrenergic modulators, dual reuptake inhibitors, and serotonin antagonist/reuptake inhibitors.

This chapter has also briefly explored the mood stabilizers for mania, and has touched upon the use of electroconvulsive therapy and psychotherapy for the treatment of depression.

Although the specific pragmatic guidelines for use of these various therapeutic agents for depression have not been emphasized, the reader should now have a basis for the rational use of antidepressant and mood stabilizing drugs founded on application of principles discussed earlier in this text, namely drug actions on neurotransmission via actions at key receptors and enzymes.

CHAPTER 7

ANXIOLYTICS AND SEDATIVE-HYPNOTICS

In this chapter and the following chapter we will discuss the anxiety disorders and antianxiety drugs as well as insomnia and the sedative-hypnotic drugs (i.e., sleeping pills). We will emphasize generalized anxiety in this chapter, and take up specific anxiety disorders such as panic disorder and obsessive compulsive disorder in the following chapter. Here we will sketch a simple outline of the clinical features and the biological basis of anxiety and insomnia in order to provide background for understanding the actions of antianxiety (i.e., anxiolytic) as well as sedative-hypnotic drugs. The reader is referred to standard references for details on diagnostic criteria for the various specific disorders of anxiety and sleep because here we will emphasize only general principles and concepts about the emotion of anxiety and the phenonena of sleep.

Our discussion of antianxiety and sedative-hypnotic treatments will attempt to develop the psychopharmacological concepts underlying how such treatments work. We will thus describe the pharmacology of gamma-amino-butyric acid (GABA) neuron and GABA receptors linked to benzodiazepine receptors. We will also build upon the pharmacological principles already introduced in our earlier discussions of serotonin (5HT) and norepinephrine (NE) neurons and receptors. However, we will not provide pragmatic guidelines on how to use anxiolytics or sedative-hypnotics in clinical practice. We may therefore omit important details, facts, or exceptions in order to emphasize the general psychopharmacological principles of antianxiety and insomnia treatments. The reader is referred to standard handbooks of drug treatment for specifics of drug dosing and side effects.

Clinical Description of Generalized Anxiety

Anxiety is a normal emotion under circumstances of threat and is thought to be part of the evolutionary "fight-or-flight" reaction of survival. Whereas it may be normal or even adaptive to be anxious when a saber-tooth tiger (or its modern day equivalent) is attacking, there are many circumstances in which the presence of anxiety is maladaptive and constitutes a psychiatric disorder. The idea of anxiety as a psychiatric disorder, however, has undergone considerable change in recent years.

The original concept in the 1960s was to separate anxiety and its drug treatments generally from depression and its drug treatments, as discussed in the preceding chapter on antidepressants (see Fig. 5-1). This concept had the effect of lumping all forms of anxiety together, and was useful from a clinical point of view, as the newly discovered benzodiazepines were shown to reduce anxiety in a general and global manner.

These diagnoses of anxiety neurosis and generalized anxiety disorder (GAD) were probably applied too widely and benzodiazepines prescribed too broadly in the early days of this concept, leading to cries of the "overmedicated society," as Valium and Xanax became some of the most widely prescribed drugs in the world. Partly in reaction to this, and partly because different types of anxiety states came to be recognized as differentially responsive to various antianxiety medications, the concept of GAD began to fragment (Fig. 7-1).

As will be discussed in further detail in Chapter 8, panic disorder became differentiated from GAD, and then social phobia became differentiated from panic disorder. Also, obsessive compulsive disorder, and posttraumatic stress disorder became well differentiated from generalized anxiety disorder. Furthermore, short-lasting anxiety due to recognizable stressors that resolves in a few months is now recognized as an adjustment disorder that is self-limiting and therefore also delineated from GAD, which is conceived as being a chronic condition. All these developments have contributed to the ultimate effect of fragmenting GAD into a residual diagnosis

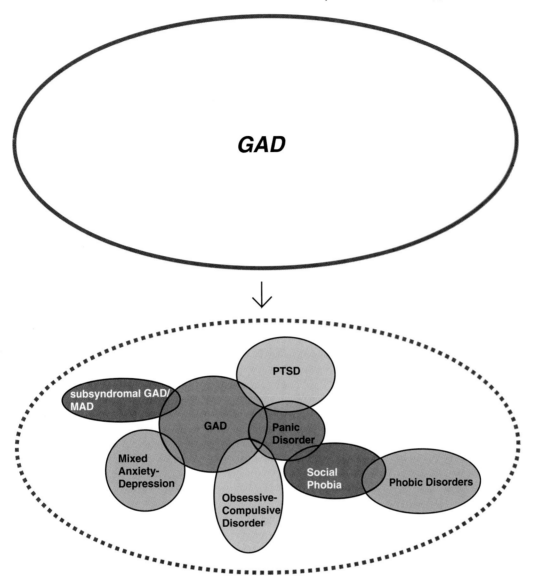

FIGURE 7–1. This figure shows the original concept of **generalized anxiety disorder (GAD)**, which lumped various types of anxiety disorders together (*top*) fragmenting into various anxiety disorder subtypes (*bottom*). The anxiety disorder subtypes that fragmented from the classical description of GAD (which was also called **anxiety neurosis**) created a new residual category of GAD (*bottom*), with the following disorders extracted from it: **panic disorder, obsessive compulsive disorder, social phobia, phobic disorders, mixed anxiety depression (MAD), subsyndromal GAD/MAD,** and **posttraumatic stress disorder (PTSD).**

(i.e., anxiety that is disabling but not caused by any of the other known anxiety disorder syndromes) (see Fig. 7–1).

The usefulness of this now residual category of GAD is under intense debate in the international psychiatric community, with different views in different parts of

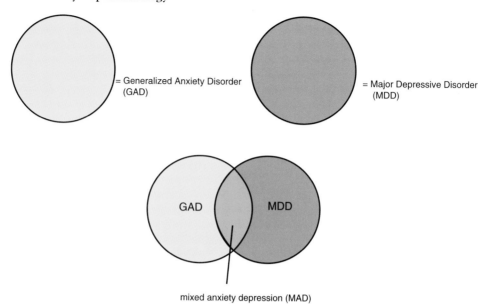

FIGURE 7–2. In the top of this figure, **generalized anxiety disorder (GAD)** is separated as a concept from **major depressive disorder (MDD)** as two distinct syndromes with no overlap. In the bottom of the figure, GAD and MDD are shown as two syndromes that overlap, thereby creating a third disorder, namely **mixed anxiety depression (MAD)**.

the world. Some work is now clarifying that individuals with GAD frequently have a second (comorbid) psychiatric disorder also present, particularly depression or another anxiety disorder.

Other work is trying to clarify the boundary between anxiety and depression, with the "splitters" arguing for sharper distinctions and the "lumpers" arguing for a middle category between anxiety and depression, sometimes termed mixed anxiety depression (MAD) (Fig. 7–2). Yet another concept is that MAD should be defined as subsyndromal (i.e., the presence of symptoms of anxiety and depression but not of sufficient severity to meet the formal diagnostic criteria for full-blown GAD or major depressive disorder) (Fig. 7–3).

Most concepts of anxiety largely define it at a single point in time, whether as a single entity, or a combination entity with depression (Fig. 7–4). Increasingly, disorders of anxiety are being defined over the course of time and with a variety of long-term outcomes. Thus, one idea is that some sufferers with subsyndromal anxiety have a chronic condition that never reaches the threshold of current definitions for a mental disorder (Fig. 7–3). More likely, however, chronic anxiety is not a stable condition. Thus, subsyndromal anxiety may alternate with states of relative normality (Fig. 7–5) or with episodes of full-blown GAD (Fig. 7–6). The latter patients follow a course similar to that already discussed in Chapter 5 on depressive disorders, and resembles the "double depression" syndrome described in Figure 5–7. Therefore, subsyndromal anxiety alternating with episodes of GAD can be considered a "double anxiety" syndrome (Fig. 7–7).

Subsyndromal anxiety may not only decompensate to GAD, but GAD may further decompensate to panic disorder (Fig. 7–8). Subsyndromal MAD may also be a har-

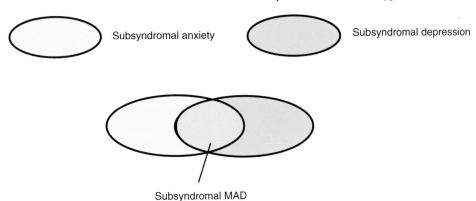

FIGURE 7−3. Shown here is the concept of symptoms of anxiety that do not reach the threshold for the diagnosis of an anxiety disorder (**subsyndromal anxiety**); also shown is the concept of symptoms of depression that do not reach the threshold for the diagnosis of major depressive disorder (**subsyndromal depression**). If these symptoms overlap, they create mixtures of anxiety and depression that also do not meet the diagnostic criteria for an affective or an anxiety disorder; this is called subsyndromal MAD (**subsyndromal mixed anxiety depression**).

binger for decompensating to a full syndrome of anxiety or depression under stress (Fig. 7−9).

Biological Basis of Anxiety

Three neurotransmitter systems are implicated in the biological basis of anxiety: the GABA−benzodiazepine receptor complex, the locus coeruleus−norepinephrine system, and serotonin. These neurotransmitter systems may mediate "normal" anxiety as well as pathological anxiety. The biological basis of anxiety in general will be discussed here. The biological basis for anxiety in the specific disorders of panic, obsessive compulsive disorder, and phobias will be discussed in Chapter 8.

GABAergic Neurons

Understanding the actions of anxiolytic drugs requires background knowledge on the pharmacology of GABAergic neurotransmission. GABAergic neurons use GABA as their neurotransmitter. GABA is synthesized from the amino acid precursor glutamate via the enzyme glutamic acid decarboxylase (Glu-AD) (see Fig. 7−10). Glutamate is derived from intraneuronal stores of amino acids. It is a nonessential amino acid and is the most abundant free amino acid in the central nervous system (CNS). Glutamate also participates in multiple metabolic functions and can be synthesized from numerous precursors (see discussion of glutamate neurons in Chapter 11).

The GABA neuron has a presynaptic transporter (reuptake pump; Fig. 7−11) similar to those that have already been described for NE, dopamine (DA), and 5HT in Chapter 5. This transporter terminates the action of synaptic GABA by removing it from the synaptic cleft for restorage or for destruction by the enzyme GABA T (GABA transaminase) (see Fig. 7−11).

Receptors for GABA also regulate GABAergic neurotransmission. There are two known subtypes of GABA receptors, known as GABA A and GABA B (Fig. 7−12).

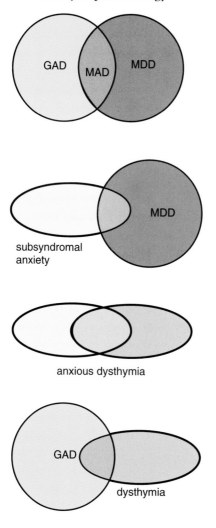

FIGURE 7–4. Anxiety and depression can be combined in a **wide variety of syndromes**. Already shown in Figure 7–2 is the concept of generalized anxiety disorder (**GAD**) overlapping with major depressive disorder (**MDD**) to form mixed anxiety depression (**MAD**). Already shown in Figure 7–3 is the concept of subsyndromal anxiety overlapping with subsyndromal depression to form subsyndromal mixed anxiety depression, sometimes also called **anxious dysthymia**. MDD can also overlap with subsyndromal symptoms of anxiety to create **anxious depression**; GAD can also overlap with symptoms of depression such as dysthymia to create **GAD with depressive features**. Thus, a **spectrum of symptoms and disorders** is possible, ranging from pure anxiety without depression, to various mixtures of each in varying intensities, to pure depression without anxiety.

GABA A receptors are the ones that are gatekeepers for a chloride channel (Figs. 7–12 and 7–13). GABA A receptors are *allosterically modulated* by a potpourri of nearby receptors. This includes the well-known benzodiazepine receptor (Fig. 7–13). The concept of allosteric modulation of one receptor by another has already been introduced in Chapter 3.

The fundamental neurobiological importance of the GABA A receptor is underscored by observations that even more receptor sites exist at or near this complex (Fig. 7–14). This includes receptor sites for the convulsant drug picrotoxin, for the anticonvulsant barbiturates, and perhaps even for alcohol. Could this receptor complex be responsible for mediating such wide-ranging CNS activities as seizures, anticonvulsant drug effects, and the behavioral actions of alcohol as well as the known anxiolytic, sedative-hypnotic, and muscle relaxant effects of the benzodiazepines?

Thus, there appear to be many locations, receptors, and points of modulation of this key GABA A receptor complex: GABA itself as the gatekeeper for the chloride

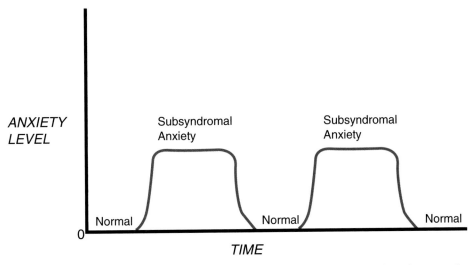

FIGURE 7–5. Some patients with **subsyndromal anxiety** have an intermittent clinical course that **waxes and wanes over time** between a normal state and a state of subsyndromal anxiety.

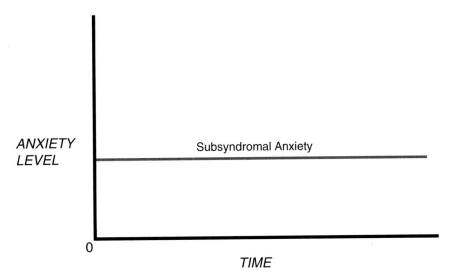

FIGURE 7–6. In contrast to Figure 7–5, other patients with subsyndromal anxiety have a chronic and relatively stable yet **unremitting clinical course** over time.

channel, and benzodiazepines, convulsants, anticonvulsants, and alcohol as allosteric modulators, all capable of manifesting their unique behavioral and neurological actions presumably through differing actions at a constellation of differing and unique receptors arranged at this complex. Many exciting therapeutic opportunities are unfolding as the pharmacology of the GABA A receptor complex becomes better understood.

Each GABA A receptor appears to be composed of several molecular subunits working together (Fig. 7–15). Many different forms of each subunit exist (molecular

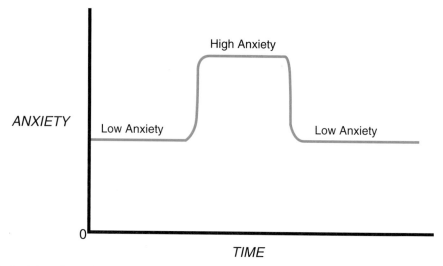

FIGURE 7–7. Subsyndromal anxiety can also be a **harbinger** of a full generalized anxiety disorder (GAD) episode. Such patients may have an intermittent clinical course that waxes and wanes over time between subsyndromal anxiety and GAD. Decompensating to full GAD with recovery only to a state of subsyndromal anxiety over time can also be called the "**double anxiety syndrome**."

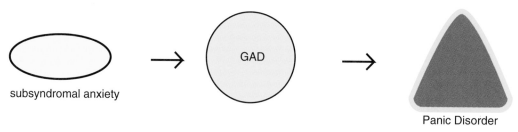

FIGURE 7–8. **Subsyndromal anxiety** may be a harbinger not only for decompensation to generalized anxiety disorder (**GAD**) as shown in Figure 7–7, but GAD in turn may be a harbinger for decompensation to **panic disorder** in some patients.

isoforms) so that a multitude of combinations of various versions of each of these subunits can be assembled in different neurons in different parts of the brain. It is not clear how this heterogeneity affects function, but it is likely that there are functional differences in some of the molecular isoforms.

The combination of an alpha and a beta subunit of the GABA A receptor appears to be adequate to create the binding site for GABA itself. However, a third subunit gamma appears to be necessary to join alpha and beta parts of the GABA site in order to create a binding site for benzodiazepines (Fig. 7–15). Several of these combined units are arranged concentrically and thereby create a channel in the middle (Figs. 7–12 through 7–15). This is the chloride channel that binding of GABA and benzodiazepines are able to modulate, as discussed throughout this chapter. This discussion of the molecular configuration of the GABA A receptor complex is oversimplified. Advances in molecular neuroscience are constantly reconfiguring and rearranging the pieces to the puzzle as new discoveries unfold. The concept to

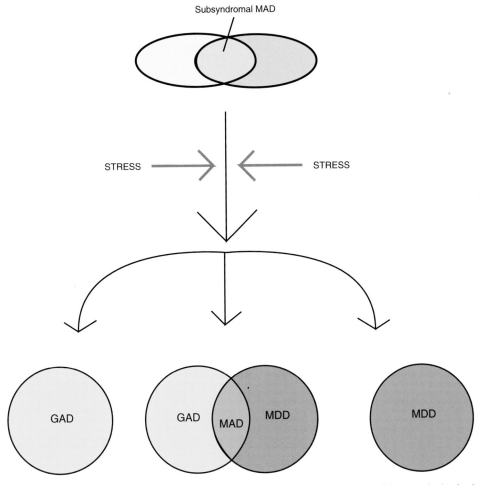

FIGURE 7–9. Subsyndromal mixed anxiety depression (**MAD**) may be an **unstable psychological state**, characterized by **vulnerability to decompensating** to more severe psychiatric disorders under stress. Such disorders may include the decompensation of subsyndromal MAD to generalized anxiety disorder (**GAD**), to full syndrome **MAD**, or to major depressive disorder (**MDD**).

grasp here is that molecules and bits of molecules cooperate to control neurotransmission at this ligand-gated ion channel.

The second GABA receptor subtype is called the *GABA B receptor* (Fig. 7–12). This receptor is not allosterically modulated by benzodiazepines, but binds selectively to the muscle relaxant baclofen. Its physiological role is not well known yet, but appears not to be closely linked to anxiety disorders or to anxiolytics.

Benzodiazepine receptors. Discovery of receptors for the powerful antianxiety and sedative-hypnotic drugs of the benzodiazepine class has thus led to an explanation for how such agents work (Fig. 7–13). Clearly, benzodiazepines bind to their receptors, and the consequence of this is to boost the actions of the fast inhibitory neurotransmitter GABA acting at GABA A receptors.

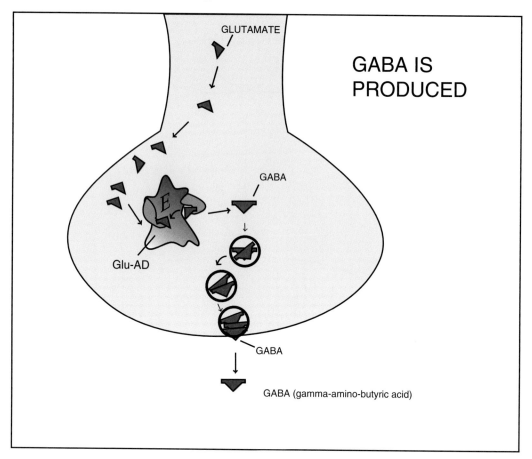

FIGURE 7–10. **Gamma-amino-butyric acid (GABA)** is **produced** by synthesis from the precursor amino acid **glutamate** by the enzyme glutamic acid decarboxylase (**Glu-AD**).

There are multiple molecular forms of benzodiazepine receptors, and there is continuing debate about how differences in the amino acid composition of benzo-diazepine receptors may lead to pharmacological differences in ligand binding and in functional activity. There may be at least five benzodiazepine receptor subtypes, including three with distinct pharmacological profiles. For example, benzodiazepine-1 (sometimes called omega-1) receptors are preferentially abundant in the cerebellum and contain recognition sites with high affinities both for benzodiazepines and for agents with different chemical structures. Anxiolytic action as well as sedative-hyp-notic actions seem to be mediated mostly through the benzodiazepine 1 receptor subtype. Benzodiazepine-2 (omega-2) receptors, on the other hand, are located pre-dominantly in the spinal cord and striatum. These receptors may be involved in mediating the muscle relaxant actions of benzodiazepines. Finally, the benzodiazepine 3 receptor, also known as the "peripheral" type (i.e., outside of the CNS) is abundant in the kidney. Its role in anxiolytic actions remains unclear.

Actions at benzodiazepine receptors are thus thought to underlie virtually all the pharmacological actions of the benzodiazepines, both those that are desirable as well

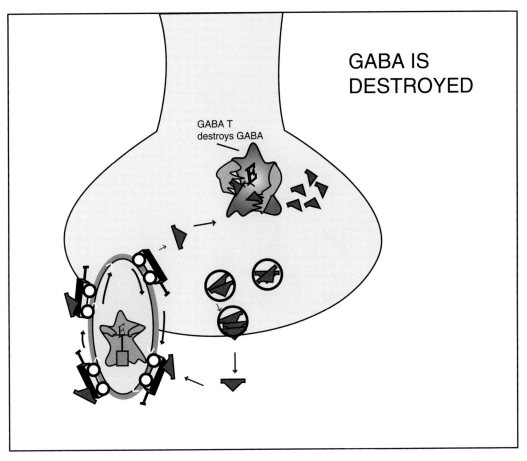

GABA IS DESTROYED

GABA T
destroys GABA

FIGURE 7–11. The action of **gamma-amino-butyric acid (GABA)** is **terminated** either by **enzymatic destruction** by GABA transaminase (**GABA T**) or by removal from the synaptic cleft by the **GABA transporter**. Following transport back into the presynaptic neuron, GABA can be re-stored in synaptic vesicles for reuse during a subsequent neurotransmission, as already pointed out for the norepinephrine, dopamine, and serotonin neurons.

as those that are undesirable. This includes the desirable *therapeutic* actions of benzodiazepines as anxiolytics, as sedative-hypnotics, as well as anticonvulsants and muscle relaxants. It also includes their undesirable *side effects* as amnestic agents and as agents that cause adaptations at the benzodiazepine receptor with chronic administration thought to underlie the production of dependence on and withdrawal from these agents (see Chapter 12).

Benzodiazepines are listed in Table 7–1. Because they act at a naturally occurring receptor in brain, it has led to speculation that the brain may make its own benzodiazepine, or "endogenous Valium." Identification of a naturally occurring ligand for the benzodiazepine receptor, however, is yet incomplete. Modulation of the GABA–benzodiazepine receptor complex is therefore thought to underlie not only the pharmacological actions of antianxiety drugs; it is also theorized as serving as the vehicle for mediating the emotion of anxiety itself. It has been speculated, for example, that reduced actions of GABA and the postulated endogenous benzodiaz-

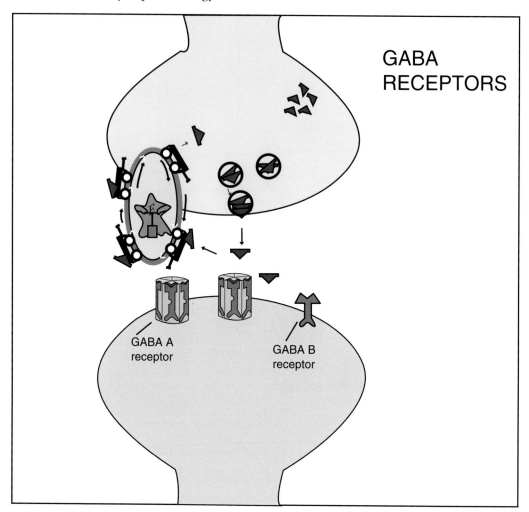

FIGURE 7–12. Various receptors for gamma-amino-butyric acid (GABA) are shown here at the GABA synapse. On the presynaptic side, there is the **GABA transporter**, the receptor linked to an active transport pump that removes GABA from the synaptic cleft thus terminating its actions there. On the postsynaptic side, there are two subtypes of GABA receptors shown. The first is the **GABA A receptor**, which is a member of the superfamily of ligand-gated ion channel receptors. The second is the **GABA B receptor**.

epines at this receptor complex may be associated with the emotion of anxiety, whether the emotion is normal or pathological.

Positive allosteric interactions between GABA A receptors and benzodiazepine receptors. Put in technical language, the benzodiazepines are positive allosteric modulators of fast inhibitory neurotransmission by GABA at GABA A receptors. The inhibitory neurotransmitter GABA is the gatekeeper neurotransmitter that interacts selectively with its GABA A receptor, the primary receptor site of this GABA–benzodiazepine chloride channel receptor complex shown in Figure 7–13. Thus, this complex is an

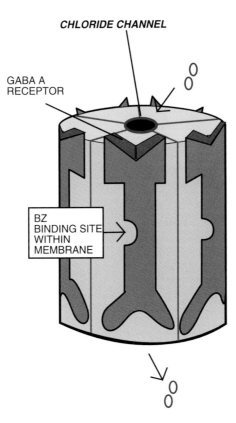

CHLORIDE CHANNEL

GABA A
RECEPTOR

BZ
BINDING SITE
WITHIN
MEMBRANE

FIGURE 7–13. The **GABA A receptor** is shown here. It acts as a gatekeeper for a **chloride channel**. It also has a key **allosteric modulatory site** nearby, known as the **benzodiazepine (BZ) binding site**.

example of the superfamily of receptors already discussed in Chapter 3 (see Figs. 3–3 through 3–14) and known as *ligand-gated receptor complexes*. In the case of the GABA–benzodiazepine receptor complex, this particular superfamily complex acts to control a chloride ion channel mediating fast neurotransmission (see discussion in Chapter 1 and Fig. 1–6).

The GABA A receptors are arranged as helical columns around a chloride channel, which itself is a column of columns, as mentioned in Chapter 3 and as shown in Figures 3–6 through 3–12 as well as in Figures 7–12 through 7–15. Following occupancy of the GABA A receptor site by GABA molecules, the GABA A receptor columns in turn interact with the chloride channel to open it a bit (Fig. 7–16). The increased chloride conductance into the neuron that results occurs quickly (i.e., fast neurotransmission; see Chapter 1 and Fig. 1–6) and is inhibitory to the firing of that neuron.

Nearby the receptor site for GABA is not only the chloride channel, but also another neurotransmitter receptor binding site, namely the benzodiazepine receptor binding site (Fig. 7–13) as has already been mentioned. It was originally thought that the benzodiazepine receptor binding site was located on an entirely different receptor protein molecule than the GABA A receptor. However, it is now conceptualized that the benzodiazepine receptor binding site is on the *same* protein molecule, only at a different location on that protein from where the GABA receptor binding site is located (see Fig. 7–15).

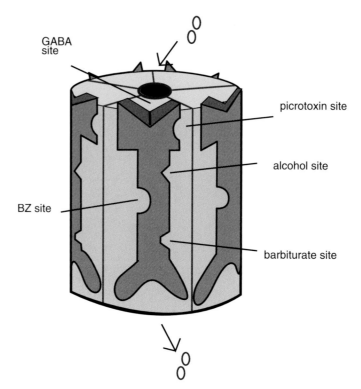

GABA
site

picrotoxin site

alcohol site

BZ site

barbiturate site

FIGURE 7–14. Multiple modulatory sites nearby the **GABA A receptor** are shown here. These include not only the **benzodiazepine (BZ) receptor** already shown in Figure 7–13 but also sites for the convulsant drug **picrotoxin**, for the anticonvulsant **barbiturate**, and possibly for **alcohol** as well. These nearby receptors suggest how GABA may be involved in modulating such diverse physiological actions as anxiety, seizures, and even the actions of alcohol.

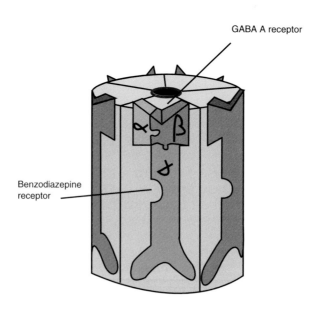

GABA A receptor

Benzodiazepine
receptor

FIGURE 7–15. The **GABA A receptor** is composed of **three molecular subunits**. Two subunits (**alpha, beta**) together are sufficient for forming the GABA A receptor binding site, but a third subunit (**gamma**) is required to form the **benzodiazepine receptor** site.

Table 7–1. *Some of the major benzodiazepines*

Alprazolam (Xanax)
Clonazepam (Klonopin)
Diazepam (Valium)
Chlordiazepoxide (Librium)
Lorazepam (Ativan)
Oxazepam (Serax)
Prazepam (Centrex)
Clorazepate (Tranxene)
Triazolam (Halcion)
Temazepam (Restoril)
Flurazepam (Dalmane)
Midazolam (Versed)
Quazepam (Doral)
Flumazenil (Romazicon)
Mitrazepam
Lormetazolam
Loprazolam
Clobazam
Flunitrazepam (Rohypnol)
Brotizolam

Benzodiazepine receptor binding sites also affect the conductance of chloride through the chloride channel. However, the benzodiazepine receptor binding site does not do this by directly modulating the chloride channel, but by *allosterically* modulating the GABA A receptor binding site, which in turn modulates the chloride channel.

Thus, when a benzodiazepine binds to its own benzodiazepine receptor site, a neighbor of the GABA A receptor binding site, nothing happens if GABA is not also binding to its own GABA A receptor site (Fig. 7–17). On the other hand, when GABA is binding to its GABA A receptor site, and there is simultaneous binding of benzodiazepine to its benzodiazepine binding site ("allosteric" other site), this causes a large amplification in GABA's ability to increase the conductance of chloride through the channel (Fig. 7–18).

Why is this necessary? It turns out that GABA working by itself can increase chloride conductance through the chloride channel only a certain extent (Fig. 7–16). Benzodiazepines cannot increase chloride conductance at all when working by themselves (Fig. 7–17). However, allosteric modulation is the mechanism to maximize the chloride conductance beyond that which GABA alone (as in Fig. 7–16) can accomplish. Thus, GABA can increase chloride conductance through the chloride channel much more dramatically when a benzodiazepine receptor binding site is helping it allosterically than it can when it is working to modulate the chloride channel by itself (Fig. 7–18).

In other words, benzodiazepines *allosterically modulate* GABA neurotransmission by potentiating GABA's ability to increase conductance of chloride through its channel. That is, GABA plus benzodiazepines, or $1 + 0 = 2$, not 1. This mechanism

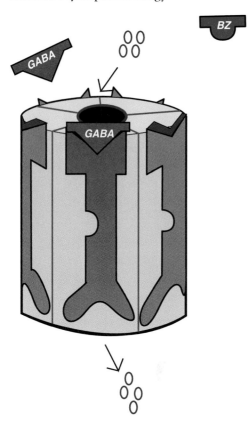

FIGURE 7–16. **GABA** is the ligand that acts at the **GABA A receptor site** to participate in opening the molecular gate for an inhibitory chloride channel. Thus, when GABA alone binds to the GABA A receptor, it **opens the chloride channel** so that more chloride can now enter the cell and cause inhibitory neurotransmission. Also shown is a **benzodiazepine (BZ) ligand** which is **not** binding to the benzodiazepine receptor in this example (but see the following examples in Figs. 7–17 and 7–18).

greatly expands the scope for the neuron to be able to regulate its fast inhibitory neurotransmission with chemical ligands.

Inverse agonists, partial agonists, and antagonists at benzodiazepine receptors. For a further degree of regulatory control of GABA neurotransmission, the concept of allosteric modulation can be combined with the concept of inverse agonists. Inverse agonists have already been introduced (see Chapter 3 for discussion). Thus, *positive* allosteric modulation of benzodiazepines upon GABA A receptors occurs because the benzodiazepines are *full agonists* at the benzodiazepine site (Fig. 7–18). However, *negative* allosteric modulation can occur when an *inverse agonist* binds to the benzodiazepine site. Instead of *increasing* the chloride conductance that GABA provokes (Fig. 7–17), the inverse agonist *decreases* it (Fig. 7–19).

This can translate into opposite behavioral actions for agonists versus inverse agonists. For example, benzodiazepine full agonists *reduce* anxiety by increasing chloride conductance as shown in Figure 7–18. However, a benzodiazepine inverse agonist *causes* anxiety, and does this by decreasing chloride conductance as shown in Figure 7–19. Benzodiazepine inverse agonists would not only be expected to be anxiogenic (create anxiety) but also to be proconvulsant (increase the likelihood of seizures), activating (opposite of sedation), and promnestic (memory promoting, the opposite of amnesia; see Fig. 7–20). The latter promnestic actions have even been considered as a possible therapeutic strategy for memory disorders such as Alzhei-

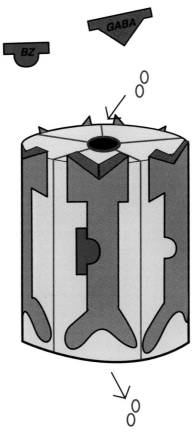

FIGURE 7–17. Shown here is a benzodiazepine (**BZ**) ligand binding to the **benzodiazepine receptor** on the GABA A receptor complex. Note that **GABA** itself is **not** binding to the GABA A receptor site in this example. Note also that the chloride channel is **not opening**. This example is thus in contrast to the previous example (Fig. 7–16) where GABA alone was binding to the GABA A receptor. In the current example where **BZ ligand alone** binds to the GABA A receptor, essentially **no more chloride can enter** the cell to cause inhibitory neurotransmission. However, see the contrast in the following example (Fig. 7–18) when both GABA and benzodiazepine bind to the GABA A receptor complex.

mer's disease (see Chapter 11). However, these agents are potentially dangerous if they would simultaneously promote anxiety and seizures. Indeed, early clinical testing in man has produced some severe anxiety reactions to inverse benzodiazepine agonists.

Consequently, the pharmacological properties of agonists and inverse agonists reveal that there can be obvious and dramatic clinical and behavioral distinctions across the agonist – antagonist – inverse agonist spectrum (Figs. 3–14 and 7–20) that can be explained by the principles of allosteric modulation of receptors.

An intermediate in the agonist spectrum (Fig. 7–20) is a partial agonist. Partial agonists have the theoretical possibility of separating the desired effects (i.e., anxiolytic) from the undesired effects (i.e., daytime sedation, ataxia, memory disturbance, dependency, and withdrawal) (see also Fig. 7–20). That is, full agonists theoretically

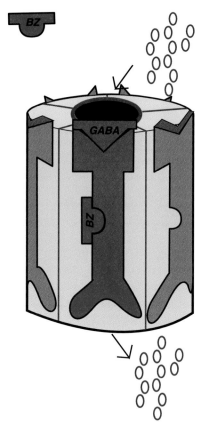

FIGURE 7–18. In this example, **both GABA and benzodiazepine (BZ) ligands** are binding to their respective receptor sites on the **GABA A receptor complex**. This causes **far more opening of the chloride channel** than can be done by GABA acting alone. Thus, it can be said that benzodiazepine ligands **allosterically modulate** GABA's ability to open the chloride channel. It is this positive allosteric modulation of the BZ receptor by benzodiazepine drugs that is thought to account for their **anxiolytic actions**.

exert the full portfolio of benzodiazepine actions, whereas a partial agonist would separate those actions thought to require only partial agonism (i.e., anxiolytic effects) from those thought to require full agonism (i.e., sedation and dependency; see Fig. 7–20). A wide variety of partial agonists for the benzodiazepine receptor have been synthesized and tested. The results to date are generally disappointing, since too much partial agonism fails to distinguish such agents from the full agonists already marketed, and too little partial agonism is associated with too little clinical efficacy in anxiety. However, this idea of a partial agonist is a conceptually attractive one, based upon the promise of such agents from preclinical testing and from theoretical considerations.

Pharmacological manipulations of benzodiazepines have advanced to the point that an antagonist, flumazenil, has been developed that can block the actions of the benzodiazepines and reverse their actions (e.g., after anesthesthesia or after an overdose) (Fig. 7–21).

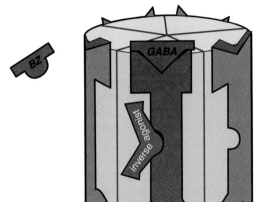

FIGURE 7–19. Shown here is what happens when an **inverse agonist** for the benzodiazepine (BZ) receptor influences GABA binding at the **GABA A receptor**. In this example, the inverse agonist **closes the chloride channel**. Thus, an inverse BZ agonist **allosterically modulates GABA in the opposite direction** of a normal BZ full agonist such as that shown in the previous example (Fig. 7–18). Consequently, a benzodiazepine inverse agonist increases anxiety (i.e., it is **anxiogenic** rather than anxiolytic).

Interestingly, as predicted from the pharmacology of the agonist spectrum (Fig. 7–20), the benzodiazepine antagonist flumazenil is also able to reverse the actions of inverse agonists (Fig. 7–22). This underscores the pharmacological principles developed in Chapter 3 showing how drugs can influence a neurotransmitter system in a very broad range when a spectrum of agents can work on the one hand from full agonist through partial agonist to neutral antagonist, and on the other hand from neutral antagonist to partial inverse agonist to full inverse agonist (Figs. 3–14 and 7–20).

Locus coeruleus and norepinephrine. A second biological substrate for anxiety is the norepinephrine neuron (see Figs. 5–16 through 5–18), which has its cell body in the brainstem in an area known as the locus coeruleus (Fig. 7–23). Electrical stimulation of the locus coeruleus to make it overactive creates a state in experimental animals analogous to anxiety. Thus, overactivity of norepinephrine neurons is thought to underlie anxiety states. Indeed, examples of symptoms of anxiety consistent with adrenergic overactivity include tachycardia, tremor, and sweating (Fig. 7–23).

The locus coeruleus noradrenergic cell bodies as well as their presynaptic nerve terminals throughout the brain are populated with alpha 2 adrenergic receptors (Fig. 7–24). When located on the noradrenergic cell body in the locus coeruleus, they function as somatodendritic autoreceptors (Fig. 7–25). This is analogous to the situation for the serotonin neuron already shown in Figures 5–25 and 5–26.

When alpha 2 adrenergic receptors are located on the presynaptic nerve terminal, they act as terminal autoreceptors (Fig. 7–26). Analogous receptors on the serotonin neuron have already been discussed (see Figs. 5–27 through 5–30).

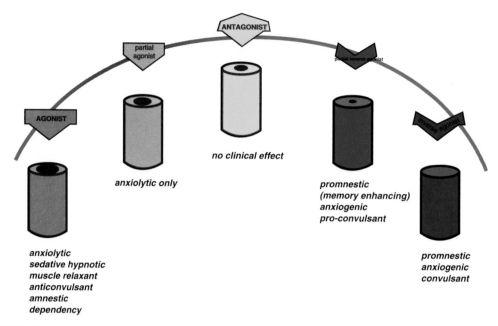

anxiolytic
sedative hypnotic
muscle relaxant
anticonvulsant
amnestic
dependency

promnestic
anxiogenic
convulsant

FIGURE 7–20. This figure reveals that there is a whole spectrum of agonist activities at the benzodiazepine receptor, ranging from **full agonist actions** through **antagonist actions** all the way to **inverse agonist actions**. These actions have already been introduced in Figure 3–14. **Full agonists** (far left of the spectrum) not only have **desired** therapeutic actions (anxiolytic, sedative-hypnotic, muscle relaxant, and anticonvulsant) but also **undesired** side effects (amnesia and dependency). Theoretically, a **happy medium** might be possible halfway between a full agonist and an antagonist as a **partial agonist** that might be **anxiolytic without causing dependency**, for example. **Antagonists** (middle of the spectrum) have no clinical effects by themselves, but may reverse the actions of any ligand at the benzodiazepine site, including the actions of both agonists as well as inverse agonists (see Figs. 7–21 and 7–22). **Full inverse agonists** (far right of the spectrum) cause essentially the **opposite** clinical effects as full agonists, and therefore potentially **desirable** memory-enhancing effects (promnestic), but **undesirable** side effects of causing anxiety and promoting seizures. Perhaps a **happy medium** could also be attained here by finding a **partial inverse agonist** that could still enhance memory without causing anxiety or seizures.

Since somatodendritic and terminal alpha 2 receptors are negative feedback receptors, they act as brakes to the flow of norepinephrine out of these neurons. When occupied by norepinephrine, they turn off the release of this neurotransmitter (Figs. 7–25 and 7–26). By contrast, blocking somatodendritic alpha 2 autoreceptors (Fig. 7–27) or terminal alpha 2 autoreceptors (Fig. 7–28) has the effect of cutting the brake cable, and the release of norepinephrine is promoted.

As we have already shown, overactivity of the locus coeruleus noradrenergic neurons is associated with anxiety (Fig. 7–23). Therefore, when alpha 2 blockers are administered, it creates in man and in experimental animals a state of anxiety and fear as it creates a physiological state analogous to stimulation of the locus coeruleus (see Figs. 7–27 and 7–28).

Not surprisingly, administering an alpha 2 agonist causes alpha 2 receptors to be occupied just as if norepinephrine itself was acting there, and this can reduce anxiety (Fig. 7–29). In fact, the alpha 2 agonist clonidine has some known anxiolytic actions

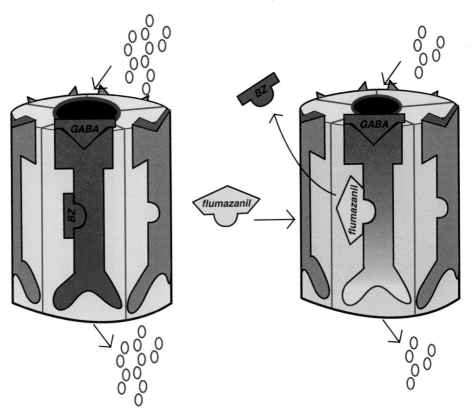

FIGURE 7–21. The **benzodiazepine (BZ) receptor antagonist flumazenil** is able to reverse a full agonist benzodiazepine acting at the benzodiazepine receptor of the **GABA A receptor complex.** This may be helpful in **reversing** the sedative effects of full agonist benzodiazepines when administered for anesthetic purposes or when taken in an overdose by a patient.

in patients with anxiety. Clonidine is especially useful in blocking the noradrenergic aspects of anxiety (i.e., tachycardia, dilated pupils, sweating, and tremor). However, it is less powerful in blocking the subjective/emotional aspects of anxiety. These same adrenergic blocking properties of clonidine have been successfully applied to reducing the adrenergic symptoms that are provoked during detoxification of patients from alcohol, barbiturates, heroin, or benzodiazepines (see Chapter 12).

Overactivity of noradrenergic neurons creates too much postsynaptic norepinephrine at noradrenergic receptors, particularly at beta receptors (Fig. 7–30). Consistent with the hypothesis of a state of norepinephrine excess in anxiety, it is possible to reduce symptoms of anxiety in some cases by blocking beta receptors with beta adrenergic blocking drugs (Fig. 7–31). This may be especially useful in some cases of social phobia as is discussed in Chapter 8.

Serotonin

This next section is somewhat complicated and may not be appropriate for the novice in psychopharmacology, who may wish to skip ahead to the subsequent section on

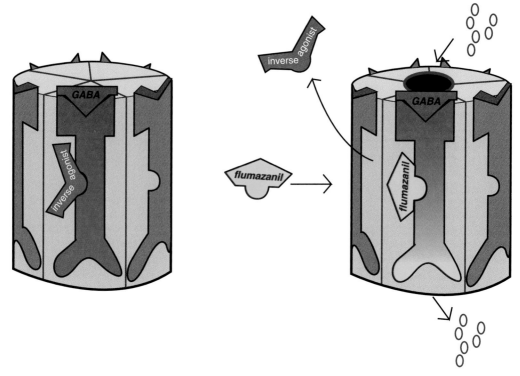

FIGURE 7–22. The **benzodiazepine (BZ) receptor antagonist flumazenil** is also able to reverse inverse agonist benzodiazepines acting at the benzodiazepine receptors of the **GABA A receptor complex**.

drug treatments of anxiety. Here we will explore various contemporary theories linking the function of serotonin and its receptors to the actions of *anxiolytic* drugs. This will be an amplification of the discussion in Chapter 6 (Figs. 6–21 through 6–25) on how serotonin and its receptors are linked to the actions of *antidepressant* drugs.

The mechanisms discussed here are just hypotheses, and may be outdated quickly as new knowledge unfolds rapidly in this area. However, these receptor-related mechanisms illustrate how pharmacological rationale can evolve from knowledge of how drugs affect receptors acutely, to how acute effects can be converted by the neuron into some type of adaptive neurobiological effect that is therapeutic to the patient. In fact, the exact role of serotonin in anxiety remains elusive and these theories are yet unproven. Nevertheless, psychopharmacologists are increasingly seeking explanations for the delayed therapeutic effects of their drugs in delayed neurobiological mechanisms. The following discussion is an example of this approach to explaining drug mechanisms of action.

Serotonin excess in anxiety? A general role of serotonin in anxiety has long been suspected because, in general, pharmacological manipulations that enhance serotonin also enhance anxiety, whereas pharmacological manipulations that reduce serotonin may also reduce anxiety. As was discussed in Chapter 6, this is essentially the opposite of depression, in which pharmacological manipulations that enhance serotonin

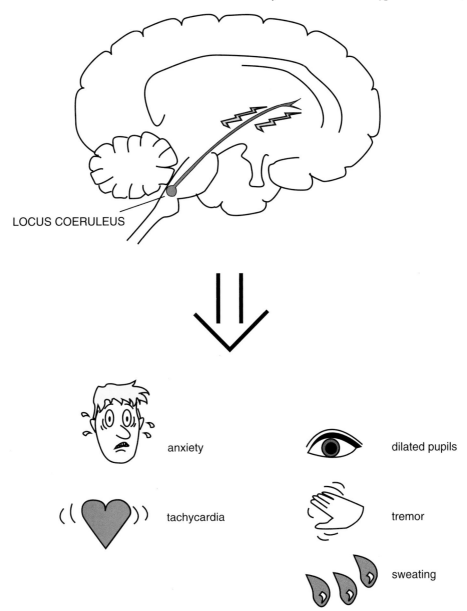

FIGURE 7–23. **Overactivity of norepinephrine neurons** is associated with **anxiety** and may mediate the autonomic symptoms associated with anxiety such as **tachycardia, dilated pupils, tremor,** and **sweating**. Shown here are hyperactive norepinephrine neurons with their axons projecting forward to the cerebral cortex from their cell bodies in the **locus coeruleus**.

often reduce depression. Such early formulations of the role of serotonin in anxiety as a "serotonin excess syndrome" and in depression as a "serotonin deficiency syndrome" are naive oversimplifications and very imprecise, although they do have some heuristic value for the student just being introduced to the pharmacology of serotonin in anxiety and depression (see Fig. 7–32). Thus, we will use the oversimpli-

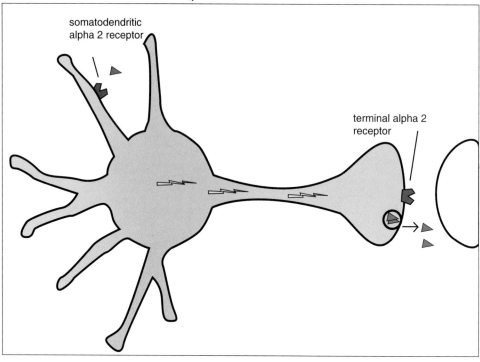

FIGURE 7–24. An enlargement of a norepinephrine neuron projecting from the locus coeruleus to the cerebral cortex is shown here. On the cell body (soma) and dendrites in the locus coeruleus are **somatodendritic alpha 2 receptors**. Also shown are **terminal alpha 2 receptors**, located on the presynaptic axon terminals projecting to the cerebral cortex. The functions of these two receptors are shown in the next two figures (Figs. 7–25 and 7–26).

fication as a starting point for explaining certain theories of how serotonin-modulating drugs might be acting as anxiolytics, recognizing that the actual role of serotonin in the actions of anxiolytic agents is likely to be far more complex.

Partial agonists both for serotonin excess and for serotonin deficiency? As explained in Chapter 3, partial agonists can function either as agonists or as antagonists, depending upon the amount of endogenous ligand present (see Fig. 3–18). In the case of serotonin neurons and their functioning in anxiety and depression, when serotonin is absent (depression), a partial serotonin agonist will be a net agonist (Fig. 7–33). When serotonin is present in excess (anxiety), the same partial agonist will, however, be a net antagonist (Fig. 7–33). Thus, a partial serotonin agonist would theoretically boost deficient serotonergic activity yet block excessive serotonergic activity.

To the extent that serotonin excess is linked to anxiety, this theory predicts that a serotonin partial agonist should be an anxiolytic. To the extent that serotonin deficiency is linked to depression, this theory predicts that a serotonin partial agonist could also be an antidepressant. How can this be so?

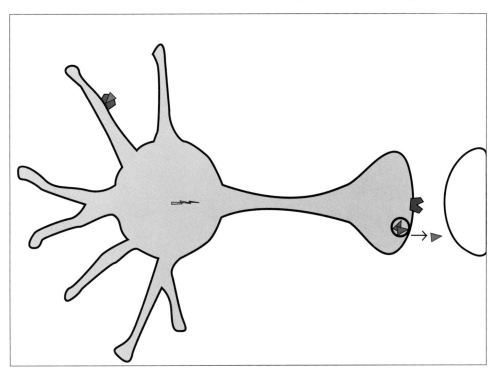

FIGURE 7–25. When **norepinephrine (NE)** occupies the **somatodendritic autoreceptors**, it is **inhibitory** to neuronal impulse flow and NE release from axon terminals. Thus, this receptor acts as a **brake** to stop NE neurotransmission when NE occupies these alpha 2 noradrenergic receptors on the cell body and dendrites in the locus coeruleus.

Returning to the light switch analogy introduced in Chapter 3 (see Figs. 3–15 through 3–17), a room will be dark when agonist (serotonin) is missing (i.e., the light switch is off). This can serve as a metaphor for depression, when serotonin is depleted. A room will be brightly lighted when it is full of natural serotonin agonist (i.e., the light switch is fully on). This serves as a metaphor for anxiety, associated with excessive serotonin activity.

If partial agonists act like a rheostat, they would act to turn the lights on partially, but not fully. Each partial agonist has its own degree of partiality built into the molecule and will light the room to a certain extent, no matter what dose is used, depending only on its intrinsic partial agonist properties. Adding a partial serotonin agonist to the dark (depressed) room where there is no serotonin will turn the lights up (presumed antidepressant action), but only as far as the partial serotonin agonist works on the serotonin receptor rheostat.

On the other hand, adding a partial serotonin agonist to the fully lighted (anxiety) room will have the effect of turning the lights down to the level of lower brightness on the serotonin rheostat. This is a net antagonistic effect relative to the fully lighted room and a presumed anxiolytic action.

Thus, after adding partial serotonin agonist to the dark (depressed) room and to the brightly lighted (anxiety) room, both rooms will be equally lighted. The degree of brightness is that of being partially turned on as dictated by the properties of

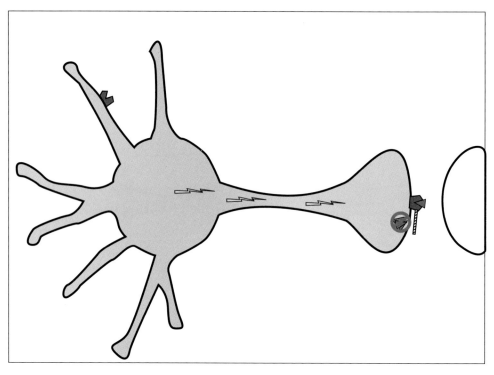

FIGURE 7−26. When **norepinephrine (NE)** occupies the **terminal alpha 2 receptors** located on presynaptic axon terminals in the cerebral cortex, it **inhibits the further release of NE**. Thus, this receptor also acts as a **brake** to stop NE neurotransmission when these alpha 2 terminal autoreceptors are occupied by NE.

the partial agonist. However, in the dark room, the partial agonist has acted as a net agonist, whereas in the brightly lighted room, the partial agonist has acted as a net antagonist.

An agonist and an antagonist in the same molecule is quite a new dimension to therapeutics. In our serotonin example, this concept has led to proposals that serotonin partial agonists could treat not only states that are theoretically deficient in serotonin (such as depression) but also states that are theoretically in excess of serotonin (such as anxiety) (see Fig. 7−33). To some extent, this has in fact been demonstrated for the marketed serotonin 1A (5HT1A) partial agonist buspirone. Investigators in some countries are, however, somewhat skeptical yet about how powerful the anxiolytic effects of buspirone are compared to those of the benzodiazepines. Several other 5HT1A compounds have shown promising efficacy both in major depression and in generalized anxiety disorder. Such agents may be particularly useful in mixed states of anxiety and depression (see Figs. 7−2 through 7−9). What is not yet known is what degree of partiality is optimal. In the case of serotonin agonists, an entire potency series of partial agonists, with a spectrum of partiality, is in clinical testing, and may yield the answer to this in due course.

Serotonin receptor adaptations as mediators of anxiety? A corollary to the hypothesis of serotonin excess in anxiety is that the 5HT receptors adapt to this excess of 5HT

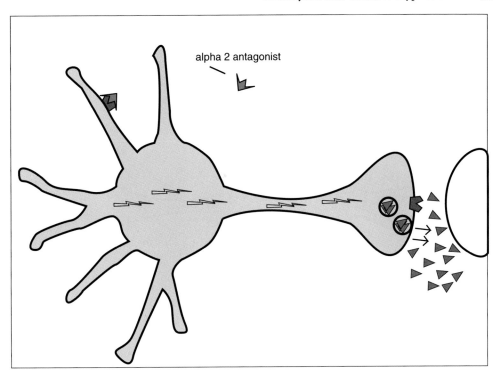

alpha 2 antagonist in somatodendritic autoreceptor increases firing of neuron and release of NE

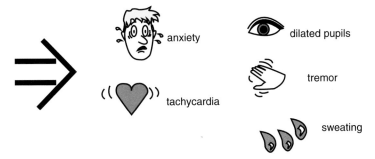

FIGURE 7–27. **Alpha 2 antagonists** acting at **somatodendritic autoreceptors** block the ability of norepinephrine **(NE)** to act as a brake for neuronal impulse flow. This has the effect of "**cutting the brake cable.**" Therefore, this action of alpha 2 antagonists will have the effect of increasing both the firing of the NE neuron and the release of NE from its axon terminals. This causes **overactivity of the NE neuron,** and therefore **anxiety** as well as its associated autonomic symptoms of **tachycardia, dilated pupils, tremor,** and **sweating.**

(Fig. 7–34). Thus, the excessive serotonin state of anxiety (Fig. 7–32) could theoretically be accompanied by down-regulation of 5HT1A receptors (Fig. 7–34) in order to counter this excess, in the neuron's futile attempt to shut down excessive neuronal impulse flow (see also the anxiety icon in Fig. 7–33).

This is the *opposite* to what has already been discussed for depression, where one expects that the deficiency of 5HT causes the 5HT1A receptors to up-regulate in a

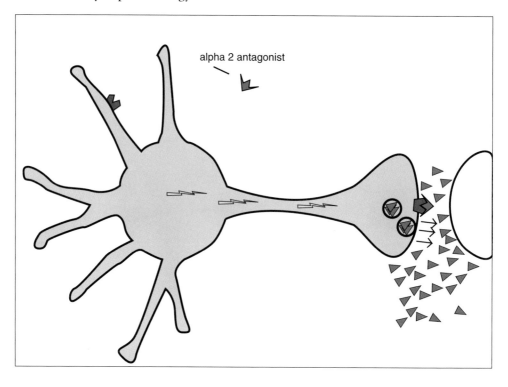

alpha 2 antagonist in presynaptic terminal autoreceptor leads to an increase in the release of NE

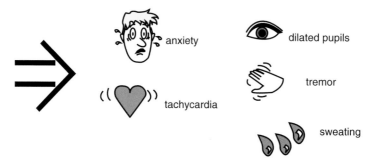

FIGURE 7–28. **Alpha 2 antagonists** can also act at **terminal autoreceptors,** blocking the ability of **norepinephrine (NE)** to shut off its own release at axon terminals. The action shown here at terminal autoreceptors is additive to the action of alpha 2 antagonists at somatodendritic autoreceptors shown in Figure 7–27. The terminal autoreceptor inhibition also has the effect of allowing much more NE to be released at the axon terminals, with consequent **overactivity of the NE neuron,** and therefore **anxiety** as well as its associated autonomic symptoms of **tachycardia, dilated pupils, tremor,** and **sweating.**

similarly unsuccessful attempt to enhance neuronal impulse flow in the 5HT neuron (see Fig. 6–21 for previous discussion as well as Fig. 7–34 and the depression icon in Fig. 7–33). These latter adaptations of 5HT receptors in depression are discussed in detail in Chapters 5 and 6 and shown graphically in relationship to the mechanism of action of antidepressant drugs in Figures 6–21 through 6–25.

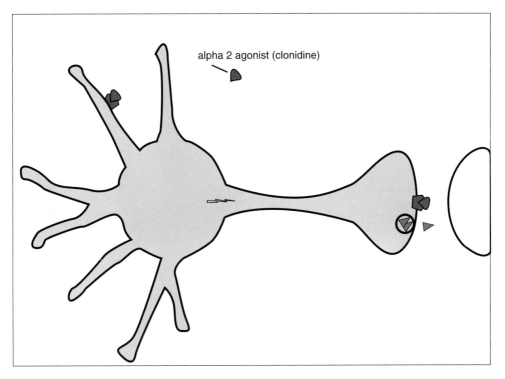

alpha 2 agonist occupies autoreceptors which decreases firing and decreases release
of NE, which has an anxiolytic effect

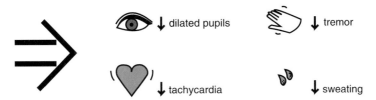

FIGURE 7–29. If an **alpha 2 agonist** is administered, such as clonidine, this will have much the same action as **norepinephrine (NE)** itself at both somatodendritic alpha 2 autoreceptors as well as at terminal alpha 2 autoreceptors. This action is that of **reducing** both **neuronal impulse in NE neurons**, and **release of NE** from noradrenergic axon terminals. This is opposite, of course, to the actions of alpha 2 antagonists at these same receptors shown in Figures 7–28 and 7–29. Thus, **alpha 2 agonists** will **decrease** the symptoms associated with **anxiety**, especially the autonomic symptoms of **dilated pupils, tachycardia, tremor,** and **sweating.**

More recent evidence on the role of serotonin in anxiety suggests the **involvement** of serotonin receptor subtypes in a variety of anxiety disorder subtypes, **especially** obsessive compulsive disorder (OCD) and perhaps panic disorder and social **phobia** as well. This is reviewed in Chapter 8 in our discussions on these anxiety disorder subtypes. In terms of generalized anxiety, what is clear is that the usefulness of **the** serotonin 1A receptor partial agonist buspirone in certain animal models of **anxiety**

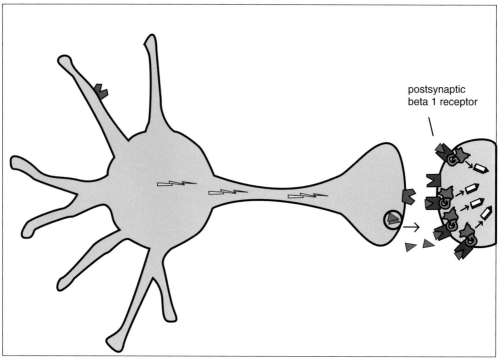

Overactivity at the postsynaptic beta receptors increases anxiety

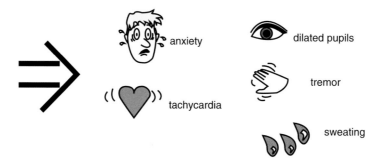

FIGURE 7–30. The **overactivity of norepinephrine (NE)** neurons and **excess release of NE** from nerve terminals that occurs in **anxiety** also causes events to occur at postsynaptic NE receptors as well. In this case, excess NE activity causes an excess of NE occupying **postsynaptic beta adrenergic receptors**. This in turn causes an excess in the postsynaptic signaling via second and subsequent messenger systems. These excess signals via postsynaptic beta adrenergic receptors mediate the autonomic symptoms associated with anxiety, including **tachycardia, dilated pupils, tremor, and sweating**.

and in generalized anxiety disorder point to some important role of 5HT1A receptors in mediating anxiety symptoms.

Do partial agonists work as anxiolytics by causing serotonin receptor adaptations? According to the hypothesis of serotonin dysfunction in anxiety, the adaptations of the 5HT1A

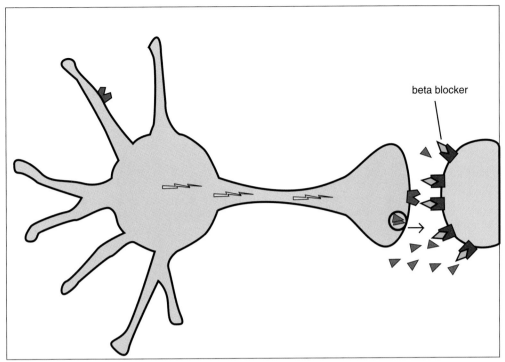

Blocking the postsynaptic beta receptors decreases anxiety

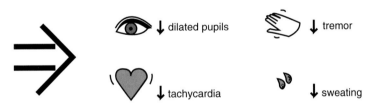

FIGURE 7–31. If **excessive activity of norepinephrine (NE)** at **postsynaptic beta adrenergic receptors** shown in Figure 7–30 can be **blocked**, so can the symptoms of anxiety that are mediated by the beta receptors. Shown here is a **beta adrenergic blocker**, or antagonist, which is preventing the excess activity of NE neurons and excess NE release to cause a corresponding excess in the stimulation of postsynaptic beta adrenergic receptors. This antagonist action at beta receptors can **decrease the autonomic symptoms associated with anxiety** such as dilated pupils, tremor, tachycardia, and sweating.

somatodendritic autoreceptors (Fig. 7–34) are not capable of overriding the excess in 5HT (Figs. 7–32 and 7–33), and cannot correct the state of anxiety. However, 5HT1A partial agonists may act upon serotonin receptors and help the neuron to correct not only the hypothesized imbalances in serotonin but also the hypothesized dysregulation of its receptors (Fig. 7–33). Such actions of the 5HT1A partial agonists cause delayed adaptations in 5HT1A receptors, which may also explain the delay in onset of anxiolytic effects of these drugs. Contrast this with the benzodiazepines, which act almost immediately, suggesting that it is their acute changes in

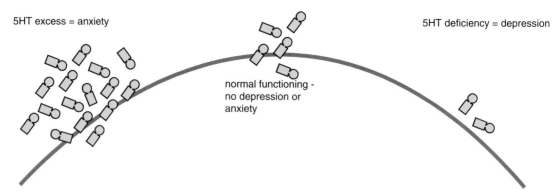

5HT excess = anxiety

5HT deficiency = depression

normal functioning -
no depression or
anxiety

FIGURE 7–32. A simplified notion of how **serotonin** may be implicated in **anxiety and depression** is depicted here. Anxiety may be associated with 5-hydroxytryptamine (5HT; serotonin) excess, and depression with 5HT deficiency.

chloride conductance and not delayed receptor adaptation that accounts for their immediate therapeutic effects.

In terms of serotonin receptors, in the anxious state, presynaptic somatodendritic 5HT1A autoreceptors may be down-regulated (Figs. 7–33 through 7–35), and serotonin may be in excess at these receptors (Figs. 7–32, 7–33, and 7–35). The down-regulated receptors are unable, however, to compensate adequately for the excessive amount of 5HT available, and the patient is therefore anxious. Neuronal cell firing may be increased and 5HT release increased from such neurons (Figs. 7–33 and 7–35).

When a 5HT1A agonist is given acutely to an anxious patient, it competes with serotonin for the 5HT1A receptors (Fig. 7–36). Instead of maximal stimulation of 5HT1A receptors by excess serotonin, the addition of a 5HT1A partial agonist causes a net reduction in the action at these receptors, because the partial agonist is acting at these receptors in a partial and weaker manner than serotonin itself (Fig. 7–36). One might predict that such an action would cause a sudden reduction in anxiety, but this is not what happens. There is simultaneously an acute replacement of 5HT by 5HT1A agonist postsynaptically as well, and the net effect seen by the postsynaptic neuron at first is no change in net 5HT activity at postsynaptic 5HT1A receptors (Fig. 7–36).

However, if the 5HT1A receptor partial agonist continues to exert net antagonistic actions with chronic treatment, this theoretically causes 5HT1A somatodendritic receptors to return to a normal state (Fig. 7–37). This readaptation of somatodendritic autoreceptors in turn restores the ability of the 5HT neuron to shut off its 5HT neuronal impulse flow and thereby causes anxiety to be relieved (Fig. 7–38). Interestingly, it does not appear that chronic drug treatment alters the sensitivity of postsynaptic 5HT1A receptors (Fig. 7–38).

Can 5HT1A agonists also work as antidepressants by causing mirror image adaptations in serotonin receptors? In the case of 5HT1A partial agonists administered for the treatment of depression, their actions can be conceived as mirror images of their actions in anxiety (shown graphically in Figs. 7–35 through 7–38). It is interesting to note that these 5HT1A partial agonist effects in depression are virtually the same as the

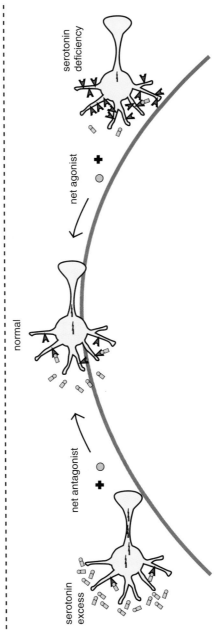

FIGURE 7–33. Serotonin 1A (5HT1A) partial agonists may have both anxiolytic and antidepressant actions. In the case of **anxiety**, an excess of serotonin and perhaps a down-regulation of 5HT1A receptors will experience a 5HT1A partial agonist as a **net antagonist**, leading to a normalization of serotonin levels and receptors and a **reduction in anxiety**. In the case of **depression**, a deficiency of serotonin and perhaps an up regulation of 5HT1A receptors will experience a 5HT1A partial agonist as a **net agonist**, leading to a normalization of serotonin levels and receptors and a **reduction in depression**.

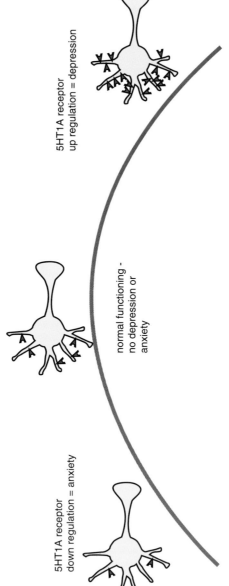

5HT1A receptor
down regulation = anxiety

5HT1A receptor
up regulation = depression

normal functioning -
no depression or
anxiety

FIGURE 7–34. In the **anxious state**, serotonin (5HT) 1A somatodendritic autoreceptors may be **down-regulated** in a futile attempt to compensate for **excessive serotonin** (left end of the spectrum). In the **depressed state**, 5HT1A autoreceptors may be **up-regulated** in a similarly futile attempt to compensate for deficient serotonin (right end of the spectrum).

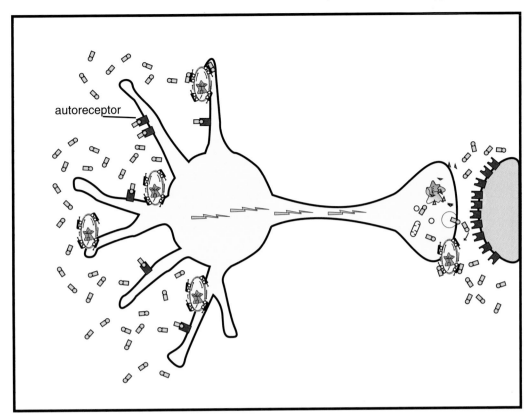

FIGURE 7–35. Depicted here is the 5HT (**serotonin**) **neuron in the anxious state**: namely, high levels of 5HT, overactive 5HT neuronal firing and transmission, and down-regulated somatodendritic presynaptic 5HT1A autoreceptors.

actions of serotonin selective reuptake inhibitors (SSRIs) in depression (discussed in Chapter 6 and shown graphically in Figs. 6–21 through 6–25).

Thus, in the depressed state, presynaptic somatodendritic 5HT1A autoreceptors may be up-regulated, and serotonin may be deficient at these receptors (Fig. 7–39). As already stated, this is the mirror image of the status of these receptors hypothesized for anxiety (i.e., Fig. 7–35; see also opposite ends of the spectrum in Figs. 7–33 and 7–34). Up-regulated receptors are unable to compensate adequately for the reduced amount of 5HT available, and the patient is therefore depressed. Neuronal cell firing is diminished and 5HT release is decreased from such neurons.

In the case of the SSRIs, the SSRI is acting *indirectly* on the 5HT1A receptor. That is, an SSRI acts directly at the reuptake pump and increases serotonin. It is this increased serotonin that acts in turn directly on 5HT1A somatodendritic autoreceptors (Fig. 6–22). In the case of a 5HT1A partial agonist, however, it acts *directly*, as a type of substitute for serotonin at the 5HT1A receptor (Fig. 7–40).

The postulated deficiency of serotonin in depression means that the direct agonist actions of 5HT1A partial agonists at up-regulated somatodendritic autoreceptors might first decrease neuronal impulse flow as would be predicted from the function of this receptor. In fact, this has been demonstrated with 5HT1A agonists in ex-

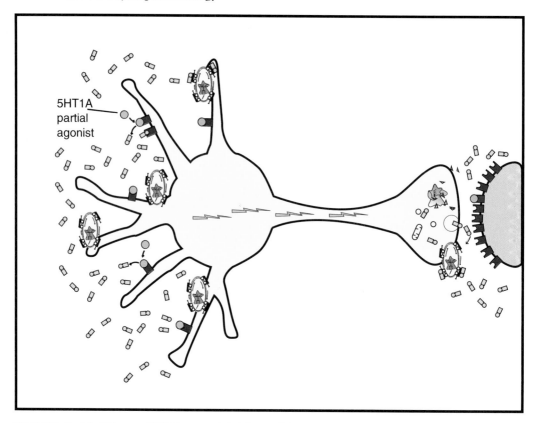

FIGURE 7–36. When a 5HT (serotonin) 1A **partial agonist** is administered **acutely** to a neuron in the **anxious state**, the somatodendritic presynaptic autoreceptors will experience an **acute antagonist effect**. That is, substitution of 5HT1A partial agonist for 5HT itself at these receptors will be weaker than the actions of 5HT itself. This could also be occurring at postsynaptic 5HT1A receptors, essentially cancelling the presynaptic actions of 5HT1A partial agonist, at least at first. This may explain why there is no immediate anxiolytic effect of 5HT1A partial agonists.

perimental animals. While this might be predicted to make depression even worse, it appears that 5HT impulse flow may already be so deficient that this is not observed, either with SSRIs or with 5HT1A partial agonists in depressed patients. Also, there is simultaneously an acute replacement of 5HT by 5HT1A agonist postsynaptically, and the net effect seen by the postsynaptic neuron at first is essentially no change in net 5HT activity (Fig. 7–40).

However, maintaining stimulation of 5HT1A somatodendritic autoreceptors with chronic 5HT1A partial agonist treatment leads to functional down-regulation of these receptors (Fig. 7–41), and neuronal impulse flow theoretically is turned on (Fig. 7–42). In experimental animals, the acute suppression of neuronal impulse flow caused by a 5HT1A agonist is lost upon chronic treatment with the 5HT1A agonist as the autoreceptors are desensitized. This could theoretically cause a delayed increase in serotonin release at the synapse (Fig. 7–42), and perhaps even down-regulation of postsynaptic 5HT2A receptors, just as the case for SSRI treatment (Fig. 6–25). Interestingly, postsynaptic 5HT1A receptors do not seem to be desen-

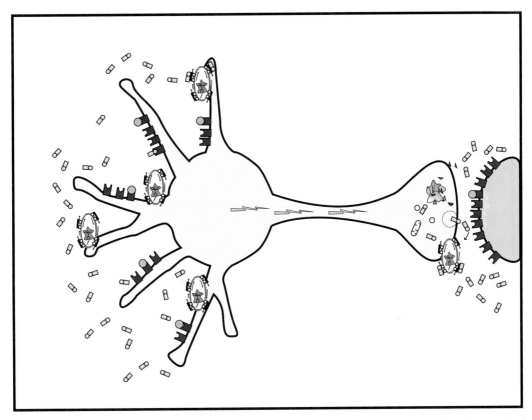

FIGURE 7–37. If 5HT (serotonin) 1A **partial agonists** are administered **chronically**, the sustained actions would cause a **resensitization of the somatodendritic autoreceptors back to normal.**

sitized by chronic treatment with 5HT1A partial agonists, only the presynaptic somatodendritic 5HT1A autoreceptors. The 5HT1A agonist is also competing for 5HT postsynaptically, somewhat mitigating the effects of increased 5HT release from enhanced neuronal impulse flow, but the net action of increased 5HT release swamps this effect, resulting in the bottom line that there is a boost in 5HT at postsynaptic receptors, and relief of depression (Fig. 7–42).

This theory thus supports the notion of a pharmacological cascading mechanism whereby both 5HT1A agonists as well as SSRIs may exert their therapeutic actions: it is hypothetically due to the down-regulation of somatodendritic 5HT1A autoreceptors, thus restoring neuronal impulse traffic in the 5HT neurons and perhaps causing an increase in 5HT release in axon terminal synapses with consequential postsynaptic 5HT2 receptor down-regulation. In the case of the 5HT1A agonists, they work directly at the somatodendritic autoreceptor. In the case of the SSRIs, they cause 5HT to increase so that 5HT itself down-regulates the somatodendritic autoreceptor.

This theoretical mechanism of action of antidepressants on serotonin receptors — and its mirror image corollary for anxiety — is still a theory. It nevertheless shows how pharmacological rationale can evolve from knowledge of how drugs affect receptors acutely, and then how those acute effects could be transposed by the neuron

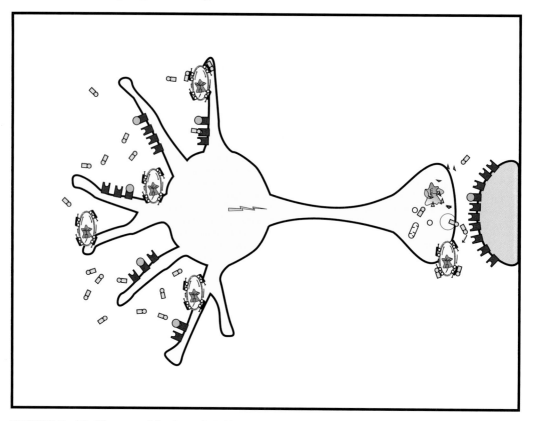

FIGURE 7–38. The resensitization of 5HT (serotonin) 1A somatodendritic autoreceptors by chronic administration of **5HT1A partial agonists** allows the neuron to **slow down its neuronal impulse flow** and to **diminish its release of serotonin.** Theoretically, this would be associated with a normalization of function and a **reduction in the symptoms of anxiety.**

into some type of adaptive neurobiological effect that is therapeutic to the patient. In fact, the exact role of serotonin in anxiety remains elusive and these theories are yet unproved.

Drug Treatments of Anxiety

Early Drug Treatments

Barbiturates. The very earliest treatments for generalized anxiety were sedating barbiturates. These agents had little in the way of a specific antianxiety action: they merely reduced anxiety in direct proportion to their ability to sedate. Due to serious dependency and withdrawal problems (see Chapter 12), and lack of a favorable safety profile, especially when mixed with other drugs or in overdose, the barbiturates fell out of favor as soon as the much more selective and less dangerous antianxiety agents of the benzodiazepine class were discovered.

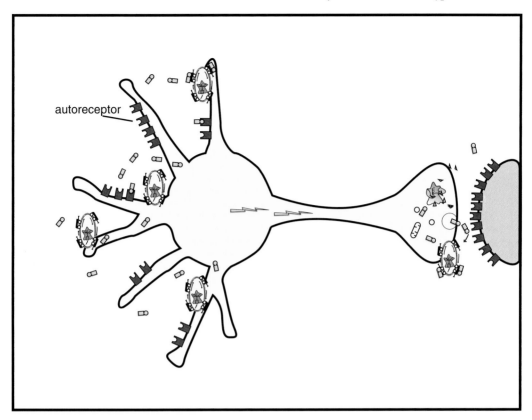

FIGURE 7–39. In the **depressed state**, 5HT (serotonin) 1A somatodendritic autoreceptors may be **up-regulated** in a futile attempt to compensate for **deficient serotonin** neurotransmitter.

Meprobamate. Meprobamate (Miltown) and tybamate (no longer available in the United States) are members of a chemical class called propanediols, and are pharmacologically very similar to the barbiturates. No advantage of meprobamate over barbiturates has been demonstrated and, although popular during the 1950s as an antianxiety agent in the United States, has fallen into disfavor and is infrequently prescribed due to its liability to abuse and withdrawal symptoms, similar to those of the barbiturates and much more severe than for the benzodiazepines.

Benzodiazepines

Early days. These agents revolutionized the treatment of anxiety when they were introduced in the 1960s. Previous agents treated anxiety essentially by substituting sedation for anxiety. Thus, the older agents acted by using sedation to crudely mask anxiety. When the benzodiazepines were introduced, however, truly selective anti-anxiety actions were observed for the first time, since reduction of symptoms of anxiety was not associated with simple masking by sedation. It is true that some benzodiazepines are more sedating than others. However, the sedating benzodiazepines are used to promote and induce sleep as sedative-hypnotics rather than to be

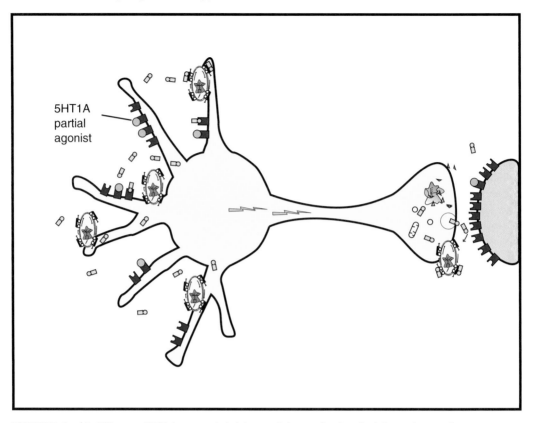

5HT1A
partial
agonist

FIGURE 7–40. When a 5HT (serotonin) 1A **partial agonist** is administered **acutely** to a neuron in the **depressed state**, the somatodendritic presynaptic autoreceptors will experience an **acute agonist effect**. That is, substitution of 5HT1A partial agonist for 5HT itself at these receptors will be a type of serotonin substitute there, and will be stronger than the deficiency of 5HT at these receptors. This could also be occurring at postsynaptic 5HT1A receptors, essentially cancelling the presynaptic actions of 5HT1A partial agonist, at least at first. This may explain why there is no immediate antidepressant effect of 5HT1A partial agonists.

employed as anxiolytics. Those benzodiazepines used as anxiolytics are truly anxio-selective; that is, they produce antianxiety effects by a means other than by producing sedation.

Benzodiazepines also have other properties including anticonvulsant and muscle relaxant, and some of these agents are employed for these clinical uses as well. Thus, the benzodiazepines as a group have four principal therapeutic actions: not just anxiolytic but also anticonvulsant, muscle relaxant, and sedative-hypnotic (see Fig. 7–20). Of the more than 12 agents introduced into clinical practice over the years, some agents are used predominantly for one of these four actions over the others. Often, this seems to be more of a marketing decision rather than a scientific one. However, all agents share these four pharmacological properties to some extent.

The original observation of anxiolytic effects in man caused great excitement because it was clear that the benzodiazepines were far more effective and far safer than the barbiturates that they replaced. Upon introduction into clinical practice,

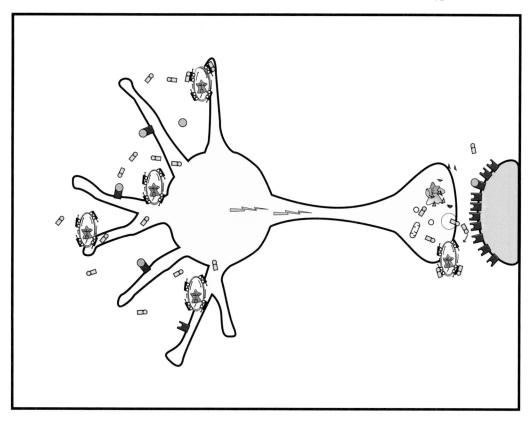

FIGURE 7–41. If 5HT (serotonin) 1A **partial agonists** are administered **chronically**, the sustained actions would cause a **resensitization (i.e., down-regulation) of the somatodendritic autoreceptors back to normal**.

the benzodiazepines were found to be true breakthrough drugs, as they truly relieved anxiety to a degree never seen previously, and they did it without the dangers – some lethal – of the short-acting barbiturates they replaced. This led to very widespread use of the benzodiazepines, as their powerful clinical usefulness for an ever-widening range of applications was coupled with a safety profile not previously seen with the earlier agents they came to replace.

Use of benzodiazepines in GAD. Using benzodiazepines for generalized anxiety disorder also involves the need to know how to balance the risks of these agents rationally against their benefits, and to compare this formula to other available therapeutic interventions. Thus, the long-term indiscriminate-use style of the 1970s is no better than the irrational "avoidance-of-benzodiazepines-as-a-form-of-heroin" myth of the 1980s. For short-term anxiety-related conditions such as an adjustment disorder with onset after a stressful life event, benzodiazepines can provide rapid relief with little risk of dependence or withdrawal if use is limited to several weeks to a few months. For conditions likely to last longer than 6 months, such as generalized anxiety

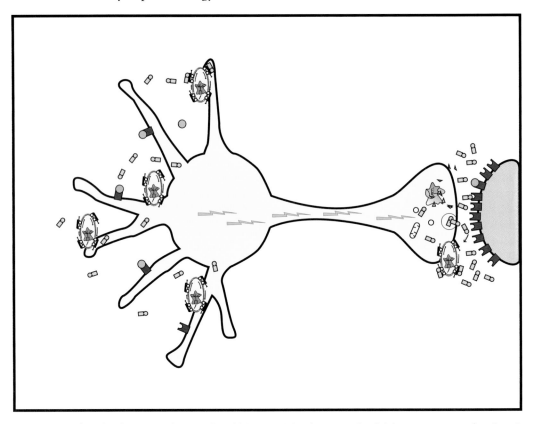

FIGURE 7–42. The down-regulation of 5HT (serotonin) 1A somatodendritic autoreceptors by chronic administration of **5HT1A partial agonists** allows the neuron to **turn back on its neuronal impulse flow** and to **increase its release of serotonin**. Theoretically, this would be associated with a normalization of function and a **reduction in the symptoms of depression**.

disorder or panic disorder, the risks of dependence and withdrawal must be weighed against the risks of the underlying disorder in light of the other treatment options.

For generalized anxiety disorder, the underlying illness is chronic by definition. Looking at GAD longitudinally suggests that indeed it is not trivial. That is, patients with GAD in psychiatric practice appear to have about the same degree of occupational and social dysfunctioning associated as experienced by patients with depression. The disability of depression is comparable to the physical and social disability associated with advanced coronary artery disease. GAD is also associated with frequent suicide attempts.

In terms of treatment effectiveness, many GAD patients "respond" to anxiolytic treatments by improving to just below the threshhold for the diagnostic criteria for GAD only to relapse to a full syndrome in several months (i.e., a "double anxiety syndrome"; see Fig. 7–7). Thus, the treatment success of GAD over time may not restore full occupational and social functioning, especially for those patients with such a waxing and waning double anxiety syndrome; that is, waxing from subsyndromal anxiety (anxious dysthymia) to full GAD and waning only back to subsyndromal anxiety but not to full remission.

When one defines recovery from either major depressive disorder or GAD as reduction to only one or two symptoms with a subjective sense of returning to normal self, major depressive disorder has an 80% rate of recovery in 2 years, whereas GAD has only a 20% chance of recovery. Thus, patients with GAD may have not only a chronic state of symptomatic impairment but also a waxing and waning course just above and just below the diagnostic threshhold over long periods of time despite current treatment regimens (Fig. 7–7). Other studies even suggest that a state of longstanding GAD may be a harbinger for panic disorder (Fig. 7–8).

Although short-term treatment studies of anxiolytic medications show that symptoms can be reduced short term, little is known about whether chronic treatment can alter the natural history of GAD; that is, by keeping it at the level of subsyndromal symptoms, rather than progressing to bouts of full syndrome GAD, major depression, or panic disorder (Figs. 7–7 through 7–9). Very little is also known about the use of specific psychotherapies for GAD in terms of outcome or comparability to anxiolytic drug treatments, especially in terms of altering long-term outcomes.

These considerations must be borne in mind when contemplating treatment of GAD patients. Short-term stabilization of symptoms in GAD and prn (as needed) use for sudden surges in symptoms are usually well-justified uses for benzodiazepines. On the other hand, long-term treatment of GAD must encompass consideration of other interventions first before long-term use of benzodiazepines is generally indicated. Thus, lifestyle changes can be the cornerstone of long-term treatment for this condition, including stress reduction techniques, exercise, healthy diet, appropriate work situation, and adequate management of interpersonal affairs.

Other agents such as the 5HT1A agents may have a safer long-term use profile if effective and well tolerated. Depression must be recognized and treated appropriately if associated with the GAD. If all such interventions fail, it may then be justified to use benzodiazepines in this condition long term.

Partial agonists at benzodiazepine receptors. All of the marketed benzodiazepines are essentially full agonists at the GABA–benzodiazepine receptor complex. It is theoretically possible to improve upon the actions of full agonists if a partial agonist of optimal partiality could be identified (see Fig. 7–20). Animal models predict that a partial agonist would still be anxiolytic but would have less sedation and less propensity for dependence and withdrawal. Attempts to identify a partial agonist for use in man are still underway, either using benzodiazepine-type agents or other unique chemical structures that are not benzodiazepines. Some of the partial agonists tested in GAD to date have been too partial and not robust enough as anxiolytics to be effective anxiolytics for marketing.

Serotonin 1A Partial Agonists

A class of anxiolytic agent newer than the benzodiazepines is that of the 5HT1A partial agonists. These have already been discussed extensively in this chapter. The first agent introduced into clinical practice is buspirone, a member of the azapirone chemical class that has been first introduced into clinical practice and clinical testing.

Buspirone is available in many countries, and several chemically related compounds are in testing worldwide (gepirone, tandospirone, and ipsapirone). More recently, experimental agents not sharing the azapirone structure have begun clinical testing including flesinoxan and CP93-393, among others.

Buspirone is the prototypical agent for the 5HT1A class of anxiolytics. It is currently marketed worldwide for GAD, although several studies also suggest efficacy in major depressive disorder, or in MAD (Figs. 7–2 through 7–4). Its disadvantages compared to the benzodiazepines are a delay in the onset of action, similar to the delay in therapeutic onset for the antidepressants. This has led to the belief that 5HT1A agonists exert their therapeutic effects by virtue of adaptive neuronal events and receptor events, rather than simply by the acute occupancy of 5HT1A receptors by the drug as discussed extensively above. In this way, the presumed mechanism of action of 5HT1A partial agonists appears to be analogous to the antidepressants (which are also presumed to act by adaptations in neurotransmitter receptors) and different from the benzodiazepine anxiolytics (which act relatively acutely by occupancy of benzodiazepine receptors).

Many of the 5HT1A partial agonists in clinical testing for GAD and major depressive disorder are administered using modern drug delivery technologies, controlling the release of drug so that tolerability is improved and dosing frequency can be decreased. Side effects associated with peak blood levels and three-times-daily dosing are both disadvantages of the currently marketed buspirone. Also, higher dosing in controlled release may allow greater efficacy to be manifest.

The advantages of 5HT1A partial agonists over the benzodiazepine agents include lack of drug interactions with alcohol, benzodiazepines, and sedative-hypnotics, and lack of production of dependence or withdrawal effects.

Adjunctive Treatments

Numerous adjunctive treatments are available for the treatment of generalized anxiety disorder. These agents are considered not only to be second-line agents with inferior efficacy but also to work essentially by producing sedation, rather than a specific anxiolytic effect. These include the sedating antihistamines, beta adrenergic blockers, and clonidine. The beta blockers may have some efficacy in social phobia (see Chapter 8), and the alpha 2 agonist clonidine may also be helpful in anxiety associated with hyperadrenergic states.

Long-Term Prospects

1. Cholecystokinin (CCK) antagonists are in clinical testing in anxiety disorder, especially in panic disorder (see Chapter 8).
2. Corticotrophin releasing factor (CRF) is a neuropeptide that may mediate some anxiety behaviors in experimental animals. This has led to the proposal that CRF antagonists may be anxiolytic. Numerous CRF antagonists are being developed and tested for anxiety, and are in the very earliest stages of development.
3. Neuroactive steroids are molecules based upon a steroid chemical structure, which interact with the GABA–benzodiazepine receptor complex. As some of these agents are naturally occurring, it is hoped that analogues may be

effective anxiolytics, with perhaps more "natural" actions than the marketed benzodiazepine anxiolytics. Such agents are in early development.

4. Just as multiple mechanisms are being targeted for novel antidepressants, so is this the case for certain new anxiolytic candidates. For example, some agents combine 5HT1A partial agonist properties with 5HT2 antagonist properties, with the hope that this would make a more powerful and perhaps more rapidly acting anxiolytic than the 5HT1A partial agonists. Other combinations of 5HT receptors are being targeted with intramolecular polypharmacy, and numerous such agents are in early development.

5. Given that GAD is chronic and in many cases lifelong, one approach to treatment is to combine current benzodiazepines or buspirone with psychotherapies. The hope is that psychotherapy will be synergistic with medication, lead to carry-over after discontinuation of treatments, and allow a parsimonious "medication-sparing" strategy to be pursued for the lifelong or chronic treatment of GAD.

Clinical Description of Insomnia and Sleep Disorders

Insomnia is a complaint, and not a disease. Some experts classify insomnia as predominantly due to a psychiatric disorder such as depression, anxiety, or psychosis. Other investigators conceptualize insomnia as a primary disorder of sleep that can be diagnosed with an electroencephalogram (EEG) taken during sleep (polysomnograph). Examples of primary sleep disorders that can cause insomnia according to this latter classification include sleep apnea and nocturnal myoclonus. Insomnia can also frequently be caused by drugs (alcohol, sedatives, stimulants, and others) or by a variety of medical disorders (such as pain, problems breathing at night from various causes, renal disorders, and endocrine disorders).

No matter what the cause or classification of insomnia, it can be treated symptomatically by various sedative-hypnotic drugs. Whether it is wise to do this is a subject of intense debate, as it may often make more sense to treat the underlying psychiatric or medical condition, rather than to induce sleep pharmacologically.

Insomnia may also be classified according to its duration as a symptom. Thus, *transient insomnia* occurs in normal sleepers who have traveled to another time zone (i.e., "jet lag"), who are sleeping in an unfamiliar surrounding, or who are under acute situational stress. Often, treatment is not required, and insomnia is reversed with time alone. *Short-term insomnia* can be experienced by one who is generally a normal sleeper but who is under a stress that does not resolve within a few days, such as divorce, bankruptcy, lawsuit, etc. Such individuals may not meet the criteria for a psychiatric disorder other than an adjustment disorder, yet may require short-term symptomatic relief of their symptom of insomnia in order to function optimally. Finally, *long-term insomnia* is not only persistent but disabling. Studies suggest that almost all of these patients have either an associated psychiatric disorder, an associated drug use/abuse/withdrawal problem, or an associated medical disorder. As mentioned above, treatment of these associated disorders may be sufficient to treat the insomnia as well. However, if the underlying disorder is not treatable, or if there is a requirement to relieve the symptom of insomnia before the underlying condition can be relieved, it may be necessary to treat the symptom of insomnia symptomatically with a sedative-hypnotic agent.

Drug Treatments for Insomnia

Assuming that insomnia cannot be adequately treated by addressing directly an underlying problem responsible for causing the insomnia, then sedative-hypnotic drugs can be used to induce sleep pharmacologically. Such treatments have become increasingly controversial in recent years due to abuse of such agents, the growing recognition of complications from treatment of insomnia with such agents, and the possibility that treating insomnia symptomatically removes the impetus to diagnose and relieve any underlying condition(s). One cannot deny, however, the widespread incidence of the complaint of insomnia in the general population, the perceived disruption of functioning and the disability that this symptom produces, and the strength of the demands of patients for drug treatments for this complaint.

Over-the-Counter Agents

Numerous nonprescription agents ("sleeping pills") are popular with the general public. Although there are numerous trade names that differ widely from time to time and from country to country, essentially all over-the-counter sleeping pills contain one or more of three active ingredients: (1) the anticholinergic agent scopolamine; (2) an antihistamine that also has anticholinergic properties; and (3) an aspirin-like salicylate, which is a mild pain reliever.

Antihistaminergic and anticholinergic properties have already been discussed in relationship to tricyclic antidepressants in Chapter 6 and shown in the icons for the tricyclic antidepressants (TCAs) in Figures 6–13, 6–16, and 6–17. In fact, the sedative properties associated with blocking either of these two receptors is exploited by drugs that share these properties, and applied to the treatment of insomnia. Thus, an unwanted side effect in one situation (such as the treatment of depression) can be turned into a virtue in another situation (such as when nighttime sedation is desired in the case of insomnia). The sedative properties associated with blockade of histamine and muscarinic cholinergic receptors demonstrate why nonprescription products containing such properties can induce sleep. Of course, they do it at the expense of the same side effects shown in Figures 6–16 and 6–17, namely dry mouth, blurred vision, and constipation. They can even cause confusion or memory problems, particularly in the elderly. However, they are not truly dependence forming, do not cause severe sleep problems when withdrawn, and are generally safe in the doses available over the counter.

Antidepressants with Sedative-Hypnotic Properties

There are also numerous drugs available only by prescription that share the same properties of the over-the-counter agents just mentioned, but are more potent. Not surprisingly, the TCAs are also good sleeping pills because they have the property of causing sedation due to the antihistaminergic and anticholinergic actions just described. Thus, skillful use of a TCA in a depressed patient with insomnia can turn the liability of unwanted sedation into an asset of relief of insomnia if the TCA is given at bedtime. This property, as discussed in Chapter 6, has nothing to do, however, with the reason that TCAs are antidepressants (shown in Figs. 6–14 and 6–15).

There is conflicting evidence on how powerful the hypnotic properties of antihistamine agents are, as they probably produce little if any change in the objective EEG parameters of sleep. Also, since such agents are generic and therefore inexpensive, their use is not promoted heavily by the pharmaceutical industry.

Another antidepressant, namely trazodone, also has significant sedating properties. This may be due to its antihistaminergic properties (Fig. 6–30). Given at bedtime, trazodone can be a very powerful sedative agent.

Sedative-Hypnotic Benzodiazepines

The benzodiazepines are the group of drugs most widely prescribed for the treatment of insomnia. These agents have been extensively discussed above in terms of their use in anxiety. Their mechanism of action in insomnia is the same as for anxiety (see Figs. 7–18 and 7–20). The decision to be promoted for use in insomnia versus anxiety often seems to be based more upon marketing than upon science. Thus, any benzodiazepine can be used either for the treatment of anxiety or for the treatment of insomnia (see Fig. 7–20).

Theoretically, benzodiazepines with short half-lives might be better as sedative-hypnotics, and benzodiazepines with long half-lives might be better as anxiolytics. This is because an ideal sedative-hypnotic would have rapid onset of sedative effects that dissipate completely once the patient no longer needs to be asleep. On the other hand, an ideal anxiolytic would have rapid onset but last for many hours, so that it would relieve anxiety all day long. Not surprisingly, therefore, some of the benzodiazepines promoted for use as sleeping pills have shorter half-lives than those promoted for use as anxiolytics.

There are several problems with using benzodiazepines for the treatment of insomnia. Short-term difficulties associated with benzodiazepine use for insomnia are usually related to giving too high a dose for an individual patient. In such cases, there are carry-over effects the morning after administration, including not only a "drugged feeling" and the persistence of sedation when the patient wants to be alert but also interference with memory formation once the patient is awake. These problems can usually be handled by reducing the dose of the benzodiazepine, particularly in elderly patients.

Longer term difficulties associated with benzodiazepine use for insomnia come from observations that many patients develop tolerance for these agents, so that they stop working after a week or two. To avoid this, patients must take a sleeping pill only a few times within several days, or for only about 10 days in a row followed by several days or weeks with no drug treatment. Furthermore, if patients persist in taking benzodiazepines as sedative-hypnotics for several weeks to months, there can be a withdrawal syndrome caused once the medications are stopped, particularly if they are stopped suddenly. This is discussed in further detail in Chapter 12.

Discontinuation of benzodiazepines as sedative-hypnotics in patients who have been taking them for a prolonged period of time can cause a condition called "rebound insomnia," where a patient has worsening of insomnia as soon as benzodiazepines are stopped. Although this condition can be avoided by the short-term or only intermittent use of benzodiazepines as sedative-hypnotics, this condition is often masked in long-term benzodiazepine users until they suddenly stop their medication. Treatment of those who have grown tolerant to the use of sedative-hypnotic benzodiazepines involves a program of tapered withdrawal, and is discussed in detail in Chapter 12.

In order to prevent both the short- and long-term problems associated with the use of benzodiazepines as sedative-hypnotics, there has been an effort to discover new agents that lack these problems by expoiting the concept of partial agonists. This has already been discussed in relationship to anxiolytics (see Fig. 7–20). The idea is the same here, namely that a partial agonist at benzodiazepine receptors may induce a desired degree of mild sedation without producing short-term memory problems, carry-over effects to the next day, or the development of tolerance and dependence and withdrawal effects upon chronic use. One such agent that attempts to meet this profile is zopiclone. This is a nonbenzodiazepine in chemical structure that nevertheless interacts at the benzodiazepine receptor (see Fig. 7–18). Zopiclone has a short half-life, is a mild sedative-hypnotic; and may produce less tolerance, dependence, and withdrawal compared to full agonist benzodiazepine sedative-hypnotics. Zolipidem is another nonbenzodiazepine available for use in some countries.

Nonbenzodiazepine Sedative-Hypnotics

Various older agents have an extensive prior history of use as sedative-hypnotics, including barbiturates and related compounds such as ethclorvynol and ethinamate; chloral hydrate and derivatives; and piperidinedione derivatives such as glutethimide and methyprylon. Because of problems of tolerance, abuse, dependence, overdose, and several withdrawal reactions far more severe than those associated with the benzodiazepines, barbiturates and piperidinedione derivatives are rarely prescribed as sedative-hypnotics today. Chloral hydrate is still somewhat commonly used because it can be an effective short-term sedative hypnotic, and is inexpensive. However, it is generally to be avoided in patients with severe renal, hepatic, and cardiac disease, or in those who are taking numerous other drugs, due to its ability to affect hepatic drug-metabolizing enzymes. The potential of chloral hydrate to induce tolerance, physical dependence and addiction requires (1) cautious use in those with histories of drug or alcohol abuse problems and (2) only short-term use in any patient.

Summary

In this chapter we have provided clinical descriptions of anxiety and insomnia. We have also described the biological basis for anxiety and insomnia, emphasizing three neurotransmitter systems: GABA-benzodiazepines, serotonin, and norepinephrine. Finally, we have discussed the treatments for anxiety and insomnia and how they play upon these three neurotransmitter systems.

In discussing the GABA neurotransmitter system, we have shown how benzodiazepines are allosteric modulators of GABA A receptors and, in turn, of inhibitory chloride channels. The benzodiazepine receptor may be involved both in the mediation of the emotion of anxiety as well as in the mechanism of anxiolytic drug action.

In terms of the noradrenergic system, this chapter has described the locus coeruleus as that part of the brain that contains the noradrenergic neurons that mediate some of the symptoms of anxiety through alpha 2 and beta adrenergic receptors.

Our discussion has also extended to the role of serotonin in anxiety, which appears to be key yet quite complex and incompletely understood. One current theory developed in this chapter is the notion that serotonin excess may lead to compensatory desensitization of somatodendritic 5HT1A autoreceptors. Anxiolytic drugs that act at 5HT1A receptors may readapt the sensitivity of these receptors back to normal and thus restore a normal amount of nerve cell firing and serotonin release from serotonin neurons.

CHAPTER 8

DRUG TREATMENTS FOR OBSESSIVE COMPULSIVE DISORDER, PANIC DISORDER, AND PHOBIC DISORDERS

Some of the most dramatic advances in clinical psychopharmacology in recent years have been in the treatment of anxiety disorders. In fact, significant new treatments have had a large hand in the remaking of diagnostic criteria for subtypes of anxiety disorder. Thus, the tasks of clarifying the clinical descriptions, epidemiologies, and natural histories of obsessive compulsive disorder, panic disorder, and social phobia were greatly facilitated once dramatic new treatments became available over the past decade.

The anxiety disorders as a group are the most common psychiatric disorders, and are therefore very important for the psychopharmacologist to understand and treat effectively. Knowledge about the anxiety disorders is advancing at a rapid pace and new treatments and diagnostic criteria are still evolving. To equip the reader with the necessary foundation to keep up with the pace of change in the anxiety disorders, this chapter will set forth the psychopharmacological principles underlying contemporary treatment strategies. The details are likely to change rapidly, so this chapter will emphasize underlying concepts rather than specific facts about drug doses and pragmatic prescribing information. The reader is referred to standard reference sources for such data. Here we will emphasize those therapeutic agents, and their pharmacological mechanisms of action for the treatment of three of the most prominent anxiety disorders in psychopharmacology, namely obsessive compulsive disorder, panic disorder, and social phobia.

Obsessive Compulsive Disorder

Clinical Description

Obsessive compulsive disorder (OCD) is a syndrome characterized by obsessions and/ or compulsions that together last at least an hour a day and are sufficiently bothersome that they interfere with one's normal social or occupational functioning. *Obsessions* are experienced internally and subjectively by the patient as thoughts, impulses or images. According to standard definitions in the *Diagnostic and Statistical Manual of Mental Disorders* (DSM-IV), obsessions are intrusive, inappropriate, and cause marked anxiety and distress. Common obsessions are listed in Table 8–1.

Compulsions, on the other hand, are repetitive behaviors or purposeful mental acts that are sometimes observed by family members or clinicians, whereas it is not

Table 8–1. *Common obsessions*

Contamination
Aggression
Religion (scrupulosity)
Safety/harm
Need for exactness or symmetry
Somatic (body) fears

Table 8–2. *Common compulsions*

Checking
Cleaning/washing
Counting
Repeating
Ordering/arranging
Hoarding/collecting

possible to observe an obsession. Patients are often subjectively driven to perform their compulsions either in response to an obsession, or according to rigid rules aimed at preventing distress or some dreaded event. Unfortunately, the compulsions are not realistically able to prevent the distress or the dreaded event, and at some level the patient generally recognizes this. Common compulsions are listed in Table 8–2.

Interest in OCD skyrocketed once clomipramine was recognized throughout the world to be an effective treatment in the mid 1980s. Originally thought to be a rare condition, recent epidemiological studies now suggest that OCD exists in the adult population in about 1 out of every 50 adults, and in about 1 out of every 200 children. Thus, as news that OCD is common and treatable emerged, intense research efforts began to identify that the serotonin selective reuptake inhibitors (SSRIs) and certain forms of behavioral therapy are also effective treatments for OCD. The initial euphoria of the 1980s is somewhat balanced today by the sobering reality that treatments ameliorate but do not eliminate OCD symptoms in many patients, and that relapse is very common after discontinuing treatments for OCD.

Biological Basis

Despite a great deal of work in this area, the biological basis for OCD remains unknown. Some data suggest a genetic component to the etiology of OCD, but abnormal genes or gene products have yet to be identified. Some evidence implicates abnormal neuronal activity in OCD patients as well as alterations in neurotransmitters in OCD patients, but it is not known whether this is a cause or an effect of OCD. There is also a longstanding belief of a neurological basis for OCD that derives mainly from data implicating the basal ganglia in OCD plus the relative success of psychosurgery in some patients.

The serotonin hypothesis of OCD. Although it is unlikely that one neurotransmitter system can explain all the complexities of OCD, recent efforts to elucidate the pathophysiology of OCD have centered largely around the role of the neurotransmitter 5-hydroxytryptamine (5HT). The serotonin hypothesis of OCD, which states that OCD is linked to 5HT dysfunction, stems largely from pharmacological treatment studies.

It has been known for more than 25 years that clomipramine, a potent serotonin reuptake inhibitor, is effective in reducing OCD symptoms. Since then, numerous studies have confirmed the superiority of clomipramine over placebo in OCD patients, whereas other antidepressant medications with less potent inhibitory effects on serotonin reuptake (e.g., amitriptyline, imipramine, desipramine) seem to be ineffective in OCD. Development of the SSRIs fluoxetine, sertraline, paroxetine, and fluvoxamine and their demonstrated anti-OCD actions support the hypothesis that the antiobsessional effects of these various pharmacological agents is due to their potent serotonergic reuptake blocking activity.

The hypothesis that SSRIs work in OCD by a serotonergic mechanism is also supported by studies showing a strong positive correlation between improvement in obsessive-compulsive symptoms during clomipramine treatment and drug-induced decreases in cerebrospinal fluid (CSF) levels of the serotonin metabolite 5-hydroxyindoleacetic acid (5-HIAA) and platelet serotonin concentrations. Thus, peripheral markers of 5HT function link the symptomatic improvement in OCD symptoms produced by SSRIs to changes in 5HT function. However, these markers do not consistently highlight a 5HT abnormality in untreated patients with OCD.

Dopamine and OCD. Up to 40% of OCD patients do not respond to SSRIs. Also, at least some OCD patients fail to demonstrate convincing dysregulation in serotonin function. Therefore, other neurotransmitters may be involved in the pathophysiology of OCD in at least some OCD patients.

Several lines of evidence show that dopamine (DA) is implicated in the mediation of some obsessive compulsive behavior. Animal studies demonstrate that high doses of various dopaminergic agents, such as amphetamine, bromocriptine, apomorphine, and L-DOPA induce stereotyped movements in animals that resemble compulsive behaviors in OCD patients. Increased dopaminergic neurotransmission may be responsible for this. Human studies consistently report that abuse of stimulants such as amphetamine can cause seemingly purposeless, complex, repetitive behaviors that resemble behaviors occurring in OCD. Cocaine can also worsen compulsive symptoms in patients with chronic motor tic disorders such as Tourette's syndrome (TS).

The strongest support for a role of DA in mediating OCD symptoms comes from the relationship of OCD symptoms and several neurological disorders associated with dysfunction of DA in the basal ganglia (i.e., Von Economo's encephalitis, TS, and Sydenham's chorea).

The most intriguing is the link between TS and obsessive compulsive symptoms. TS is a chronic neuropsychiatric disorder characterized by multiple motor and vocal tics. Between 45% and 90% of TS patients also have obsessions and compulsions. If OCD symptoms were considered alone, a high percentage of TS patients would

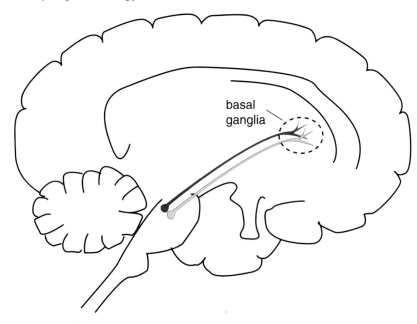

FIGURE 8–1. **Serotonin-dopamine projections to the basal ganglia.** Serotonin neurons from the midbrain raphe project to the basal ganglia (shown here as yellow neurons). Dopamine neurons from the substantia nigra in the brainstem also project to the basal ganglia (shown here as blue neurons). The axon terminals and the interactions between the serotonin and dopamine neurons there are shown in Figure 8–2.

meet diagnostic criteria for OCD. Family genetic studies show that TS and OCD are linked, leading to proposals that a common genetic factor may manifest itself as tics in some individuals and as obsessions and compulsions in others. Put differently, perhaps "tics" are the behavioral manifestations of a genetically based basal ganglia dysfunction, with TS being manifested as "tics of the body" and OCD as "tics of the mind."

Also supportive of dopamine involvement in the pathophysiology of OCD are observations that adjunctive neuroleptic therapy (which blocks DA receptors) added to ongoing SSRI treatment reduces the severity of OCD symptoms in OCD patients resistant to SSRI treatment alone, especially in those with concomitant TS.

Serotonin-dopamine hypothesis of OCD. On the basis of the studies on both 5HT and DA in OCD, it seems possible that at least in some forms of OCD (e.g., OCD with a history of TS) both 5HT and DA transmitter systems may be involved in the pathophysiology of symptoms. It is not clear whether the primary abnormality is in 5HT function, DA function, or in serotonin-dopaminergic balance. This hypothesis is supported by many preclinical data that suggest that important anatomical and functional interactions exist between serotonergic and dopaminergic neurons (Figs. 8–1 and 8–2). (This will also be discussed in Chapter 9 on antipsychotic drugs that work simultaneously on DA and 5HT receptors).

Thus, it may be that decreases in serotonin tonic inhibitory influences on DA neurons could lead to increased dopaminergic function due to the functional con-

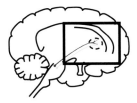

Normally, 5HT inhibits DA release

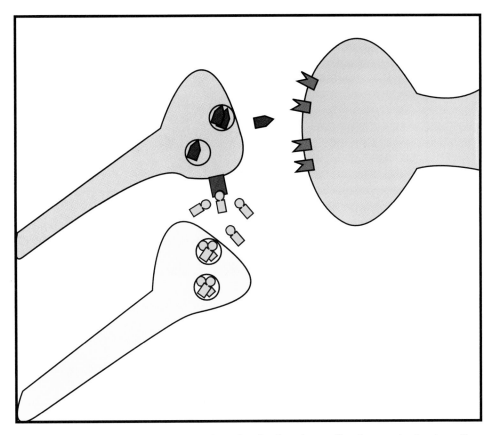

FIGURE 8–2. **Serotonin-dopamine interactions in the basal ganglia.** Serotonin in the yellow neurons normally has the ability to **inhibit dopamine release** in the blue neurons. This type of interaction may be via serotonin axons interacting with dopamine axons in an axoaxonal synapses. Alternatively, serotonin receptors on presynaptic dopamine axon terminals may be able to interact with serotonin that diffuses there from serotonin axons, but in a chemically addressed fashion rather than at a synapse (see explanation in Fig. 1–5). Some evidence suggests that this serotonin interaction at dopamine neurons occurs via 5HT2 receptors.

nections between DA and 5HT neurons in the basal ganglia (Fig. 8–3). OCD patients with a history of TS may thus represent a subtype of the disorder with two neurotransmitters and the balance between them involved in the pathophysiology of their symptoms.

In summary, the hypothesis that an abnormality in neurotransmitter functioning might underlie OCD has generated numerous studies of 5HT, and DA neuronal systems. To date, no compelling or consistent neurotransmitter dysfunction has been

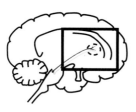

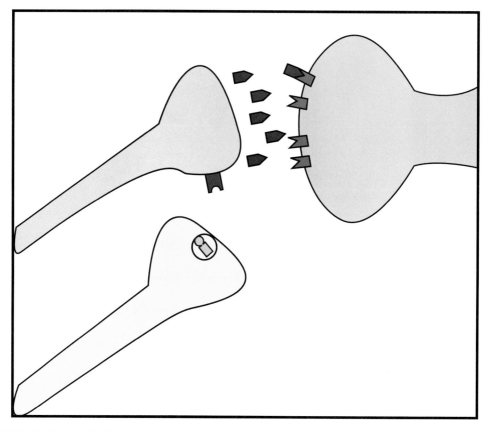

FIGURE 8–3. **Serotonin-dopamine interactions in the basal ganglia in obsessive compulsive disorder (OCD).** In OCD, a deficiency of serotonin may lead to a deficiency in the normal inhibitory actions of serotonin on dopamine release. In this case, dopamine release would be unopposed by serotonin, and therefore present in excess. This could explain the association of Tourette's syndrome – which may be characterized by dopamine excess – with OCD, which may be characterized by serotonin deficiency.

described that can adequately explain the neurobiological basis for OCD. However, it seems clear that changes in 5HT neuronal systems are caused by the known therapeutic agents for OCD, suggesting an important role for 5HT in mediating treatment responses in OCD.

Neuroanatomy in OCD. Abnormalities on positron emission tomography (PET) scans of neuronal activity of cortical projections to the basal ganglia have been confirmed by a number of investigators in OCD patients. Specifically, projections from the orbitofrontal cortex may be implicated in OCD. Such PET-demonstrated abnormalities in cortical projections to the basal ganglia may even be linked to the severity of symptoms in OCD patients, since they diminish as OCD patients improve, whether that improvement occurs after drug treatment or after behavioral therapy.

Drug Treatments

Serotonin reuptake inhibitors. Clomipramine is a tricyclic antidepressant first recognized more than 20 years ago as an effective treatment for depression. It has only been recognized widely and on a worldwide basis for the treatment of OCD since the mid 1980s. Originally, the efficacy of clomipramine in OCD was debated because depression is frequently present in OCD patients, leading some researchers to propose that clomipramine was only effective in treating the depressive symptoms and not the obsessions and compulsions in OCD patients. Others suggested that clomipramine was only effective in treating core OCD symptoms if symptoms of depression were also present. However, it is now clearly recognized that clomipramine has unique anti-OCD effects independent of its antidepressant effects in OCD patients.

Since clomipramine is a potent inhibitor of serotonin reuptake, it is hypothesized that the anti-OCD effects of clomipramine are linked to its serotonin reuptake blocking properties. However, clomipramine is also metabolized to a norepinephrine (NE) reuptake blocker, so the role of NE reuptake blockade in the mechanism of action of clomipramine remained unexplained until recently. That is, the somewhat NE-selective reuptake inhibitor desipramine has virtually no anti-OCD efficacy compared to clomipramine. Furthermore, the SSRIs, which lack entirely NE reuptake blocking properties, are all proven to have anti-OCD efficacy.

Although some similarities exist between the treatment of OCD with SSRIs and the treatment of depression with SSRIs, there are also some important differences. In general, doses for SSRIs in OCD are greater than doses for the treatment of depression. Also, onset of therapeutic effects may be even more delayed in OCD (i.e., 12 weeks or longer) than it is in depression (i.e., 4 to 8 weeks) following SSRI administration.

There are also differences in treatment responses between OCD and depression following SSRI treatment. Whereas many patients with depression recover completely after SSRI treatment, the average response of an OCD patient is about a 35% reduction in symptoms after 12 weeks of treatment. Relapse rates are less well studied in OCD, but appear to be much higher in OCD than in depression. One other important difference in the mechanism of SSRIs in OCD versus depression is that the therapeutic response in OCD may be less dependent upon the immediate availability of 5HT than is the therapeutic response in depression. Thus, when tryptophan is depleted from depressed patients, and 5HT synthesis is suddenly diminished, patients who have responded to SSRIs with an antidepressant response transiently deteriorate until 5HT synthesis is restored. By contrast, when tryptophan is depleted from OCD patients who have responded to SSRI treatment, their OCD symptoms are not worsened. This may suggest that SSRIs work via a different mechanism in OCD than they do in depression.

In summary, SSRIs undoubtedly improve symptoms in OCD, just as they improve symptoms in depression. However, compared to the use of SSRIs in depression, OCD responses to SSRIs specifically require 5HT and not NE reuptake inhibition, the OCD responses are generally slower, less robust, more likely to relapse after SSRI discontinuation, and are not as immediately dependent upon synaptic 5HT availability.

Adjunctive treatments. SSRIs are the foundation of treatment for OCD. However, many patients are refractory to SSRI treatment, or their responses are incomplete and unsatisfactory. This has led to a variety of strategies to augment SSRIs to attain a more satisfactory therapeutic response. Augmentation strategies include those directed at serotonergic functioning, those that are pharmacological but directed at other neurotransmitter systems, and those that are nonpharmacological.

SEROTONERGIC AUGMENTATION STRATEGIES   Since SSRIs do not work well for all OCD patients, and do not work at all as monotherapies for other OCD patients, psychopharmacologists have attempted to boost the effectiveness of SSRIs with various agents capable of augmenting serotonergic action. Three of these will be discussed here: buspirone, fenfluramine, and trazodone/nefazodone.

As SSRIs depend upon the presence of 5HT itself to down-regulate receptors and to be released once neuronal impulse flow is restored (Figs. 6−21 through 6−25), what do you do if 5HT is depleted (Fig. 8−4)? In that case, the SSRIs will be ineffective, since there is no 5HT available. If no 5HT is present, inhibition of reuptake is useless. In other words, SSRIs cannot enhance what is not there (Fig. 8−4). It is not known if 5HT depletion is a cause of refractoriness to SSRI treatment, but some augmentation therapies are directed towards this possibility.

Thus, the task would be to replete serotonin so that an SSRI can now work. How to do that? One possibility is via precursor loading with the amino acid tryptophan (see Fig. 5−22). This is not available for implementing as a strategy today, since tryptophan use has been associated with a potentially lethal immunological and muscular disorder known as eosinophilia myalgia syndrome (EMS), and is not generally considered to be a safe approach to this problem.

Another possibility is to shut the serotonin neuron off for a while, or to slow its firing down so that neuronal impulses are stopped or slowed. This would cause less serotonin to be released so that it could theoretically build back up in the neuron. Serotonin stores would be repleted by continued synthesis of 5HT. Slowing neuronal impulse flow can be accomplished by the use of 5HT1A partial agonists such as buspirone as discussed in Chapter 7. Thus, administration of buspirone with an SSRI may allow the neuron to replete its stores of 5HT to the point that the SSRIs get a boost in their efficacy (Figs. 8−5 and 8−6). It is not certain whether such a mechanism can account for the observations that buspirone can boost SSRI actions in depression, OCD, and panic, but it is indeed sometimes useful to administer both drugs in combination.

What if the neuron is incapable of releasing its serotonin (Fig. 8−7)? In that case, the SSRIs would also be incapable of working, since 5HT would sit in the presynaptic terminals, and not in the synapse. Thus, an SSRI would have no synaptic 5HT whose reuptake it could block and would therefore be ineffective. A serotonin releaser is fenfluramine, a halogenated amphetamine derivative more selective for

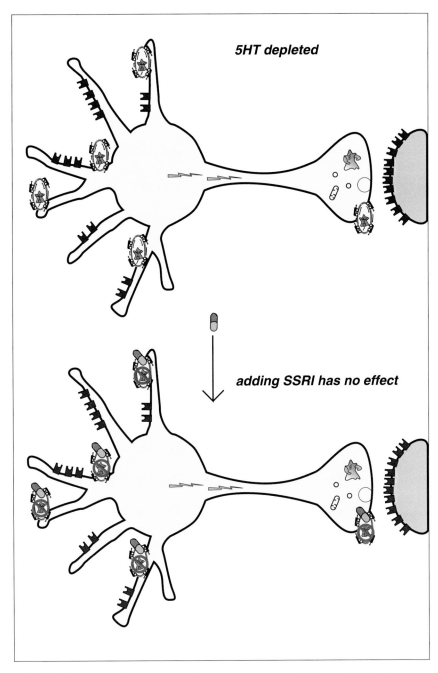

FIGURE 8–4. **Ineffectiveness of serotonin selective reuptake inhibitor (SSRI) therapy when serotonin (5HT) is depleted.** If 5HT is depleted from the 5HT neuron, then essentially no 5HT can be released from 5HT neurons. Since SSRIs are dependent upon the presence of 5HT released from 5HT neurons, they will be incapable of having an adequate therapeutic action on a 5HT-depleted neuron.

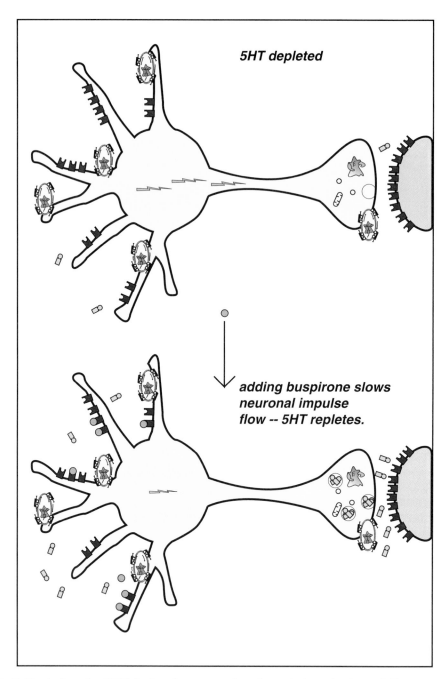

FIGURE 8–5. **Repleting the 5HT-depleted neuron**. One theoretical mechanism of allowing 5HT to reaccumulate in the 5HT-depleted neuron is to shut down neuronal impulse flow. If 5HT release is essentially turned off for a while so that the neuron retains all the 5HT it synthesizes, this may allow repletion of 5HT stores. A 5HT1A agonist such as buspirone is able to act on somatodendritic autoreceptors to inhibit neuronal impulse flow, possibly allowing repletion of 5HT stores. Also, buspirone could boost actions directly at 5HT1A receptors in order to help the small amount of 5HT available in this scenerio accomplish the targeted down-regulation desired at these receptors.

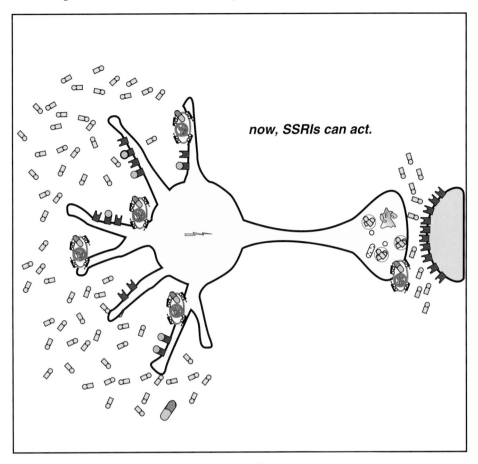

now, SSRIs can act.

FIGURE 8–6. **5HT1A partial agonists potentiate ineffective serotonin selective reuptake inhibitors (SSRIs).** The combination of 5HT1A agonists plus SSRIs may be more effective together in treating OCD, depression, or panic disorder than are SSRIs alone. This could be due to the mechanisms demonstrated in Figure 8–5.

releasing 5HT than DA. Thus, administration of fenfluramine could cause the stubborn neuron to release its 5HT (Fig. 8–7), whereupon the SSRI could grab the released 5HT and block its reuptake (Fig. 8–8). Again, it is not certain that lack of 5HT release can account for refractoriness of SSRIs in OCD, but it has been observed that fenfluramine can boost the clinical usefulness of the SSRIs.

Finally, it is possible that the postsynaptic 5HT2 receptors are not responding to the enhanced 5HT release (Fig. 8–9) accomplished after down-regulation of somatodendritic autoreceptors depicted in Figures 6–21 through 6–25. The serotonin might need a helper that acts by another mechanism to make the postsynaptic 5HT2 receptors respond with adequate down-regulation. This could theoretically be accomplished with a serotonin-2 antagonist/reuptake inhibitor (SARI) such as trazodone or nefazodone (Fig. 8–9). These SARIs act by blocking 5HT2 receptors, which causes 5HT2 receptor down-regulation in its own right (Fig. 8–9). Thus, an SSRI plus an SARI could work as partners to provoke down-regulation by two different

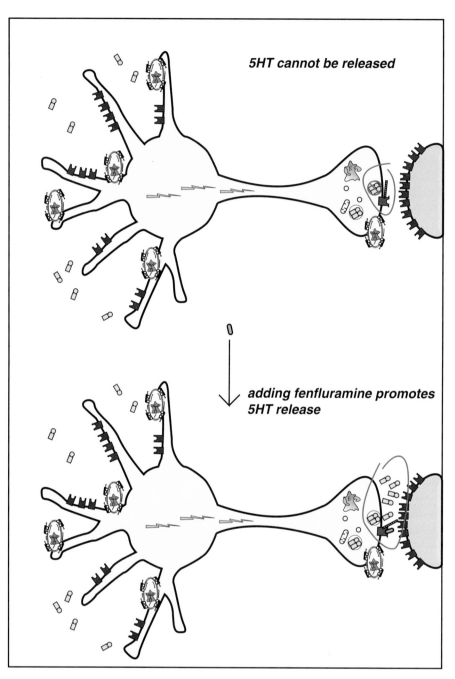

5HT cannot be released

adding fenfluramine promotes 5HT release

FIGURE 8–7. SSRIs would also be ineffective at 5HT neurons **incapable of releasing their 5HT**. If 5HT cannot be released, SSRIs would be incapable of working, since 5HT would sit in the presynaptic terminals, and not in the synapse. Thus, an SSRI would have no synaptic 5HT whose reuptake it could block and would therefore be ineffective. A serotonin releaser is fenfluramine, and administration of fenfluramine causes the 5HT neuron to start releasing its 5HT.

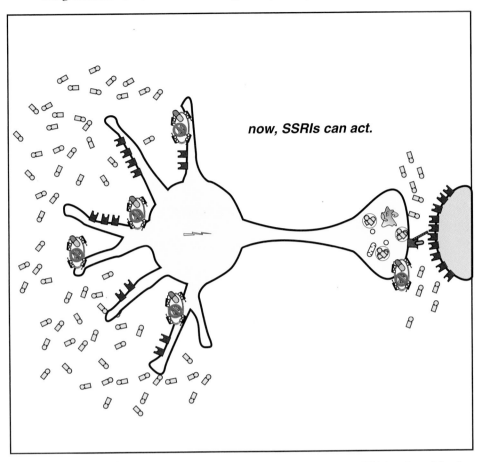

now, SSRIs can act.

FIGURE 8–8. **Potentiation of ineffective SSRIs by fenfluramine**. Once 5HT is released by fenfluramine through the mechanism discussed in Figure 8–7, an SSRI can now act to block the reuptake of the now-released 5HT.

pharmacological mechanisms, leading to the desired pharmacological adaptation (Fig. 8–9). It is not known whether lack of down-regulation of postsynaptic 5HT2 receptors is a cause of refractoriness to SSRIs, or whether boosting this down-regulation is accomplished by the coadministration of an SARI with an SSRI. However, it has been observed, for example, that trazodone addition to an SSRI can boost antidepressant, anti-OCD, and even antipanic efficacy of the SSRIs. SSRI augmentation strategies are thus summarized in Figures 8–4 through 8–9.

NEUROTRANSMITTER COMBINATION STRATEGIES   Rather than boosting the SSRI with a pharmacological intervention aimed at helping the SSRI at the serotonergic neuron, it is also possible that adding another neurotransmitter mechanism to the SSRI action at the serotonin neuron would boost the SSRI action indirectly. At least two such strategies have proven useful in some OCD patients whose response to SSRIs is unsatisfactory.

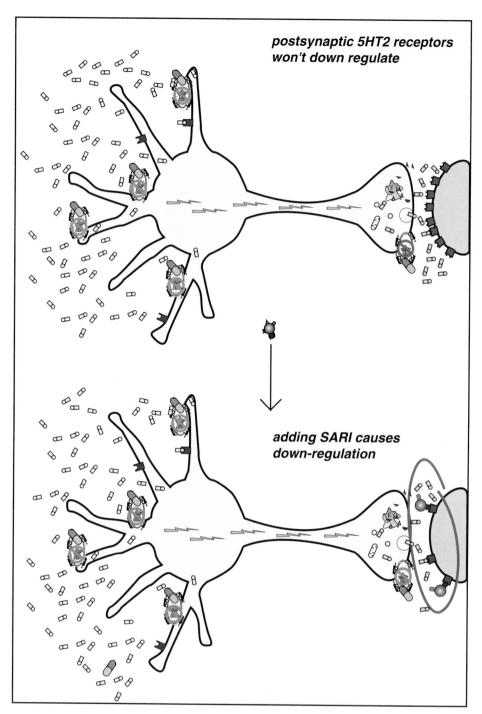

FIGURE 8–9. **Lack of sufficient down-regulation of postsynaptic 5HT2 receptors by SSRIs.** It is possible that some patients not responding to SSRI treatments have postsynaptic 5HT2 receptors that are not responding to the enhanced 5HT release accomplished after down-regulation of somato-dendritic autoreceptors. The serotonin might need a helper that acts by another mechanism to make the postsynaptic 5HT2 receptors respond with adequate down-regulation. This could theoretically be accomplished with a serotonin-2 antagonist/reuptake inhibitor (SARI) such as trazodone or nefazodone. SARIs act by blocking 5HT2 receptors, which causes 5HT2 receptor down-regulation in its own right. Thus, an SSRI plus an SARI could work as partners to provoke down-regulation by two different pharmacological mechanisms, leading to the desired pharmacological adaptation.

As discussed above, the addition of a neuroleptic that blocks DA receptors can be useful in some cases of OCD, particularly those with concomitant TS. Other cases of OCD, including those who have associated schizophreniform-type symptoms, or whose obsessions border on delusions without any insight, may also respond to the boosting effect of a neuroleptic agent.

Another possibility for boosting the SSRIs is to add a benzodiazepine, especially clonazepam. The SSRI boosting effect of clonazepam may be mediated partially by allowing a high dose of SSRI to be tolerated, partially by reducing nonspecific anxiety symptoms associated with OCD, and partially due to a direct serotonin-enhancing action of clonazepam itself.

BEHAVIORAL THERAPY   The most common concomitant therapy to the use with SSRIs is behavioral psychotherapy. Used by itself for selected cases, behavioral therapy can be as effective as SSRIs, and may last longer after discontinuation of treatment than the SSRIs do after they are stopped. Little is known from formal studies combining SSRIs with behavioral therapy, but it is well known from anecdotal clinical experience that this combination can be much more powerful than the use of SSRIs or behavioral therapy alone.

PSYCHOSURGERY   For extremely severe cases refractory to all these treatments alone and in combination, there is the possibility to gain some relief from a neurosurgical procedure cutting the neuronal loop connecting the cortex with the basal ganglia. Few centers have any experience with this procedure in OCD, and long-term outcomes are yet unknown. However, early results in very severe, very refractory OCD cases are encouraging.

A summary of OCD treatments is shown in Figure 8–10 and combination therapies are depicted graphically in Figure 8–11.

New prospects. Given that there are at least five serotonin reuptake blockers available to treat OCD, and that each is roughly comparable to the other in efficacy, it does not seem likely that much more therapeutic ground will be gained merely by developing yet another SSRI for OCD. On the other hand, it is not clear what pharmacological mechanism to target other than serotonin reuptake blockade in order to make an effective anti-OCD therapy.

It is theoretically possible that novel agents combining the actions of single agents used in combination and discussed above (Fig. 8–11) might be more powerful than a drug that is merely a selective inhibitor of serotonin reuptake. However, this is purely hypothetical at the moment because the mechanisms of action of the combinations described above are not proven.

It is also possible that certain novel agents acting uniquely upon serotonin and other neurotransmitter systems, and being tested as antidepressants or antipsychotics, will also prove to be anti-OCD agents. It is therefore logical to test the anti-OCD actions of the novel antidepressant nefazodone, a serotonin-2 receptor modulator and a weak SSRI (Figs. 6–30 and 6–31), as well as the potential anti-OCD actions of the dual reuptake inhibitor venlafaxine (Figs. 6–28 and 6–29). Also, the novel antipsychotic agent risperidone, which blocks both 5HT2 and DA2 receptors, is also worthy of investigation as a potential anti-OCD agent (see Chapter 10 and Figs. 10–8, 10–11, and 10–12). Other possibilities include the pure 5HT2 antagonists,

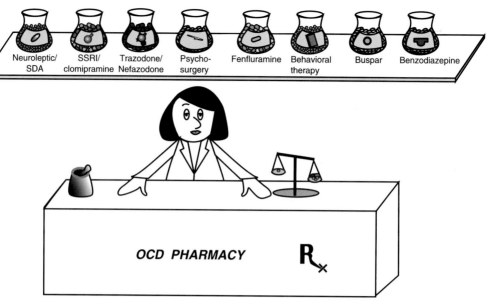

FIGURE 8–10. Shown here are the variety of therapeutic options for treating obsessive compulsive disorder (OCD).

as well as agents acting as agonists or antagonists of other serotonin receptors, either single receptors or combinations of receptors.

Panic Attacks and Panic Disorder

Clinical Description

A panic attack is a discrete episode of unexpected terror accompanied by a variety of physical symptoms. Associated symptoms include fear and anxiety as well as catastrophic thinking with a sense of impending doom or the belief that loss of control, death, or insanity is imminent. Physical symptoms can be neurological, gastrointestinal, cardiac, or pulmonary, and therefore may mimic many different types of medical illnesses. Panic attacks have therefore sometimes been called "the great medical imposters." Behaviors associated with panic attacks typically include an attempt to flee the situation and eventually to avoid anxiety-producing situations, or any situation that has previously been associated with a panic attack.

A panic attack usually lasts from 5 to 30 minutes, with the symptoms peaking at about 10 minutes, but attacks have been reported to last for hours. A person must have at least 4 of the 13 symptoms listed in Table 8–3 for an episode to be classified as a panic attack. Panic attacks may occur during sleep, in which case they are known as nocturnal panic attacks. These attacks may wake the person from sleep but are otherwise similar in symptoms to daytime panic attacks. A majority of patients with panic disorder will experience nocturnal panic, but only a few patients describe having the majority of their panic attacks at night.

It is common to confuse panic attacks with panic disorder. Many psychiatric disorders can have panic attacks associated with them (see Table 8–4). However, to

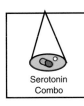

Serotonin Combo   SSRI   +   buspirone/fenfluramine/trazodone/nefazodone

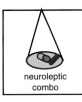

neuroleptic combo   SSRI   Neuroleptic

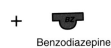

Benzo Combo   SSRI   +   Benzodiazepine

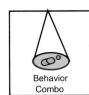

Behavior Combo   SSRI   +   Behavioral therapy

FIGURE 8–11. Various treatments can be given in combination for obsessive compulsive disorder (OCD). The basis of all combination treatments is an SSRI (or clomipramine). Added to this basis may be a neuroleptic (neuroleptic combo), a benzodiazepine (benzo combo), or behavioral therapy (behavior combo). The serotonin combo used for treating depression can also be used here to treat OCD.

Table 8–3. *Symptoms of a panic attack*

Palpitations, pounding heart, or accelerated heart rate
Sweating
Trembling or shaking
Sensations of shortness of breath or smothering
Feeling of choking
Chest pain or discomfort
Nausea or abdominal distress
Feeling dizzy, unsteady, lightheaded, or faint
Derealization (feelings of unreality) or depersonalization (being detached from oneself)
Fear of losing control or going crazy
Fear of dying
Paresthesias
Chills or hot flushes

Table 8–4. *Not all panic attacks are panic disorder*

Diagnosis	Spontaneous Panic Attacks	Situational Panic Attacks	Anticipatory Anxiety	Symptoms of Autonomic Arousal	Phobic Avoidance
Panic disorder	+++	+/−	+++	+++	+
Agoraphobia	+/−	+/−	+++	++	+++
Social Phobia	−	++	++	++	+++
Specific Phobia	+/−	+++	++	++	+++
PTSD	+/−	+	+/−	+++	+
GAD	+/−	+/−	+/−	+	+/−

+, ++, or +++ = present.
− = not usually present.
+/− = frequently present but not needed for diagnosis.

qualify for the diagnosis of panic disorder itself, patients must have some panic attacks that are entirely *unexpected*. Panic attacks can also be reproducibly triggered by certain specific situations for various individuals, and therefore can be *expected* (see Table 8–4). Situations that frequently act as triggers for panic attacks include driving or riding in a vehicle, especially in heavy rain or over bridges, shopping in crowded stores, and waiting in lines. The perception of lack of control or feeling "trapped" is a common theme in situational triggers.

As already emphasized, not all who have panic attacks have panic disorder (Table 8–4), and the distinguishing factor is the type of panic attacks. Patients with social phobia, posttraumatic stress disorder, or specified phobia will frequently experience panic attacks that are *expected*, since they are in response to specific situations or stimuli. However, such patients do not experience *unexpected* panic attacks. Unexpected panic attacks are thus uniquely characteristic of panic disorder.

Panic disorder, therefore, is the presence of recurrent unexpected panic attacks followed by at least a 1-month period of persistent anxiety or concern about recurrent attacks, consequences of attacks, or significant behavior changes related to the attacks. The presence of persistent anxiety or behavior changes is important because 10% of the normal population report having had panic attacks at some time in their life; however, since they do not develop persistent anxiety and do not modify their behavior, they do not develop panic disorder.

Panic disorder affects about 2% of the population but less than one third receive treatment. Panic disorder typically begins in late adolescence or early adulthood but can present in childhood. Onset is rare after age 45. Panic disorder is more prevalent in women, perhaps twice the rate in men. Genetic studies demonstrate a 15 to 20% rate of panic disorder in relatives of patients with panic disorder, including a 40% concordance rate for panic disorder in monozygotic twins.

Although not generally recognized by medical or mental health practitioners, panic disorder patients have a suicide rate comparable to patients with major depression – 20 to 42% of panic disorder patients report having made suicide attempts and 44 to 60% admit to having had suicidal ideation. This high rate of suicide attempts does not appear to be caused by the presence of depression in panic disorder patients.

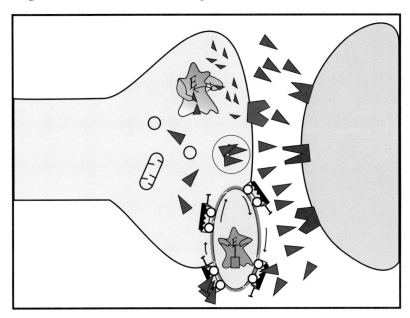

FIGURE 8–12. One theory about the **biological basis of panic disorder** is that there is an excess of norepinephrine, causing down-regulation of postsynaptic adrenergic receptors.

Panic disorder patients report a subjective feeling of poor physical and emotional health, impaired social and marital functioning, and increased financial dependency: 70% lose or quit their jobs because of their disorder, with an average length of work disability of 2.65 years and 50% are unable to drive more than 3 miles from their home. Panic disorder patients also have the highest use of emergency rooms of any psychiatric population.

Biological Basis

Neurotransmitter dysregulation. One theory about the biological basis of panic disorder is that there is an initial excess of norepinephrine, causing down-regulation of post-synaptic adrenergic receptors (Fig. 8–12). This theory is supported by evidence that panic disorder patients are hypersensitive to alpha 2 antagonists and hyposensitive to alpha 2 agonists. Thus, yohimbine, an alpha 2 antagonist, acts like a promotor of NE release by "cutting the brake cable" of the presynaptic NE autoreceptor (as shown in Fig. 7–27). The consequence of yohimbine administration is to have an exaggerated response in panic disorder patients, including the precipitation of overt panic attacks. Caffeine is also panicogenic. That is, caffeine is an adenosine antagonist that boosts second messengers for norepinephrine, and when patients are given the caffeine equivalent of four to six cups of coffee, many experience a panic attack, whereas most normals do not panic. On the other hand, panic patients have a blunted physiological response to postsynaptic adrenergic agonists, perhaps a consequence of an overactive noradrenergic system.

The neurotransmitter gamma-amino-butyric acid (GABA) and its allosteric mod-ulation by benzodiazepines have been implicated in the biological basis of panic disorder. That is, it appears that the ability of benzodiazepines to modulate GABA is out of balance. This may be due to changes in the amounts of endogenous benzodiazepines (i.e., "the brain's own Xanax" or "Valium-like compound"), or to alterations in the sensitivity of the benzodiazepine receptor itself.

Very little is known about endogenous benzodiazepine ligands, so most of the emphasis has been placed on investigating the responsivity of the benzodiazepine receptor in panic disorder patients. Nevertheless, it is possible that the brain makes less than the necessary amount of an endogenous full agonist, so that there is less ability of the brain to decrease anxiety on its own due to a postulated deficiency in a naturally occurring benzodiazepine full agonist. Alternatively, it is possible that the brain is producing an excess in anxiogenic inverse agonists, causing the panic disorder patient to have more anxiety and panic attacks due to such a postulated and unwanted increase in a naturally occurring benzodiazepine inverse agonist.

These are just theoretical possibilities, but some data do actually suggest an abnormality in the benzodiazepine receptor in panic disorder patients, in which the "set point" is shifted towards the inverse agonist conformation (Fig. 8–13). Conceptually, the resting state of the GABA A–benzodiazepine–chloride channel receptor complex is shifted to the left in the agonist spectrum already discussed (see Fig. 7–20). Thus, chloride channel conductance is already too diminished due to an altered sensitivity of the benzodiazepine receptor site (Fig. 8–13). Evidence for this comes from the fact that such patients require administration of exogenous benzodiazepine ligands (i.e., real Xanax [alprazolam] or real clonazepam) to reset the receptor complex's set point to normal. Also, flumazenil, which is neutral and without behavioral effects in normals, because it acts as a relatively pure antagonist, acts differently in panic disorder patients. In these patients, it acts as an inverse agonist due to the abnormal shift of the set point towards an inverse agonist conformation. Thus, whereas flumazenil acts as an antagonist with no behavioral effects in a normal patient, it acts as a partial inverse agonist in panic patients and provokes panic attacks in these patients.

Carbon dioxide hypersensitivity. Another theory regarding the biological substrate for panic disorder is based upon observations that panic disorder patients experience panic attacks more readily than people without panic disorder when breathing carbon dioxide or when given lactate. This has generated a theory of carbon dioxide hypersensitivity in panic disorder patients with a corollary hypothesis that panic patients demonstrate these findings because they are chronic hyperventilators.

False suffocation alarm theory. This theory proposes that panic disorder patients have a suffocation monitor located in the brainstem that misinterprets signals and misfires, triggering a "false suffocation alarm" (panic attack). Many factors are consistent with this hypothesis including the above theory of chronic hyperventilation and carbon dioxide hypersensitivity. The disorder of Ondine's curse (congenital central hypoventilation syndrome) appears to be virtually the opposite of panic disorder, and is characterized by a diminished sensitivity of the suffocation alarm, rendering sufferers of this disorder to a lack of adequate breathing, especially when asleep. These various observations support the existence of a distinct suffocation monitor, which is overly sensitive in panic disorder and not sensitive enough in Ondine's

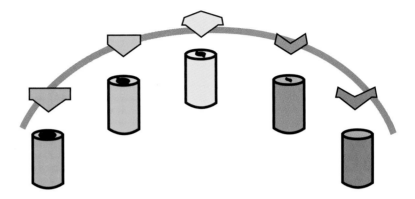

THE BENZODIAZEPINE RECEPTOR SPECTRUM

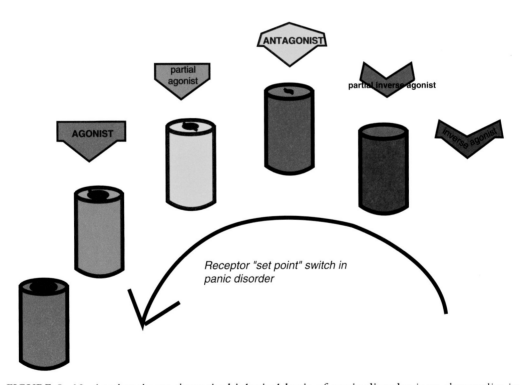

FIGURE 8–13. Another theory about the **biological basis of panic disorder** is an abnormality in the set point for benzodiazepine receptors. Perhaps the sensitivity of these receptors is switched to the left in this spectrum, rendering the receptors less sensitive to full agonists, and experiencing antagonists as inverse agonists.

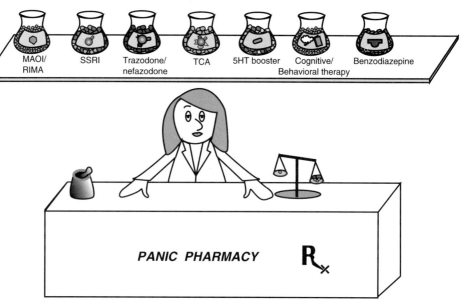

FIGURE 8–14. Shown here are the variety of therapeutic options for treating panic disorder.

curse. According to this theory, spontaneous (i.e., unexpected) panic attacks are thought to be mediated by this mechanism, whereas chronic anxiety or fear is not.

Neuroanatomical findings. Animal studies suggest that the locus coeruleus appears central to modulation of vigilance, attention, and anxiety or fear. Hypersensitivity of the limbic system has been considered a possible etiology or mechanism mediating panic disorder but few studies have been done. Lactate-sensitive patients have been found to have abnormal hemispheric asymmetry of parahippocampal blood flow on PET scans. Patients with temporal lobe epileptic foci frequently experience panic-like symptoms; however, only an extremely small minority of panic disorder patients have been found to have abnormal electroencephalograms (EEG). Nevertheless, the ictal seizure-like analogy may be useful, for panic may be tantamount to seizure-like neuronal activation in parts of the brain that mediate emotions, whereas true epilepsy may involve locations in the brain mediating movement and consciousness rather than emotions of anxiety and panic (see Fig. 4–17).

Drug Treatments (See Fig. 8–14)

Benzodiazepines. High-potency benzodiazepines (alprazolam, clonazepam) generally are more effective in panic disorder than low potency benzodiazepines (e.g., diazepam, lorazepam). Although less research has been done on the low-potency benzodiazepines, it is generally accepted that they frequently result in sedation prior to adequately treating panic attacks. The primary advantage to using benzodiazepines is rapid relief from anxiety and panic attacks. Other agents have a delayed therapeutic onset (see below). The disadvantages of benzodiazepines include sedation, cognitive clouding, interaction with alcohol, physiological dependence, and the potential for a withdrawal syndrome. Misinformation and stigma about the benzodiazepines can prevent patients from accepting appropriate treatment with these agents, and can prevent prescribers from administering these agents.

The reader is referred to the discussion of benzodiazepines in Chapter 7 for a detailed overview of mechanism of action. A critique of the issues of benzodiazepine dependence and appropriate use is given in Chapter 12. The situation in panic disorder is different in many ways than the situation for short-term states of generalized anxiety in that panic disorder may be quite chronic, require long-term, even lifelong treatment, and the consequences of inadequate treatment can be very severe loss of social and occupational functioning as well as suicide. These considerations must be weighed, as the risk/benefit ratio for benzodiazepine treatment is calculated for each patient individually.

To be fair, many practitioners adopt a "benzodiazepine-sparing strategy" for panic disorder patients. Thus, mild cases that can await the therapeutic onset of alternative treatments and for which alternative treatments are sufficiently powerful may be able to avoid benzodiazepine treatment altogether. On the other hand, if immediate therapeutic effects are required, benzodiazepines are the treatment of choice. In such cases, a second agent can be added (see Fig. 8–15) and, once the case is stabilized, the benzodiazepine can be tapered and the second agent continued. If the patient relapses on the second agent following benzodiazepine taper, this may be justification for continued use of concomitant benzodiazepines, but may allow a lower dose to be used for long-term maintenance with a second agent than was required for stabilization prior to the onset of the therapeutic actions of the second agent.

Alprazolam has been researched more extensively than any other benzodiazepine in panic disorder, and is very effective. Due to its short duration of action, it generally must be administered in three to five daily doses. A controlled-release formulation that extends the half-life, allowing for once- or twice-a-day administration, is in development and may eliminate this problem of the need for frequent daily dosing.

Clonazepam, which has a longer duration of action than alprazolam, has also been extensively investigated in panic disorder. It can generally be administered twice a day. Clonazepam is reported to have less abuse potential than alprazolam and to be easier to taper during discontinuation due to its longer half-life.

Anecdotal observations suggest that other benzodiazepines may also be effective in treating panic attacks in some panic disorder patients. In general, benzodiazepines are rapidly effective, and in many cases the benefits of treatment far outweigh the disadvantages.

Serotonin selective reuptake inhibitors. Many medications originally developed or used in treatment of depression have been found to be effective in treating panic disorder. Since many patients have coexisting depression and panic disorder, SSRIs are often considered first-line treatment for such patients. Each class of antidepressants has individual advantages and disadvantages; however, all antidepressants take 3 to 8 weeks before benefit may be noticed, and they must be started at low doses and increased slowly because of their tendency to exacerbate panic symptoms when started at normally recommended starting dosages for depression.

These medications (fluoxetine, paroxetine, sertraline, and fluvoxamine) have fewer data to support their efficacy in panic disorder than do the benzodiazepines because

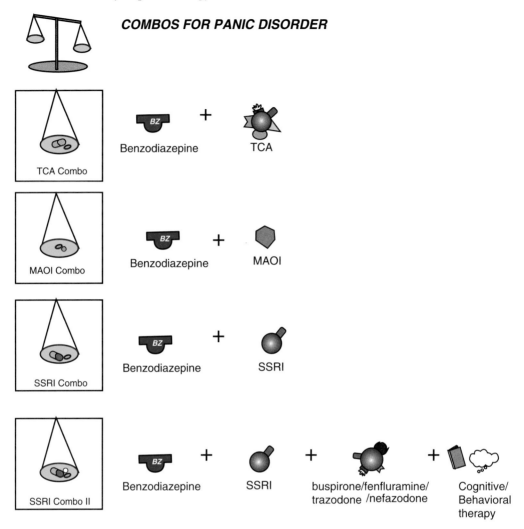

COMBOS FOR PANIC DISORDER

TCA Combo — Benzodiazepine + TCA

MAOI Combo — Benzodiazepine + MAOI

SSRI Combo — Benzodiazepine + SSRI

SSRI Combo II — Benzodiazepine + SSRI + buspirone/fenfluramine/ trazodone /nefazodone + Cognitive/ Behavioral therapy

FIGURE 8–15. Various treatments can be given in combination for panic disorder. The basis of many combination treatments is a high-potency benzodiazepine. Added to this basis may be any of a number of antidepressants, including a tricyclic antidepressant (TCA combo), an MAOI (MAOI combo), an SSRI (SSRI combo) or possibly an SSRI plus the same serotonin boosters used in combination therapy for depression and for obsessive compulsive disorder (SSRI combo I). Cognitive and behavioral psychotherapies can also be added to any of these drug treatments.

of their relatively more recent development. However, they are commonly used for the treatment of panic disorder, and are generally considered effective treatment, with the primary disadvantage being a significant worsening of anxiety on initiation of treatment. This has led to their concomitant use with benzodiazepines (see Fig. 8–15). The benzodiazepines not only appear to act synergistically to boost the efficacy of both agents used in combination but also appear to block the anxiogenic actions of the SSRIs, and lead to better tolerability as well as the ability to attain therapeutic dosing levels for the SSRIs.

Tricyclic antidepressants. Imipramine and clomipramine have been the most extensively studied in this class of medications, and both have demonstrated efficacy in treating panic disorder. Other tricyclic antidepressants that have shown some evidence of efficacy include desipramine, doxepin, amitriptyline, and nortriptyline.

The advantages to these medications include once-a-day dosing, no benzodiazepine-type of physiological dependence or withdrawal, and no dietary restrictions (necessary with monoamine oxidase inhibitors [MAOIs]). Disadvantages include anticholinergic side effects, orthostatic hypotension, and weight gain (due to actions at receptors discussed in Chapter 6). These side effects can lead to long-term noncompliance, with consequential reemergence of panic attacks once treatment with tricyclic antidepressants is discontinued.

Monoamine oxidase inhibitors. The classical irreversible MAOIs are effective in treating panic disorder, with anecdotal observations that they may be even more effective than imipramine. Clinical experience with reversible inhibitors of MAO A (RIMAs) (see Fig. 6–10) is also favorable for the treatment of panic disorder. However, the RIMAs may be somewhat less effective than the irreversible MAOIs, but this is not well established. Advantages for MAOIs include less tendency to cause activation early in treatment, no tolerance or dependence, and lower anticholinergic side effects. Disadvantages for the irreversible MAOIs include orthostatic hypotension, weight gain, sexual dysfunction, and dietary restrictions (low-tyramine diet), with the potential for a tyramine-induced hypertensive crisis. The RIMAs appear safer, with lessened potential for side effects as discussed in Chapter 6, but also with possibly less efficacy.

Cognitive and behavioral psychotherapies. These two therapies are commonly combined in the treatment of panic disorder with or without agoraphobia. Cognitive therapy focuses on identifying the cognitive distortions and modifying them, whereas behavior therapy specifically attempts to modify a patient's responses, often through exposure to situations or physiological stimuli that are associated with panic attacks. Behavioral therapy appears to be most effective in treating the phobic avoidance aspect of panic disorder and agoraphobia and does not appear as effective in treating the panic attacks. These treatments have had as high a rate of effectiveness as have the antipanic drugs. Furthermore, for those who are able to complete an adequate period of treatment with behavioral treatment, their improvements are perhaps more likely to be sustained after discontinuing treatment than are drug-induced improvements after discontinuation of antipanic drugs.

Combination therapy. This term can refer either to combination of drug therapy with cognitive-behavioral therapy, or combinations of more than one drug (Fig. 8–15). This area remains underdeveloped, since few studies have been done comparing single-mode and combination therapy. However, common clinical practice for many panic disorder patients is indeed the artful choosing of combinations of the available treatments. Tailoring a treatment program to the individual patient is becoming the state of the art, although such combinations are generally inadequately investigated in controlled clinical trials.

Many clinicians feel that some patients are so anxious or depressed initially that they are unable to participate in or receive much benefit from psychotherapy, so these patients may be excluded from psychotherapy until their symptoms improve somewhat on medication treatment. Other therapists may feel that benzodiazepines interfere significantly in cognitive-behavioral therapy, since it is true that a certain amount of anxiety must be present for behavioral therapy to be effective. Until conclusive data are reported, there is no contraindication for using combination therapy, and there may be additional benefit. Nevertheless, the combination of drugs and behavioral therapy must be individualized for the case at hand.

In terms of combining drug therapies, the two most widely used classes of drugs are a benzodiazepine plus an antidepressant. The preferred benzodiazepines are either alprazolam or clonazepam, as mentioned earlier. Although the preferred antidepressant to combine with a benzodiazepine may have originally been a tricyclic antidepressant or an MAOI, currently the emphasis is shifting to a preference for an SSRI. This is generally due to the evolving picture of efficacy of these agents, plus their generally enhanced tolerability profile compared to the older antidepressant agents. However, this differs significantly from clinician to clinician and from one country to another.

A variation on the theme of SSRI combination with benzodiazepine is the combination of an SSRI booster with an SSRI plus or minus a benzodiazepine (Fig. 8–15). The SSRI boosters were previously discussed for OCD above and shown in Figures 8–4 through 8–8. Virtually any antipanic agent can be combined with cognitive behavioral therapy in well-selected patients. A summary of available antipanic treatments is shown in Figure 8–14. A summary of combination treatments for panic disorder is shown in Figure 8–15.

Relapse after medication discontinuation. Relapse rates after discontinuation of antidepressants in the treatment of major depressive disorder have been much more thoroughly studied than have relapse rates of panic disorder in patients discontinued from antipanic agents. Although panic disorder can frequently be in remission within 6 months of beginning treatment, the relapse rate is apparently very high on the basis of existing studies, once treatment is stopped, even for patients who have had complete resolution of symptoms. When a patient has been asymptomatic on medication for 6 to 12 months, it is reasonable to have a trial off medication. If medication is discontinued, it should be done slowly, and the benzodiazepines in particular should be tapered over a period of at least 2 months and possibly as long as 6 months. More commonly now panic disorder is considered a chronic illness that requires maintenance therapy. Investigations are underway to provide much clearer guidelines for chronic therapy in panic disorder.

SSRIs for panic, OCD, and depression. The reader may be beginning to wonder why the SSRIs seem to have such a widespread utility for so many psychiatric disorders. Does this mean SSRIs work for everything that ails you? If they act indiscriminately, maybe it means they really do not work at all for anything.

There are good theoretical reasons to suggest why the SSRIs work in the three disorders of panic, OCD, and depression, and it is not because these agents are a panacea for all psychiatric suffering. Serotonin neurons project to several key areas of the brain and are able to exert a regulatory influence wherever they go. Thus, a dimension of many behaviors, and potentially of disorders of behaviors, may be

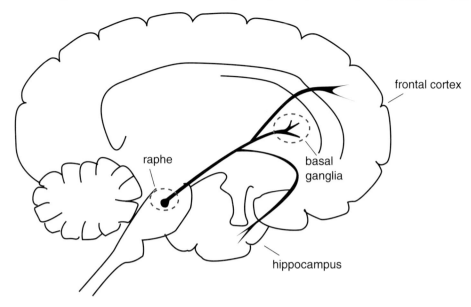

FIGURE 8–16. **Neuroanatomical hypothesis for the serotonergic basis of SSRI therapeutic actions in depression, OCD, and panic disorder**. Serotonin neurons project to several key areas of the brain and are able to exert a regulatory influence wherever they go. Thus, serotonin projections to one part of the brain may be useful in modulating mood, in another part obsessions and compulsions, and in a third part panic. Since the SSRIs act at the raphe, which is the command center for all the serotonin projections throughout the brain, it may be that every projection is modulated by SSRIs in a similar fashion. Thus, when somatodendritic 5HT1A autoreceptors down-regulate, serotonin output is enhanced in all of its projection fields. In the case of depression, OCD, and panic, perhaps only one of these is critical, and the fact that serotonin input is occurring elsewhere is irrelevant. Perhaps enhanced serotonin output in the **prefrontal cortex** may be key for **antidepressant actions**, but outputs in hippocampus and basal ganglia perhaps are irrelevant for antidepressant actions of SSRIs. On the other hand, it may be that very increase in serotonin output in **basal ganglia** that is key to therapeutic actions in **OCD** and enhanced output in **hippocampus** key for therapeutic actions in **panic**.

serotonergic. It is far from the only dimension, but rather like a single colored thread woven throughout a complex tapestry composed of many other threads.

Serotonin projections to one part of the brain may therefore be useful in modulating mood, in another part obsessions and compulsions, and in a third part panic (see Fig. 8–16). Since the SSRIs act at the raphe, which is the command center for all the serotonin projections throughout the brain, it may be that every projection is modulated by the SSRI in a similar fashion. The modulation of raphe serotonin function and receptors has been extensively discussed in Chapter 6 and shown in Figures 6–21 through 6–25.

When somatodendritic autoreceptors down-regulate, serotonin output is enhanced in all of its projection fields. In the case of depression, OCD, and panic, perhaps only one of these is critical, and the fact that serotonin input is occurring elsewhere is irrelevant. Preclinical data suggest that enhanced serotonin output in the prefrontal cortex may be key for antidepressant actions, but outputs in hippocampus and basal ganglia are perhaps irrelevant for antidepressant actions of SSRIs. On the other hand, it may be that very increase in serotonin output in basal ganglia that is key to therapeutic actions in OCD, and enhanced output in hippocampus key for therapeutic actions in panic.

Psychopharmacologists are searching for answers to why the SSRIs appear to have such pervasive actions in so many disorders of behavior. The schematic in Figure 8–16 is just one example of a modern theory to account for this.

New Prospects

Long-acting or controlled release benzodiazepines. Long-acting formulations of the leading benzodiazepine for the treatment of panic disorder, namely alprazolam, are under development.

Better documentation for SSRIs. Numerous clinical trials are ongoing to document the efficacy of SSRIs. More information is needed clarifying the onset of action and the utility of SSRIs compared to placebo as well as known antipanic agents such as benzodiazepines, tricyclic antidepressants, and MAOIs.

Partial agonists at benzodiazepine receptors. As discussed for general anxiolytic agents in Chapter 7, the partial agonists could be a theoretical advance over the marketed benzodiazepines. Partial agonists should have the same efficacy as full agonists, but less potential for sedation and dependence and withdrawal.

Nonbenzodiazepine ligands at benzodiazepine sites. This is a variation on the theme of partial benzodiazepine agonists, as these agents act at the same site as benzodiazepines, but are not structurally related to benzodiazepines. Thus, the pharmacology of nonbenzodiazepines is that of a partial agonist, but the chemistry is different from that of a benzodiazepine.

RIMAs. Clinical experience with RIMAs in those countries where these agents are approved for marketing or testing suggest potential utility as antipanic agents. Further research is required to determine the relative advantages and relative efficacy of these compounds compared to available antipanic agents.

Other novel serotonergic agents. Given the apparent importance of serotonin in mediating the therapeutic benefits of SSRIs for the treatment of panic disorder, it is theoretically possible that novel pharmacological agents acting in unique manners may also have antipanic actions. Thus, *pure serotonin-2 antagonists*, *SARIs*, and *serotonin-dopamine antagonists (SDAs)* may all have some utility in panic disorder, but as yet are not adequately tested. *Dual reuptake blockers* of serotonin and norepinephrine are appealing from a theoretical vantage, but have not been thoroughly tested. Antagonists of other serotonin receptors such as *5HT3 antagonists* as well as *5HT1A antagonists* have some hypothetical appeal as antipanic agents, but have not been sufficiently tested in panic disorder patients.

Phobic Disorders

Clinical Description

A phobia is a fear, and there are several disorders called phobias. Here we will briefly discuss agoraphobia, social phobia, and specified phobias. *Agoraphobia* literally translated means "fear of the marketplace" or essentially fear of going out from one's home. However, the diagnosis of agoraphobia more precisely refers to anxiety about being in all the different situations from which escape might be difficult or in which help may not be available in the event of having a panic attack. This anxiety leads to avoidance of such situations (called phobic avoidance), often to the extent that the patient becomes housebound. Although agoraphobia is usually seen in conjunction with panic disorder, it is a separate disorder and may be diagnosed without a diagnosis of panic disorder. About one third of panic disorder patients also have agoraphobia. Patients who have panic disorder accompanied by agoraphobia appear to have a more severe and complicated course than patients with panic disorder alone.

Specific phobias used to be called simple phobias, and included excessive and unreasonable fears of specific objects or situations such as flying in an airplane, heights, animals, seeing an injection, or seeing blood. In specific phobias, exposure to the feared situation or object causes an immediate anxiety response, even a full-blown panic attack. In *social phobia*, on the other hand, there is an intense, irrational fear of social or performance situations in which the patient is exposed to unfamiliar people or to possible scrutiny by others and anticipates humiliation or embarrassment.

There is both a generalized type and a more discrete type of social phobia. In the generalized type, the patient fears practically all social situations in which evaluation and scrutiny are possible. It is significantly more common than the discrete type, in which the individual fears a very specific social situation, usually of public speaking or public performance. Generalized social phobia is also more severe and disabling and less amenable to treatment than discrete social phobia.

Social phobia occurs in 1.3% of the population, and affects twice as many women as men. First-degree relatives of social phobics have a greater prevalence of social phobia than the normal population. Social phobia usually has an early onset, between 11 and 15 years of age, and has a chronic, unremitting course with significant lifelong disability. Children as young as 21 months of age who exhibit behavioral inhibition (intense anxiety and fear when faced with new social situations) have an increased prevalence of childhood anxiety phenomena, including social phobia–like symptoms as well as agoraphobia-like symptoms by the time they are 8 years old.

Two thirds of social phobics are single, divorced, or widowed. More than half of all patients with social phobia never completed high school. In fact, one fifth of social phobics are unable to work and must therefore collect welfare or disability benefits.

The most common fears among social phobics are speaking in front of a small group of people, speaking to strangers or meeting new people, and eating in public. More than half of social phobics will suffer at some point in their lifetime from a specific phobia as well.

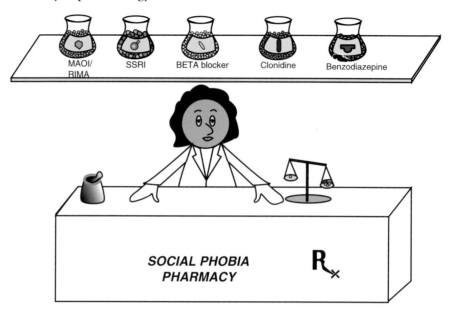

FIGURE 8–17. Shown here are the variety of therapeutic options for treating social phobia.

Social phobia and *specific phobia* can be distinguished from panic disorder by the fact that panic attacks (if present) are in response to specific situations and do not occur unexpectedly. Also, the fear in social phobia is a fear of humiliation, shame, or embarrassment instead of a fear of having a panic attack. Somatic symptoms differ between panic disorder patients with agoraphobia and social phobia, with blushing more common among social phobics. Difficulty breathing, dizziness, and syncope occur more frequently among the agoraphobics.

Posttraumatic stress disorder (PTSD) is another anxiety disorder that can be characterized by attacks of anxiety or panic, but is notably different from panic disorder or social phobia in that the initial anxiety or panic attack in PTSD is in response to a real threat (e.g., being raped) and subsequent attacks are usually linked to memories, thoughts, or flashbacks of the original trauma.

Biological Basis

The biological basis of social phobia has only recently been investigated, and appears to fit into the panic disorder spectrum, with very similar findings to date (see discussion above for panic disorder).

Drug Treatments

There are no officially approved drug treatments for social phobia, although a growing literature supports the use of a number of agents (Fig. 8–17). Treatments for social phobia derive significantly from treatments for panic disorder (Figs. 8–14 and 8–15). Most notable in the treatment of social phobia are the high potency benzodiazepines alprazolam and clonazepam, as well as SSRIs and the MAOIs. The

RIMAs may also work in social phobia, but perhaps not as fast as the irreversible MAOIs. Some but not all studies suggest that beta adrenergic blockers such as propranolol and atenolol may also be useful. The efficacy of tricyclic antidepressants in social phobia has not been adequately explored. Augmentation strategies for the treatment of social phobia are also in their infancy. It is possible that serotonin augmentation therapies might also be useful in social phobia, based upon analogies with panic disorder (Fig. 8–15), but very little has been formally researched. Other agents such as buspirone monotherapy and clonidine monotherapy have also been investigated, with no clear consensus on therapeutic utility in social phobia.

Psychotherapeutic Treatments

Psychotherapeutic treatments for social phobia are also in their relative infancy. Relaxation techniques, while sometimes advocated as part of anxiety management, are difficult to apply to patients with social phobia. Exposure therapy, on the other hand, can be successfully implemented if the anxiety-provoking stimuli are categorized into common themes and if the patient practices increasing the frequency of exposure to these stimuli throughout the day. Major cognitive distortions are maintained by social phobics during social situations. For example, they overestimate the scrutiny of others, attribute critical thoughts to others, underestimate their own social skills, and fear the responses of others to their anxiety. For such patients, cognitive restructuring can be helpful. The task is to challenge and reorganize unrealistic, emotional, and catastrophic thoughts. Cognitive and behavioral techniques in a group setting may be the best psychosocial interventions for social phobic patients, especially when combined with drug therapy. Drug treatments for social phobia are represented pictorially in Figure 8–17. They can also be combined as has been previously discussed for the treatment of depression, OCD, and panic and graphically represented in Figures 6–37, 8–11, and 8–15.

New Prospects

As social phobia is only recently becoming better recognized and researched, better documentation for the various treatments mentioned above is now evolving. Thus, clearer guidelines are emerging for the use of high-potency benzodiazepines, serotonin selective reuptake inhibitors, MAOIs, RIMAs, and various drugs in combination with second drugs or with behavioral therapies.

Under investigation are also the dual reuptake inhibitors, the serotonin-3 antagonists, and virtually every compound being studied in depression and in panic disorder.

Summary

In this chapter, we have given clinical descriptions and have also explored the biological basis and a variety of treatments for numerous anxiety disorder subtypes, including OCD, panic disorder, and social phobia.

Obsessive compulsive disorder may be linked to abnormalities of the neurotransmitters serotonin and dopamine. The neuroanatomical basis of OCD may be related to dysfunctioning in the basal ganglia. The hallmark of treatment for OCD is SSRIs plus the tricyclic antidepressant clomipramine.

Panic disorder is characterized by unexpected panic attacks, possibly linked to abnormalities in the neurotransmitters norepinephrine, GABA, or in the sensitivity of benzodiazepine receptors, or even in the sensitivity of the brain to carbon dioxide. Drug treatments include high-potency benzodiazepines, and numerous antidepressants including MAOIs, many tricyclic antidepressants, and SSRIs.

Social phobia is characterized by expected panic attacks; that is, they are expected in situations of public scrutiny because of the fear the patient has of that situation. Treatments are similar to those of panic disorder.

PSYCHOSIS AND SCHIZOPHRENIA

Psychosis is a difficult term to define and therefore has no universally accepted definition. It is frequently misused not only in the newspapers, movies, and on television but, unfortunately, among mental health professionals as well. This is due to both the lack of consensus among experts as to how to define psychosis and psychotic illnesses and to stigma and fear in lay society. Debates about diagnostic criteria lead to frequent reformulations among experts, whereas the average citizen worries about longstanding myths of "mental illness," including "psychotic killers," "psychotic rage," and the equivalence of "psychosis" with the pejorative term "crazy."

We have already discussed public misconceptions about mental illness in Chapter 5 on depression (Table 5–1). There is no area of psychiatry where misconceptions

Table 9–1. *Disorders in which psychosis is a defining feature*

Schizophrenia
Substance-induced (i.e., drug-induced) psychotic disorders
Schizophreniform disorder
Schizoaffective disorder
Delusional disorder
Brief psychotic disorder
Shared psychotic disorder
Psychotic disorder due to a general medical condition

---

are greater than in the area of psychotic illnesses. The reader is well served to develop an expertise on the facts about the diagnosis and treatment of psychotic illnesses in order to dispel unwarranted beliefs and to help destigmatize this devastating group of illnesses.

This chapter is not intended to list the diagnostic criteria for all the different mental disorders in which psychosis is either a defining feature or an associated feature. The reader is referred to standard reference sources (*Diagnostic and Statistical Manual of Mental Disorders* [DSM-IV] and *International Classification of Diseases* [ICD-10]) for that information. We will approach psychosis as a syndrome that is a target for antipsychotic drug treatment irrespective of the specific mental disorder with which it is associated.

Clinical Description of Psychosis

Psychosis is a syndrome (i.e., a mixture of symptoms) that can be associated with many different psychiatric disorders, but is not a specific disorder itself in diagnostic schemes such as DSM-IV or ICD-10. At a minimum, psychosis means delusions and hallucinations. It generally also includes symptoms such as disorganized speech, disorganized behavior, and gross distortions of reality testing.

Therefore, psychosis can be considered a set of symptoms in which a person's mental capacity, affective response, and capacity to recognize reality, communicate, and relate to others is impaired. Psychotic disorders have psychotic symptoms as their defining features, but there are other disorders in which psychotic symptoms may be present, but which are not necessary for the diagnosis.

Disorders that require the presence of psychosis (Table 9–1) as a defining feature of the diagnosis include two prominent psychotic disorders: schizophrenia and substance-induced (i.e., drug-induced) psychotic disorder. Other disorders that require psychosis as a defining feature include schizophreniform disorder, schizoaffective disorder, delusional disorder, brief psychotic disorder, shared psychotic disorder, and psychotic disorder due to a general medical condition.

Disorders that may or may not be associated with psychotic symptoms (Table 9–2) include mania and depression as well as several cognitive disorders such as Alzheimer's dementia.

Psychosis itself can be paranoid, disorganized/excited, or depressive. Perceptual distortions and motor disturbances can be associated with any type of psychosis. *Perceptual distortions* include being distressed by hallucinatory voices; hearing voices

Table 9–2. *Disorders in which psychosis is an associated feature*

Mania
Depression
Cognitive disorders
Alzheimer's dementia

that accuse, blame, or threaten punishment; seeing visions; reporting hallucinations of touch, taste, or odor; or reporting that familiar things and people seem changed. *Motor disturbances* are peculiar, rigid postures; overt signs of tension; inappropriate grins or giggles; peculiar repetitive gestures; talking, muttering, or mumbling to oneself; or glancing around as if hearing voices.

Paranoid Psychosis

In paranoid psychosis, the patient has paranoid projections, hostile belligerence, and grandiose expansiveness. *Paranoid projection* includes preoccupation with delusional beliefs; believing that people are talking about oneself; believing one is being persecuted, or being conspired against; and believing people or external forces control one's actions. *Hostile belligerence* is verbal expression of feelings of hostility; expressing an attitude of disdain; manifesting a hostile, sullen attitude; manifesting irritability and grouchiness; tending to blame others for problems; expressing feelings of resentment; complaining and finding fault; as well as expressing suspicion of people. *Grandiose expansiveness* is exhibiting an attitude of superiority; hearing voices that praise and extol; and believing that one has unusual powers, is a well-known personality, or has a divine mission.

Disorganized/Excited Psychosis

In a disorganized/excited psychosis, there is conceptual disorganization, disorientation, and excitement. *Conceptual disorganization* can be characterized by giving answers that are irrelevant or incoherent; drifting off the subject; using neologisms; or repeating certain words or phrases. *Disorientation* is not knowing where one is, the season of the year, the calendar year, or one's own age. *Excitement* is expressing feelings without restraint; manifesting speech that is hurried; exhibiting an elevated mood; exhibiting an attitude of superiority; dramatizing oneself or one's symptoms; manifesting loud and boisterous speech; exhibiting overactivity or restlessness; and exhibiting excess of speech.

Depressive Psychosis

Depressive psychosis is characterized by retardation, apathy, and anxious self-punishment and blame. *Retardation and apathy* are manifesting slowed speech; indifference to one's future; fixed facial expression; slowed movements; deficiencies in recent memory; manifesting blocking in speech; apathy toward oneself or one's problems;

slovenly appearance; low or whispered speech; and failure to answer questions. *Anxious self-punishment and blame* is the tendency to blame or condemn onself; anxiety about specific matters; apprehensiveness regarding vague future events; an attitude of self-deprecation; manifesting a depressed mood; expressing feelings of guilt and remorse; preoccupation with suicidal thoughts, unwanted ideas, and specific fears; and feeling unworthy or sinful.

This discussion of clusters of psychotic symptoms does not constitute diagnostic criteria for any psychotic disorder. It is given merely as a description of several types of symptoms in psychosis to give the reader an overview of the nature of behavioral disturbances associated with the various psychotic illnesses.

Schizophrenia

Although schizophrenia is perhaps the best known type of psychotic illness and the most common psychotic disorder, it is not synonymous with psychosis, but is just one of many causes of psychosis. Schizophrenia affects 1% of the population, and in the United States there are over 300,000 acute schizophrenic episodes annually. Between 25% and 50% of schizophrenia patients attempt suicide, and 10% eventually succeed, contributing to a mortality rate eight times greater than that of the general population.

In the United States, schizophrenic patients occupy 25% of all hospital beds and consume 40% of all long-term care days. Over 20% of all social security benefit days are used for the care of schizophrenic patients. The direct and indirect costs of schizophrenia in the United States alone are estimated to be in the tens of billions of dollars every year.

Schizophrenia by definition is a disturbance that must last for 6 months or longer, including at least 1 month of delusions, hallucinations, disorganized speech, grossly disorganized or catatonic behavior, or negative symptoms.

Delusions are erroneous beliefs that usually involve a misinterpretation of perceptions or experiences. The most common content of a delusion in schizophrenia is persecutory, but may include a variety of other themes including referential (i.e., erroneously thinking that something refers to oneself), somatic, religious, or grandiose. *Hallucinations* may occur in any sensory modality (e.g., auditory, visual, olfactory, gustatory, and tactile), but auditory hallucinations are by far the most common and characteristic hallucinations in schizophrenia.

Positive and negative symptoms of psychosis. Schizophrenia is actually a mixture of symptoms that are commonly called *positive and negative symptoms*. Positive symptoms seem to reflect an excess of normal functions, whereas negative symptoms reflect a diminution or loss of normal functions. *Positive symptoms* (Table 9–3) typically include delusions and hallucinations; they may also include distortions or exaggerations in language and communication (disorganized speech) as well as in behavioral monitoring (grossly disorganized or catatonic behavior). *Negative symptoms* (Table 9–4) include at least five types of symptoms all starting with the letter A:

Affective flattening – restrictions in the range and intensity of emotional expression
Alogia – restrictions in the fluency and productivity of thought and speech
Avolition – restrictions in the initiation of goal-directed behavior

Table 9-3. *Positive symptoms of psychosis*

Delusions
Hallucinations
Distortions or exaggerations in language and communication
Disorganized speech
Disorganized behavior
Catatonic behavior
Agitation

Table 9-4. *Negative symptoms of psychosis*

Blunted affect
Emotional withdrawal
Poor rapport
Passivity
Apathetic social withdrawal
Difficulty in abstract thinking
Lack of spontaneity
Stereotyped thinking
Affective flattening – restrictions in the range of intensity of emotional expression
Alogia – restrictions in the fluency and productivity of thought and speech
Avolition – restrictions in the initiation of goal-directed behavior
Anhedonia – lack of pleasure
Attentional impairment

Anhedonia – lack of pleasure
Attentional impairment

Negative symptoms in schizophrenia such as blunted affect, emotional with-drawal, poor rapport, passivity and apatahetic social withdrawal, difficulty in abstract thinking, lack of spontaneity, and stereotyped thinking are associated with long periods of hospitalization and poor social functioning.

Biological Basis of Positive Psychotic Symptoms

The biological basis of schizophrenia remains unknown. However, the biological basis of positive psychotic symptoms is believed to be linked to overactivity of dopamine neurons: specifically, the *mesolimbic dopamine pathway*. This system appears to account for positive psychotic symptoms whether those symptoms are part of the illness of schizophrenia, or of drug-induced psychosis, or whether positive psychotic symptoms accompany mania, depression, or dementia. The negative symptoms of schizophrenia may involve other regions of the brain such as the *dorsolateral prefrontal cortex* and other neurotransmitter systems. Indeed, the behavioral deficit state sug-gested by negative symptoms implies underactivity or even "burn-out" of some neuronal system. This may be related to excitotoxic overactivity of *glutamate systems* discussed in Chapter 4 (see Fig. 4–10 and also our discussion of neuroprotective agents in Chapter 11). In schizophrenia, the disorder can be progressive in some patients, also implying some ongoing degenerative process creating an ever-increasing deficit state.

Dopamine Hypothesis

For more than 20 years, it has been observed that diseases or drugs that increase dopamine will enhance or produce positive psychotic symptoms, whereas drugs that decrease dopamine will decrease or stop positive symptoms. For example, stimulant drugs such as amphetamine and cocaine release dopamine and, if given repetitively, can cause a paranoid psychosis virtually indistinguishable from schizophrenia. Also, all known antipsychotic drugs capable of treating positive psychotic symptoms are blockers of dopamine receptors, particularly D2 dopamine receptors. This is sometimes referred to as the dopamine hypothesis of schizophrenia. Perhaps a more precise modern designation is the mesolimbic dopamine hypothesis of positive psychotic symptoms, since it is believed that it is overactivity specifically in this dopamine pathway that mediates the positive symptoms of psychosis (Fig. 9–1). Likewise, it is blockade of the postsynaptic dopamine receptors specifically in this pathway that is thought to mediate the antipsychotic efficacy of the antipsychotic drugs and their ability to diminish or block positive psychotic symptoms (Fig. 9–2).

Four Dopamine Pathways in the Brain

The neuroanatomy of dopamine neuronal pathways in the brain can explain both the therapeutic effects and the side effects of the known antipsychotic agents. The four well-defined dopamine pathways in the brain are shown in Figure 9–3.

Mesolimbic dopamine pathway. The first of these pathways, namely the mesolimbic dopamine pathway, projects from the brainstem to limbic areas of the brain (Fig. 9–3), and is thought to control behaviors and especially to produce delusions and hallucinations when overactive (Fig. 9–1). When these pathways are shut down by blocking the postsynaptic dopamine receptors, it is hypothesized that this is what causes reduction of delusions and hallucinations (Figs. 9–2 and 9–4). When these pathways are turned on by stimulant drugs, schizophrenia, mania, depression, or cognitive disorders, the result is the same, namely delusions and hallucinations (Fig. 9–1).

Nigrostriatal dopamine pathway. Another key dopamine pathway in brain is the nigrostriatal dopamine pathway, which controls movements. When dopamine receptors are blocked in the postsynaptic projections of this dopamine system, it produces disorders of movement that can appear very much like those in Parkinson's disease, which is why these movements are sometimes called drug-induced parkinsonism (Fig. 9–4). Since the nigrostriatal pathway projects to basal ganglia, a part of the extrapyramidal neuronal system of the central nervous system, side effects associated with blockade of dopamine receptors there are sometimes also called extrapyramidal reactions (EPRs).

Descriptively, this is a type of stiff lack of movements sometimes referred to as "neurolepsis." The term "neuroleptic" was coined by the first clinicians to observe

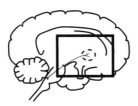

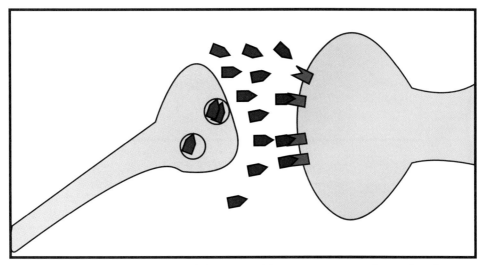

Mesolimbic overactivity = positive symptoms of psychosis

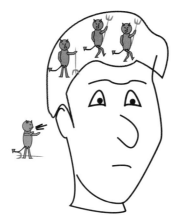

FIGURE 9–1. **The dopamine hypothesis of psychosis.** Overactivity of dopamine neurons in the mesolimbic dopamine pathway may mediate the positive symptoms of psychosis.

the behavioral syndrome caused when antipsychotic drugs were administered to patients, namely psychomotor slowing as well as emotional quieting and affective indifference. This has led to designation of the antipsychotic drugs that block dopamine receptors as "neuroleptics." In humans, neuroleptic antipsychotic drugs that block dopamine receptors in the nigrostriatal pathway cause movement disorders including akathisia (a type of restlessness), dystonia (twisting movements especially

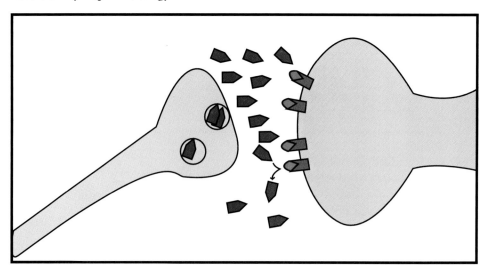

Mesolimbic pathway blocked = diminished positive
psychotic symptoms

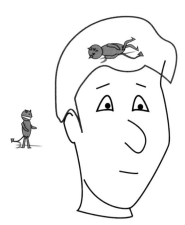

FIGURE 9–2. **The dopamine receptor antagonist hypothesis of antipsychotic drug action.**
Blockade of postsynaptic dopamine receptors in this pathway is thought to mediate the antipsychotic
efficacy of the antipsychotic drugs and their ability to diminish or block positive psychotic symptoms.

of the face and neck), tremor, rigidity, and akinesia/bradykinesia (i.e., lack of movement, or slowing of movement). Obviously, these effects of the antipsychotic neuroleptic agents are unwanted side effects, and are part of the price one has to pay
in order to get the therapeutic effects that come from simultaneously blocking the
mesolimbic dopamine pathway's postsynaptic dopamine receptors (Fig. 9–4).

Mesocortical dopamine pathway. A pathway related to the mesolimbic dopamine pathway is the mesocortical dopamine pathway (Fig. 9–4). Its role in mediating positive

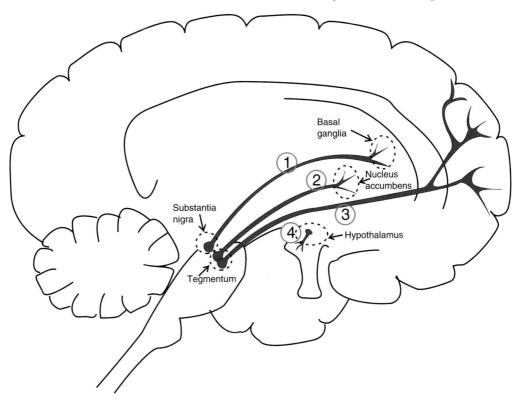

FIGURE 9–3. **Four dopamine pathways in the brain**. The neuroanatomy of dopamine neuronal pathways in the brain can explain both the therapeutic effects and the side effects of the known antipsychotic agents. (1) The **nigrostriatal dopamine pathway** projects from the substantia nigra to the basal ganglia, and is thought to control movements. (2) The **mesolimbic dopamine pathway** projects from the midbrain ventral tegmental area to the nucleus accumbens, a part of the limbic system of the brain thought to be involved in many behaviors, such as pleasurable sensations, the powerful euphoria of drugs of abuse, as well as delusions and hallucinations of psychosis. (3) A pathway related to the mesolimbic dopamine pathway is the **mesocortical dopamine pathway**. It also projects from the midbrain ventral tegmental area, but sends its axons to limbic cortex, where it may have a role in mediating positive and negative psychotic symptoms or cognitive side effects of neuroleptic antipsychotic medications. (4) The fourth dopamine pathway of interest is the one that controls prolactin secretion, called the **tuberoinfundibular dopamine pathway**. It projects from the hypothalamus to the anterior pituitary gland.

and negative psychotic symptoms and its reaction to neuroleptic antipsychotic medication is still a matter of debate. Some researchers believe that this pathway is involved along with the mesolimbic dopamine pathway in mediating positive psychotic symptoms, and perhaps negative symptoms of psychosis as well. This formulation hypothesizes that blockade of this pathway by neuroleptics is desired because it helps to reduce negative symptoms. A counter point of view is that conventional neuroleptic antipsychotic medications are not especially useful for the negative symptoms of schizophrenia, and in fact might produce blunting of emotions and various cognitive side effects due to blockade of dopamine receptors in this pathway that actually mimic negative symptoms themselves. Sometimes these cognitive side effects of neuroleptics are called the "neuroleptic-induced deficit syn-

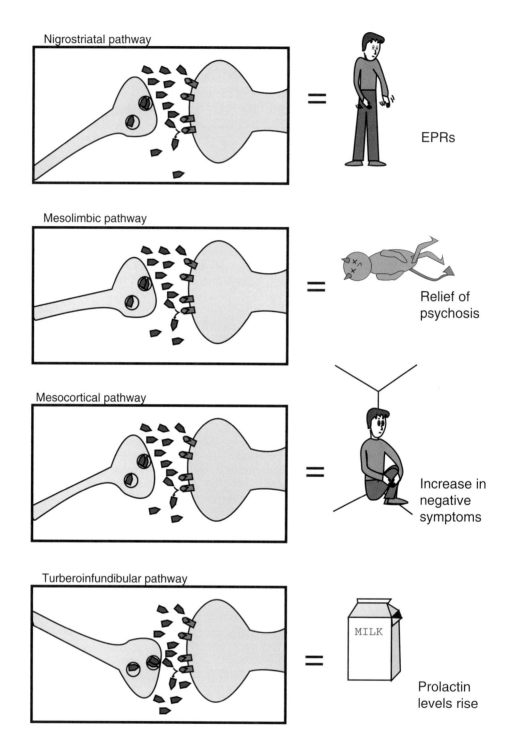

Nigrostriatal pathway

= EPRs

Mesolimbic pathway

= Relief of psychosis

Mesocortical pathway

= Increase in negative symptoms

Turberoinfundibular pathway

MILK

= Prolactin levels rise

drome," and was even recognized by the first clinicians when they coined the term neuroleptic as already mentioned. This deficit syndrome can be especially noticeable in patients who take neuroleptics and who have no underlying psychosis (such as Tourette's syndrome). The neuroleptic-induced deficit syndrome may be expressed in a schizophrenic patient who already has negative symptoms of psychosis as an exacerbation of these negative symptoms, and therefore can be easily confused with negative symptoms of psychosis.

It is easy to understand why there is so much debate about negative symptoms, dopamine activity, and the role of the neuroleptic drugs in improving or exacerbating negative symptoms of psychosis. To the extent that negative symptoms are the result of *overactivity* in the mesolimbic dopamine pathway, they should be improved by neuroleptics; to the extent that negative symptoms are the result of *underactivity and burnout* in the mesolimbic dopamine pathway, they should be worsened by neuroleptics.

Currently there is no resolution to this debate, as there is no consensus as to how well the conventional neuroleptics treat negative symptoms, the role neuroleptics have in actually producing side effects tantamount to a type of negative symptom of psychosis as the concomitant of reducing positive symptoms of psychosis, and finally whether the mesocortical dopamine pathway mediates positive or negative psychotic symptoms, or cognitive side effects of neuroleptic medication treatment. The pharmacological quandary here is what to do if one wishes simultaneously to decrease dopamine in order to treat positive psychotic symptoms theoretically mediated by the mesolimbic dopamine pathway and yet to increase dopamine to treat negative symptoms and avoid cognitive medication side effects mediated by the mesocortical dopamine pathway. This may be approachable by the use of partial dopamine agonists as will be discussed below.

Tuberoinfundibular dopamine pathway. A final dopamine pathway of interest is the one that controls prolactin secretion, called the tuberoinfundibular dopamine pathway (Fig. 9–4). When the dopamine receptors in this pathway are blocked, prolactin levels rise, sometimes so much so that women can begin lactating inappropriately, a condition known as galactorrhea.

FIGURE 9–4. Effects of dopamine receptor blocking neuroleptics in each of the four dopamine pathways. When dopamine receptors are blocked in the postsynaptic projections of the nigrostriatal pathway, it produces disorders of movement that can appear very much like those in Parkinson's disease, which is why these movements are sometimes called drug-induced parkinsonism. Since the nigrostriatal pathway projects to basal ganglia, a part of the extrapyramidal neuronal system of the central nervous system, side effects associated with blockade of dopamine receptors there are sometimes also called extrapyramidal reactions (EPRs). Shutting down the mesolimbic dopamine pathway by blocking the postsynaptic dopamine receptors there is what causes reduction of delusions and hallucinations. When dopamine receptors are blocked in the mesocortical dopamine pathway, it may produce blunting of emotions and various cognitive side effects that actually mimic negative symptoms themselves. Sometimes these cognitive side effects of neuroleptics are called the "neuroleptic-induced deficit syndrome." Finally, when the dopamine receptors in the tuberoinfundibular dopamine pathway are blocked, prolactin levels rise, sometimes so much so that women can begin lactating inappropriately, a condition known as galactorrhea.

The dopamine hypothesis of schizophrenia thus articulates not only a useful hypothesis about a neurobiological mechanism for psychosis and a psychopharmacological mechanism for antipsychotic drug action; it also describes a dilemma for the psychopharmacologist. That is, there is no doubt that the standard antipsychotic neuroleptic medications have been dramatic therapeutic agents for positive symptoms of psychosis since the 1950s, when they were first introduced. However, there are *four* dopamine pathways that exist in the brain, and it appears that blocking dopamine receptors in *only one* of them is useful, whereas blocking dopamine receptors in the remaining three pathways may be *harmful*.

Specifically, we have already emphasized that the theoretically useful action of the neuroleptics is to block mesolimbic dopamine pathways in order to reduce delusions and hallucinations (Fig. 9–4). However, the consequence of this is to block dopamine receptors in the three other dopamine pathways at a cost to the patient. Blocking tuberoinfundibular pathways means the elevation of prolactin levels and the possibility of galactorrhea (Fig. 9–4).

Blocking nigrostriatal dopamine pathways means the acute production of drug-induced parkinsonism, or EPRs, characterized by disorders of movement. As psychosis may be a chronic illness, and neuroleptics may need to be given for a long time, especially in schizophrenia, there can be long-term consequences to the blockade of dopamine receptors in the nigrostriatal pathway. The most immediate may be that the patient stops his medication to stop these highly undesirable side effects, especially akathisia, ridigity, and tremor.

Worse yet is the fact that long-term blockade of nigrostriatal dopamine receptors by chronic treatment with neuroleptics can cause a disfiguring and potentially irreversible movement disorder, namely a condition called *tardive dyskinesia*. Tardive dyskinesia is a set of hyperkinetic movements, especially of the face, neck, and extremities. This can include such movements as lip smacking, chewing, tongue protrusions, facial grimacing, and rapid limb movements. It is thought that tardive dyskinesia is caused by the consequences of long-term dopamine receptor blockade in the nigrostriatal dopamine pathway, causing the neurons there to up-regulate their postsynaptic dopamine receptors in a futile attempt to overcome drug-induced blockade of these receptors (Fig. 9–5). The consequence of this up-regulation may be tardive dyskinesia. If the receptor blockade is removed early enough, tardive dyskinesia may reverse, theoretically due to decreases in the dopamine receptors once the receptor blockers are removed. However, in long-term cases, the dopamine receptors apparently cannot or do not reset, even when neuroleptics are removed, leading to an irreversible condition of tardive dyskinesia, whether neuroleptics are administered or not.

A final problem of blocking every dopamine receptor in the brain when a neuroleptic is administered is to block mesocortical dopamine receptors. This has already been discussed and is shown schematically in Figure 9–4. Whereas we have mentioned that some evidence may suggest that this would be good, either to aid in the reduction of positive symptoms, or to decrease negative symptoms, there is other evidence to suggest that blocking dopamine receptors here is counterproductive, either by worsening negative symptoms or by producing cognitive blunting due to a neuroleptic-induced deficit state (Fig. 9–4). Since this mesocortical dopamine pathway may already be underactive and mediating negative symptoms, blocking it may well only reduce it more and produce even a greater amount of negative symptoms (Fig. 9–4).

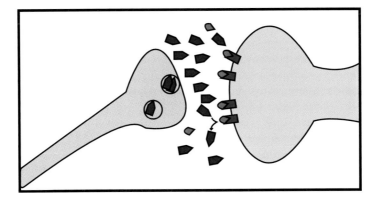

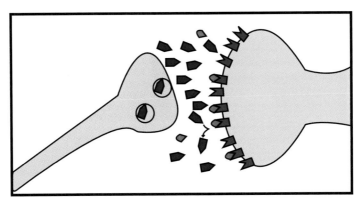

FIGURE 9–5. Long-term **blockade** of dopamine receptors in the nigrostriatal dopamine pathway (*upper panel*) may cause them to **up-regulate**. The clinical consequence of this may be the hyperkinetic movement disorder known as **tardive dyskinesia** (*lower panel*). This up-regulation may be the consequence of the neuron's futile attempt to overcome drug-induced blockade of its dopamine receptors.

Thus, there is a painful trade-off in using the neuroleptics. For patients with a malignant psychotic illness characterized by the devastation of their lives by positive symptoms of delusions and hallucinations, the neuroleptics are a merciful treatment, alleviating this type of suffering. On the other hand, the price to be paid is the simultaneous production of acute EPRs (most cases), chronic tardive dyskinesia (common), possible galactorrhea (rare), and even deterioration in negative symptoms (theoretical). There is even the possibility of a rare but potentially fatal complication called the neuroleptic malignant syndrome, associated with extreme muscular rigidity, high fevers, coma, and even death. These significant limitations to the treatment of psychosis have ignited a research effort to find better therapeutics, which will be discussed later in this volume following a description of the standard neuroleptics.

Summary

In this chapter we have given a clinical description of psychosis, with special emphasis on the psychotic illness schizophrenia. We have explained the dopamine hypothesis of schizophrenia, which is the major hypothesis for explaining the mechanism for the positive symptoms of psychosis (delusions and hallucinations).

The four major dopamine pathways in the brain have been described, including antipsychotic drug actions upon dopamine receptors in each of these pathways. The mesolimbic dopamine system may mediate the positive symptoms of psychosis; the mesocortical system, negative symptoms of psychosis or of antipsychotic agents; the nigrostriatal system, extrapyramidal muscular reactions and tardive dyskinesia; and the tuberoinfundibular system, the control of plasma prolactin levels.

CHAPTER 10

CONVENTIONAL NEUROLEPTIC DRUGS FOR SCHIZOPHRENIA AND NOVEL ANTIPSYCHOTIC AGENTS

This chapter will explore the various drug treatments of psychotic disorders, with a special emphasis on schizophrenia. Such treatments include not only the traditional antipsychotic drugs but also a look into the future at the drugs under development and those that are theoretical possibilities. The traditional treatments of psychosis are antipsychotic drugs of the neuroleptic class, which block dopamine receptors, as discussed in the Chapter 9. The specifics of antipsychotic drug treatment will differ, of course, depending upon which psychotic disorder is under treatment (i.e., schizophrenia or another psychotic disorder). Also, antipsychotic treatments can vary notably in terms of specific antipsychotic drug, dose, duration of treatment, and combinations with additional psychotropic medications. The reader is referred to standard reference manuals and textbooks for such information.

As in previous chapters, this chapter on antipsychotic drugs will emphasize basic pharmacological concepts of mechanism of action. The pharmacological concepts developed here should help the reader understand the rationale for use of antipsychotic agents. This rationale will be developed from a pharmacological perspective of how drugs for schizophrenia and the psychoses may interact with different neurotransmitter systems in the central nervous system to exert their therapeutic actions.

Antipsychotic Drugs

Treatments for schizophrenia and other psychotic illnesses have arisen both from serendipitous clinical observations and from scientific knowledge of the neurobiological basis of psychosis. These approaches are currently accelerating the pace at which new therapeutic agents for schizophrenia are being developed. Here we will review not only those classical neuroleptic antipsychotic agents already in use for the treatment of psychosis but also the wide-ranging research efforts to find new drug therapies. We will also review modern therapeutic approaches that are still concepts and have not yet led to specific drugs but which have considerable long-term promise.

Conventional Antipsychotic Treatments: The Neuroleptics

The first antipsychotic drugs were discovered by accident in the 1950s, when a drug thought to be an antihistamine (chlorpromazine) was serendipitously observed to have unique antipsychotic effects when the putative "antihistamine" was tested in schizophrenic patients. Chlorpromazine indeed has some antihistaminic activity, but also has more important activity at dopamine receptors. It even has additional but generally unwanted activity at alpha adrenergic receptors and muscarinic cholinergic receptors (Fig. 10–1). Just as is the case for the classical tricyclic antidepressants (see Fig. 6–13), the classical antipsychotic neuroleptic drugs have activities at three neurotransmitter receptors that turn out to mediate their side effects but not their therapeutic effects, namely antihistamine properties (weight gain), alpha adrenergic blocking properties (cardiovascular side effects), and muscarinic cholinergic blocking properties (dry mouth, blurred vision, and constipation) (see Fig. 10–2).

Once chlorpromazine was observed to be an effective antipsychotic agent, it was tested experimentally to try to discover its mechanism of action. Early in the testing process, chlorpromazine and other antipsychotic agents were all found to cause "neurolepsis" in experimental animals. New neuroleptics were discovered largely by their ability to produce this effect. It was not until many years later, perhaps in the late 1960s and 1970s, that it was widely recognized that all the known neuroleptics at that time shared the common property of blocking dopamine receptors, particularly dopamine-2 (D2) receptors (Fig. 10–2 and Table 10–1).

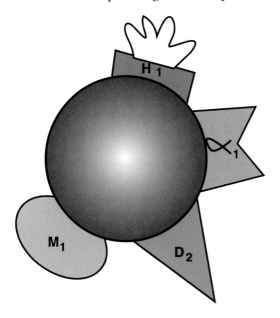

FIGURE 10–1. This figure represents a **typical neuroleptic drug**. Such drugs are conventional antipsychotic agents that have at least **four actions**: blockade of dopamine-2 receptors (**D2**), blockade of muscarinic cholinergic receptors (**M1**), blockade of alpha adrenergic receptors (**alpha** 1), and blockade of histamine receptors (antihistaminic actions [**H1**]).

The various antipsychotic agents differ in terms of their ability to block the various receptors represented in Figure 10–1. Because of this, neuroleptics differ in their side-effect profiles, but not overall in their therapeutic profiles. Some neuroleptics are more sedating than others; some neuroleptics have more ability to cause cardiovascular side effects than others; and some neuroleptics are more potent than others. However, all neuroleptics reduce psychotic symptoms – especially positive psychotic symptoms – about equally in groups of schizophrenic patients in multicenter trials. That is not to say that one individual patient might not respond better to one neuroleptic agent rather than another, but there is no recognized difference in the efficacies among all the typical neuroleptic agents when tested in large groups of patients.

All typical neuroleptic agents are capable of producing extrapyramidal reactions (EPRs) (see Fig. 9–4) and tardive dyskinesia (see Fig. 9–5), both of which derive from the dopamine-2 receptor blocking properties of the typical neuroleptics (Figs. 10–1 and 10–2). Thus, this dopamine-2 receptor antagonism mediates not only the therapeutic effects of antipsychotic agents but also some of the side effects of these very same agents, as discussed above and shown in Figure 9–4.

Some neuroleptics have a greater propensity to produce extrapyramidal side effects (mediated by dopamine-2 receptor blockade in the nigrostriatal pathway) than others. Those neuroleptics that cause more EPRs are the agents that have only *weak* anticholinergic properties. Those neuroleptics that can cause fewer EPRs are the agents that have *stronger* anticholinergic properties. Thus, anticholinergic agents are frequently given to patients who are taking neuroleptic agents in order to reduce EPRs.

How does cholinergic receptor blockade reduce the EPRs caused by dopamine receptor blockade? The reason seems to be that dopamine and acetylcholine have a reciprocal relationship to each other in the nigrostriatal pathway (see Figs. 10–3, 10–4, and 10–5). Dopamine neurons in the nigrostriatal dopamine pathway make

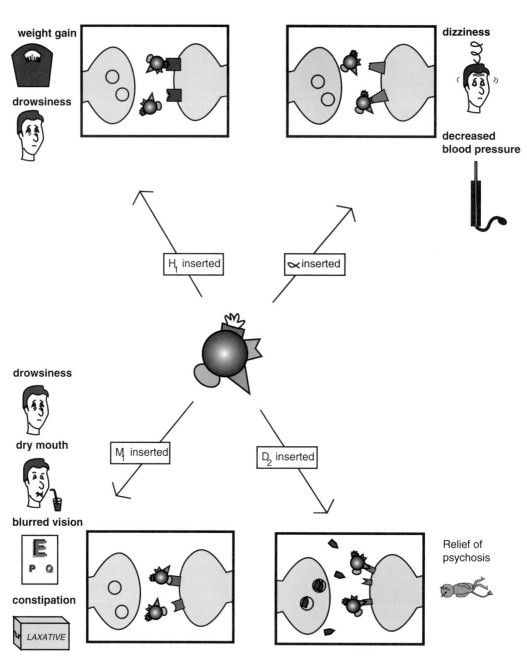

FIGURE 10–2. Shown here are the actions of a conventional antipsychotic drug in mediating both its **therapeutic actions** and its **side effects**. Thus, dopamine-2 (**D2**) antagonist properties are therapeutic and lead to **relief of psychosis**; however, side effects are mediated by the other actions of a conventional antipsychotic drug. These are the results of histamine receptor blockade (antihistaminic properties [**H1**]), causing **weight gain** and **drowsiness**; alpha 1 receptor blockade causing **dizziness** and **decreased blood pressure**; and anticholinergic (muscarinic [**M1**]) blockade causing **drowsiness, dry mouth, blurred vision,** and **constipation**.

Table 10–1. *Agents used to treat psychosis and schizophrenia in the United States*

Generic name	Trade Name	Action
Acetophenazine	Tindal	Typical neuroleptic
Carphenazine	Proketazine	Typical neuroleptic
Chlorpromazine	Thorazine	Typical neuroleptic
Chlorprothixene	Taractan	Typical neuroleptic
Clozapine	Clozaril	Atypical
Fluphenazine	Prolixin; Permitil	Typical neuroleptic
Haloperidol	Haldol	Typical neuroleptic
Loxapine	Loxitane	Typical neuroleptic
Mesoridazine	Serentil	Typical neuroleptic
Molindone	Moban; Lidone	Typical neuroleptic
Perphenazine	Trilafon	Typical neuroleptic
Pimozide	Orap	Typical neuroleptic[a]
Piperacetazine	Quide	Typical neuroleptic
Prochlorperazine	Compazine	Typical neuroleptic[b]
Risperidone	Risperdal	SDA (serotonin dopamine antagonist)
Thioridazine	Mellaril	Typical neuroleptic
Thiothixene	Navane	Typical neuroleptic
Trifluoperazine	Stelazine	Typical neuroleptic
Triflupromazine	Vesprin	Typical neuroleptic

[a]Approved in the United States for Tourette's syndrome.

[b]Approved in the United States for nausea and vomiting as well as psychosis.

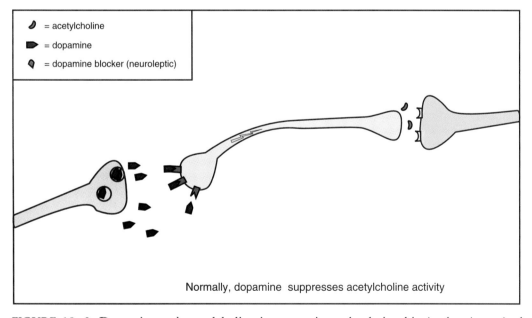

FIGURE 10–3. **Dopamine** and **acetylcholine** have a **reciprocal relationship** in the nigrostriatal dopamine pathway. Dopamine neurons here make postsynaptic connections with cholinergic neurons. Normally, dopamine suppresses acetylcholine activity.

267

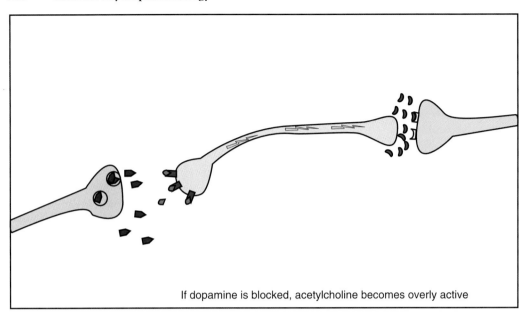

If dopamine is blocked, acetylcholine becomes overly active

FIGURE 10–4. This figure shows what happens to acetylcholine activity when **dopamine receptors are blocked**. Since dopamine normally suppresses acetylcholine activity, removal of this causes an increase in acetylcholine activity. Thus, if dopamine receptors are blocked, **acetylcholine becomes overly active**. This is associated with the production of extrapyramidal reactions (EPRs). The pharmacological mechanism of EPRs therefore seems to be dopamine deficiency and acetylcholine excess.

postsynaptic connections with cholinergic neurons (Fig. 10–3). Dopamine normally *blocks* acetylcholine release from postsynaptic nigrostriatal cholinergic neurons, thus suppressing acetylcholine activity there (Fig. 10–3). If dopamine can no longer suppress acetylcholine release because dopamine receptors are being blocked by a neuroleptic drug, then acetylcholine becomes overly active (Fig. 10–4).

One compensation for this overactivity of acetylcholine is to block it with an anticholinergic agent (Fig. 10–5). Thus, anticholinergics will overcome the excess acetylcholine activity caused by removal of dopamine inhibition when dopamine receptors are blocked by neuroleptics (Fig. 10–5).

This has led to the strategy of giving anticholinergic agents along with neuroleptics in order to reduce the EPRs caused by neuroleptics. As some neuroleptics have a bit of anticholinergic built into their molecules (Fig. 10–1), this tends to reduce the EPRs caused by the other property of dopamine receptor blockade by the same drug. Thus, depending upon the relative amounts of dopamine receptor blockade and acetylcholine receptor blockade, one neuroleptic will have a greater or lesser ability to cause EPRs.

Theoretically, other pharmacological agents that boost dopamine could also help reverse EPRs as they do in Parkinson's disease, but at the expense of increasing dopamine as well in the mesolimbic area and possibly increasing positive symptoms of psychosis. In fact, amantadine, which is an antiparkinsonian agent capable of releasing dopamine, can help reverse EPRs in drug-induced parkinsonism without

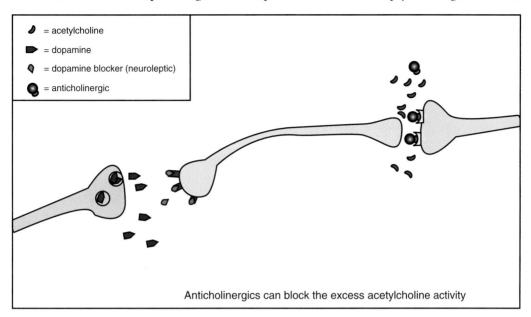

FIGURE 10–5. One **compensation** for the overactivity of acetylcholine that occurs when dopamine receptors are blocked is to block them as well with an **anticholinergic agent**. Thus, anticholinergics overcome excess acetylcholine activity caused by removal of dopamine inhibition when dopamine receptors are blocked by neuroleptics. This also means that extrapyramidal reactions (EPRs) are reduced.

necessarily causing a worsening of psychosis. In practice, anticholinergic agents are the agents most frequently used concomitantly with neuroleptics in order to increase the tolerability of the antipsychotic agents by making them cause less troublesome EPRs (Fig. 10–5). Unfortunately, this concomitant use of anticholinergic agents does not lessen the ability of these same neuroleptics to ultimately cause tardive dyskinesia (Fig. 9–5).

Long-term use of antipsychotic drugs. All of the typical neuroleptic agents show the ability to reduce positive psychotic symptoms after several weeks of treatment. Withdrawal of neuroleptic agents causes relapse of psychosis in patients with schizophrenia, at the rate of approximately 10% per month, so that 50% or more have relapsed by 6 months after discontinuation of neuroleptic agents. Consequently, long-term treatment with antipsychotics may be indicated in schizophrenia, where the illness is projected to be long term, but not in illnesses where the psychosis may be short term or intermittent.

Thus, a "neuroleptic-sparing strategy" should be taken in any case where the risks of long-term treatment are not justified. This is often true, for example, in psychotic depression, which may not require long-term neuroleptic treatment once the illness is stabilized. On the other hand, it is all too frequent in schizophrenia that the benefit of treating psychosis justifies the side effects of neuroleptics. Psychosis can be even more malignant than the risk of tardive dyskinesia, leading to the reluctant if necessary continuation of neuroleptic treatment despite the presence of short- and long-term side effects, including tardive dyskinesia.

Long-term side effects have led to the pursuit of neuroleptic treatments that would reduce or eliminate such problems yet still be powerful antipsychotic agents for positive symptoms of psychosis. Troublesome side effects also lead to noncompliance, since patients frequently wish to discontinue their medications to rid themselves of the side effects, despite high risk of relapse of psychotic symptoms.

Atypical Antipsychotics

The first attempt to improve the therapeutic profile of the classical typical neuroleptic drugs was based upon research which showed that dopamine receptors in the nigrostriatal dopamine pathway mediate the extrapyramidal side effects of neuroleptics, but that the dopamine receptors in the mesolimbic dopamine pathway are more likely to mediate the antipsychotic therapeutic actions of neuroleptics (see Fig. 9–4). Drug discovery efforts have therefore sought to find agents that are more selective for mesolimbic dopamine receptors than for nigrostriatal dopamine receptors (Fig. 10–6), in order to generate theoretically an improved side-effect profile. Hints that this might be a useful approach derive from clinical observations of certain neuroleptics already used in clinical practice. The reputedly "atypical" neuroleptics thioridazine and sulpiride, for example, seem to have less propensity to produce extrapyramidal side effects, while still showing good antipsychotic properties when compared to "typical" neuroleptic agents such as thorazine or haloperidol. Thus, the term "atypical" was coined and first applied to the concept of typical efficacy with atypical side effects.

A series of benzamide compounds structurally related to sulpiride have been synthesized and have been found to exhibit the desired "atypical profile" of preference for mesolimbic over nigrostriatal dopamine receptors in animal models (Fig. 10–6). Several of these have been tested in schizophrenia patients, and the first of these to come into clinical practice is remoxipride (Roxiam), which was introduced in Europe and Canada but then withdrawn from the market and never sold in the United States because of reports associating it with aplastic anemia. A related compound, raclopride, is more potent than remoxipride, has been a useful tool in positron emission tomography (PET) scan studies, and may eventually enter the market as an atypical neuroleptic upon completion of clinical testing now in progress.

Other atypical neuroleptics with promising profiles in animal models are melperone and zotepine. Clinical testing of these particular compounds is either incomplete or suspended; thus, they are unlikely to be marketed, at least in the United States, according to current projections.

FIGURE 10–6. This figure demonstrates the concept of **atypical neuroleptic** drugs more selective for mesolimbic pathway dopamine receptors than for nigrostriatal pathway dopamine receptors. A typical neuroleptic agent blocks dopamine receptors equally in both the nigrostriatal and the mesolimbic dopamine pathways. However, an atypical neuroleptic theoretically blocks mesolimbic pathways preferentially to nigrostriatal dopamine pathways. Thus, atypical neuroleptics should have the same efficacy of a typical neuroleptic, but less of a propensity to produce extrapyramidal side effects.

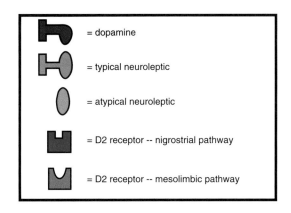

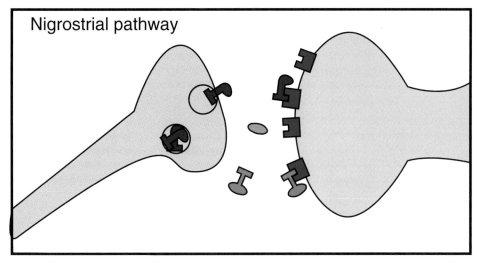

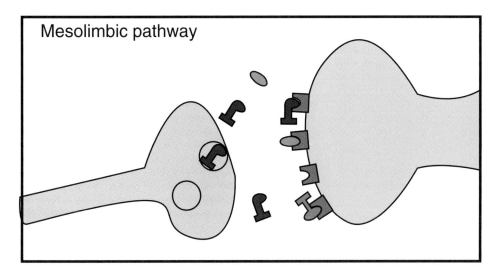

Clozapine, A Drug Class in Itself

Clozapine was recognized for its atypical clinical properties soon after its introduction into clinical practice in Europe. Clozapine is thus an atypical neuroleptic in the sense that it has few if any extrapyramidal side effects in addition to being an effective antipsychotic. Also, it does not seem to cause tardive dyskinesia.

Clozapine also came to be recognized as unusual in another key manner, namely that it can be more effective than typical neuroleptics, especially in patients who have failed to respond adequately to conventional neuroleptics. Some investigators have expanded the concept of "atypical" to being that of *enhanced efficacy* as well as *diminished side effects* compared to typical neuroleptics, and as exemplified uniquely by clozapine. However, as the atypical efficacy of clozapine was being revealed, so was its atypical risk profile, namely the possibility of developing a life-threatening and occasionally fatal complication called agranulocytosis.

These unusually favorable therapeutic properties accompanied by unusually unfavorable side effects have spawned a race for a clozapine-like compound, but which would not have clozapine's dangerous bone marrow toxicity (agranulocytosis). In order to do this, pharmacologists have been attempting to define what it is about clozapine's biochemical mechanism of action that makes it "clozapine-like" and different from other neuroleptics. Apparently, site-selective action on mesolimbic versus nigrostriatal dopamine receptors is not sufficient to explain this, since "atypical" neuroleptics such as the benzamides discussed above may have an improved side-effect profile, but there is no evidence to suggest that they have the special efficacy properties of clozapine.

Clozapine is one of the most complicated drugs in psychopharmacology. So far, it is known to have notable interactions with at least nine neurotransmitter receptors (Fig. 10–7). It is not known which of these or which combinations of these may be the mediators of clozapine's special clinical efficacy. As mentioned above, along with the good news about clozapine's efficacy is the bad news that it can cause a potentially fatal bone marrow toxicity known as agranulocytosis. This means in practice that patients' complete blood counts must be monitored vigilantly to detect the possibility of this complication developing, and stopping the drug immediately, instituting appropriate supportive therapy.

Fortunately, it does not seem that any of the nine neurotransmitter receptors mediate this serious adverse reaction to clozapine, so that it is theoretically possible to attain the same efficacy of clozapine without the agranulocytosis risk of clozapine by changing the chemical structure of the drug, but not the pharmacological properties. The quandary is which pharmacological properties of clozapine to retain for its special efficacy, and which to remove to improve the side-effect profile (such as seizures, sedation, hypotension, as well as agranulocytosis).

The efforts to find clozapine-like antipsychotic agents that retain the efficacy of clozapine but factor out the undesired side effects of clozapine will now be reviewed. Current attempts to find clozapine-like drugs can be summarized largely as variations on the theme of targeting dopamine and serotonin receptors selectively and in combinations, since six of the nine known neurotransmitter interactions of the clozapine molecules are upon dopamine or 5-hydroxytryptamine (5HT; serotonin) receptor subtypes (Fig. 10–7).

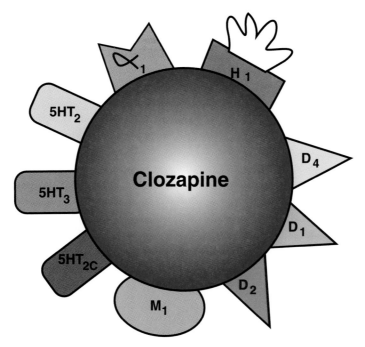

FIGURE 10–7. **Clozapine** is one of the most **complicated** drugs in psychopharmacology. So far, it is known to have interactions with at least **nine neurotransmitter receptors**. None of these nine actions seem to explain the agranulocytosis caused by clozapine in some patients. Three of the receptor actions may account predominantly for **side effects**, similar to those discussed earlier for tricyclic antidepressants (Fig. 6–13) and typical neuroleptics (Fig. 10–1), namely blockade of **alpha 1** receptors, histamine 1 (**H1**) receptors, and (**M1**) muscarinic 1 receptors. Six of the known receptor interactions for clozapine are at various dopamine and serotonin receptor subtypes. Some combination of these actions at serotonin and dopamine receptors probably accounts for the therapeutic actions of clozapine. The quandary is which pharmacological properties of clozapine account for its special efficacy in patients who do not respond to conventional antipsychotic agents.

The Search for Clozapine-like Drugs: Variations on the Theme of Targeting Dopamine and 5HT Receptor Subtypes Selectively

Serotonin-dopamine antagonists. Scientists are actively looking for the neurobiological basis of clozapine's unique clinical actions. The leading hypothesis is that some unique aspect of dopamine and serotonin pharmacology mediate clozapine's unique clinical actions. The most prominent theory is that simultaneous blockade of dopamine-2 receptors and 5HT2 receptors accounts for the unique properties of clozapine (Fig. 10–8). This possibility has already led to the clinical testing of a plethora of related drugs, now known as serotonin-dopamine antagonists (SDAs). These include risperidone, olanzepine, sertindole, ziprasidone, seroquel, iloperidone, ORG-5222, amperozide, savoxepine, among others.

The individual members within the SDA series differ from one another in the relative amounts of dopamine-2 versus 5HT2 receptors they block at a given dose. Drugs in this class also differ from one another in their blockade of additional receptors such as alpha adrenergic, muscarinic, and histaminic receptors. Generally,

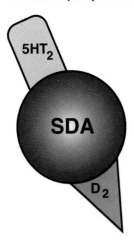

FIGURE 10–8. Serotonin-2 antagonist – dopamine-2 antagonist (SDA) agents combine a dual blocking action at these two receptors. The addition of novel serotonin-2 receptor antagonist properties to the conventional dopamine-2 receptor antagonist properties of typical neuroleptics may produce a pharmacological profile of improved efficacy for negative symptoms of schizophrenia or improved side-effect profile of reducing extrapyramidal reactions (EPRs), especially at lower doses.

these latter receptors are considered to be responsible for various side effects rather than for therapeutic effects. However, some investigators believe that alpha receptors may be involved to some extent in mediating therapeutic effects of antipsychotic agents. Clozapine is a powerful blocker of all these receptors as well, but the SDA hypothesis considers these actions of clozapine at muscarinic, alpha, and histamine receptors to be irrelevant to clozapine's desired properties. It is hoped that the SDAs can deliver the special efficacy of clozapine without the undesired bone marrow toxicity.

One of the possibilities of how SDAs may mediate the special properties of clozapine is that there may be less blockade of dopamine-2 receptors required for therapeutic action in schizophrenia when 5HT2 receptors are blocked simultaneously. PET scanning techniques (using radiolabeled neuroleptics to bind dopamine-2 sites in the caudate and 5HT2 sites in the cortex) are beginning to clarify how much blockade of dopamine-2 and 5HT2 receptors is optimal.

That is, approximately 70 to 90% of dopamine-2 receptors are blocked at therapeutic doses of typical neuroleptics (Fig. 10–9A), but only 30 to 60% of dopamine-2 receptors are blocked at therapeutic doses of clozapine (Fig. 10–10A). PET scanning studies are in progress now for some of the new SDAs in clinical trials, also attempting to explore how much 5HT2 receptor blockade is occurring simultaneously with dopamine-2 receptor blockade. Thus, 85 to 90% of 5HT2 receptors are blocked by a dose of clozapine (Fig. 10–10B) that simultaneously blocks only 20% or so of dopamine-2 receptors (Fig. 10–10A). On the other hand, essentially no serotonin receptors are blocked (Fig. 10–9B) by an antipsychotic dose of haloperidol that blocks more than 80% of dopamine-2 receptors (Fig. 10–9A). Evidently, the atypical neuroleptic thioridazine also blocks a high percentage of 5HT2 receptors, as it simultaneously blocks a high percentage of dopamine-2 receptors.

Early studies with the novel, recently marketed SDA risperidone suggest that an antipsychotic dose blocks approximately 60% of 5HT2 receptors (Fig. 10–11B) and, simultaneously, 50% of dopamine-2 receptors (Fig. 10–11A). The ability to study blockade of dopamine-2 receptors and 5HT2 receptors in vivo with PET scanning techniques in schizophrenic patients is helping to clarify what the optimal profile is for an SDA in terms of relative receptor blockade that is desired. One thing that

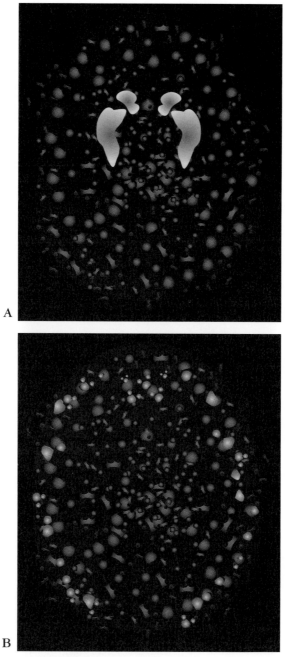

FIGURE 10–9. Simulation of PET scans demonstrating blockade of dopamine-2 (D2) receptors and serotonin-2 (5HT2) receptors by typical neuroleptics. At therapeutic doses, typical neuroleptics block 70 to 90% of D2 receptors (*A*) but virtually no 5HT2 receptors (*B*).

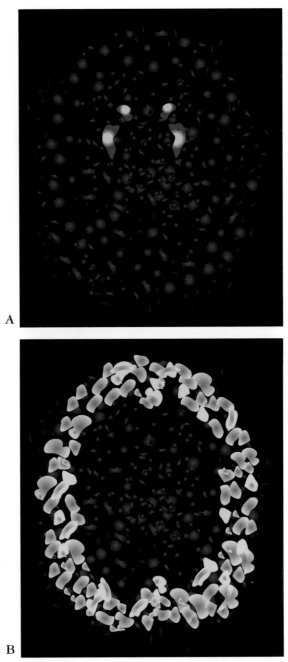

A

B

FIGURE 10–10. Simulation of **PET scans demonstrating blockade of dopamine-2 (D2) receptors and serotonin-2 (5HT2) receptors by clozapine.** In contrast to typical neuroleptics, clozapine blocks only 20 to 60% of D2 receptors (*A*) and 85 to 90% of 5HT2 receptors (*B*) at therapeutic doses.

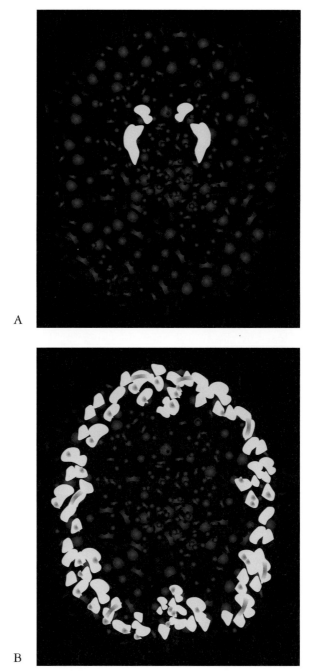

A

B

FIGURE 10–11. **Simulation of PET scans demonstrating blockade of dopamine-2 (D2) receptors (A) and serotonin-2 (5HT2) receptors (B) by serotonin-dopamine antagonists (SDAs).** Like clozapine, but unlike typical neuroleptics, SDAs block 5HT2 receptors. At therapeutic doses of SDAs, perhaps 60% of 5HT2 receptors (B) and 50% of D2 receptors (A) are blocked.

appears evident from clinical trials so far is that some degree of dopamine-2 antagonism is desired, since the pure 5HT2 antagonist ritanserin, which does not block dopamine-2 receptors at all, appears to have little efficacy in positive symptoms of schizophrenia, although it may reduce negative symptoms and not induce extrapyramidal side effects.

5HT2 receptor interactions in the basal ganglia may also explain why the SDAs apparently have less propensity to produce EPRs, especially at lower doses. This may relate to the interaction of dopamine and serotonin in the basal ganglia already discussed in relationship to serotonin selective reuptake inhibitors (SSRIs) and obsessive compulsive disorder (OCD) (Figs. 8–1, 8–2, and 8–3). In the case of SDAs, it appears that these agents may exploit the difference in the wiring of dopamine and serotonin in various parts of the brain. That is, in the basal ganglia, serotonin input to the nigrostriatal dopamine neuron causes the dopamine neuron to be inhibited by serotonin neurotransmission working through postsynaptic 5HT2 receptors on presynaptic dopaminergic nerve terminals (Fig. 8–2). This type of serotonin input appears to be lacking in the mesolimbic dopamine area.

Thus, when dopamine receptors are blocked in the mesolimbic dopamine pathway by the D2 blocking properties of the SDAs, they would theoretically reduce psychosis (see Figs. 9–2 and 9–4). When they similarly block D2 receptors in the nigrostriatal pathway, they also block the 5HT2 receptors that are also there (see Fig. 9–4). Thus, the 5HT2 blockade tends to reverse the effects of D2 blockade, but only in the nigrostriatal system (Fig. 10–12), and not in the mesolimbic system (see Figs. 9–2 and 9–4). D2 receptors are blocked everywhere in the brain by the SDAs, but the simultaneous blocking of 5HT2 only in the nigrostriatal area turns on DA release, which uniquely has the possibility of overcoming the D2 blockade in this specific area of the brain (Fig. 10–12). This may explain why SDAs have less propensity to produce EPRs than do D2 antagonists that lack 5HT2 antagonist properties. It may also explain why the 5HT2 properties do not similarly mitigate dopamine receptor blockade and therefore dilute antipsychotic efficacy in the mesolimbic DA pathway, since there is no similar 5HT neuronal input there.

Many clinical trials are now in progress for the numerous SDAs listed above, but it is too early to tell how advantageous the SDAs will be compared to clozapine or to the conventional neuroleptic antipsychotic agents. Currently, it is well established that the first drug in this class, risperidone, has clinical efficacy comparable to haloperidol in schizophrenia. There are indications of an improved side-effect profile compared to haloperidol as well, but this is not as well established as its efficacy. Also, risperidone has not yet been demonstrated to be superior to typical neuroleptics in efficacy, nor comparable to clozapine in refractory cases. Such studies are in progress now that risperidone has entered marketing in various countries including the United States. Several other SDAs are now demonstrating clinical efficacy superior to placebo and comparable to typical neuroleptics such as haloperidol, but are not yet marketed.

It is generally only after marketing that the truly unique properties of new therapeutic agents for schizophrenia are identified. The possibility that SDAs are clozapine-like is beginning to be investigated, as are other aspects, and it is hoped that the SDAs will become differentiated more clearly from the typical neuroleptics and perhaps in ways not yet recognized from clozapine.

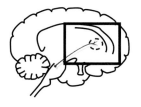

If 5HT is blocked, it increases
DA release, thus reversing the effects
of D2 blockade.

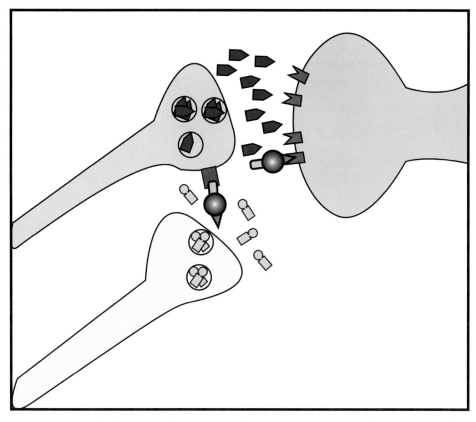

FIGURE 10–12. **Serotonin-dopamine interactions in the basal ganglia and the effects of se-rotonin-dopamine antagonists (SDAs).** Serotonin-2 (5HT2) receptor interactions in the basal ganglia may explain why the SDAs apparently have less propensity to produce extrapyramidal reactions (EPRs), especially at lower doses. Serotonin input to nigrostriatal dopamine neurons in the basal ganglia normally causes dopamine neurons to be inhibited by serotonin neurotransmission working through postsynaptic 5HT2 receptors on presynaptic dopaminergic nerve terminals (see Fig. 8–2). This type of serotonin input appears to be lacking in the mesolimbic dopamine area. Thus, when dopamine receptors are blocked in the mesolimbic dopamine pathway by the D2 blocking properties of the SDAs, they would theoretically reduce psychosis. When they similarly block D2 receptors in the nigrostriatal pathway, however, they also block the 5HT2 receptors that are there. Thus, the 5HT2 blockade tends to reverse the effects of D2 blockade, but only in the nigrostriatal system, and not in the mesolimbic system. This may explain why SDAs have less propensity to produce EPRs than do D2 antagonists, which lack 5HT2 antagonist properties. It may also explain why the 5HT2 properties do not similarly mitigate dopamine receptor blockade and therefore dilute antipsychotic efficacy in the mesolimbic dopamine pathway, since there is no similar 5HT neuronal input there.

Dopamine-4 antagonists. Receptor subtyping for dopamine receptors is proceding at a fast pace, as molecular biology is identifying unique genes for multiple subtypes. There are at least five pharmacological subtypes of dopamine receptors, each with multiple possible additional molecular isoforms. Mapping the properties of clozapine across these receptor subtypes, it appears to be a more powerful antagonist of D4 receptors than the typical neuroleptics. Interestingly, some of the SDAs also have powerful antagonist properties at D4 receptors. The hunt is now on for drugs that are selective antagonists for D4 receptors and no other receptor, to see if such agents would have special advantages in schizophrenia (Fig. 10–13).

Dopamine-1 antagonists. Clozapine also blocks D1 receptors, and queries have been posed whether a selective D1 antagonist, which has no actions at any other receptor, would be a useful treatment in schizophrenia (Fig. 10–13). The prototype agent is SCH-23390, but it has poor bioavailability and has not progressed in clinical development. It has been used as a preclinical pharmacological tool and a prototype for other agents in earlier development, such as SCH-39166. Clinical testing of selective D1 antagonists in schizophrenia is still in progress.

Dopamine partial agonists. An interesting new concept in pharmacology is that of dopamine partial agonists. These compounds mimic the naturally occurring neurotransmitter dopamine, which is a full agonist; however, the partial agonists generate only a portion of the response that the full agonist dopamine generates (thus the designation *partial* agonist). Partial agonists can exist for any neurotransmitter and have the interesting property of being either an agonist or an antagonist, depending upon the amount of naturally occurring full agonist present. This is discussed extensively in Chapter 3 on special properties of receptors, and in Chapter 7 on anxiolytics and serotonin 1A partial agonists. In an analogous sense, a dopamine partial agonist would be a *net agonist* in the absence of dopamine (such as may exist in dorsolateral prefrontal cortex for the negative symptoms of schizophrenia) and simultaneously would be a *net antagonist* when dopamine is in excess (such as postulated in the mesolimbic dopamine pathway for the positive symptoms of schizophrenia). Also, where normal dopamine activity may exist (such as in nigrostriatal neurons), a partial agonist may not generate extrapyramidal side effects as easily as would the full antagonist typical neuroleptics.

Although several dopamine partial agonists are in preclinical research, relatively little is yet known about their potential clinical activity in schizophrenia. However, there is a certain theoretical appeal to these agents as a solution to the quandary posed earlier in this chapter of how to simultaneously increase deficient dopamine activity and reduce excessive dopamine activity in different dopamine pathways of the brain at the same time.

Dopamine autoreceptor selective agonists. The presynaptic autoreceptor of the dopamine neuron is responsible for detecting the amount of synaptic dopamine and turning off release of further dopamine from the presynaptic neuron when activity becomes excessive. Dopamine itself and most known dopamine agonists are not able to distinguish between the presynaptic autoreceptor and the postsynaptic receptor. Therefore, when dopamine or dopamine agonists turn off the presynaptic neuron, this is

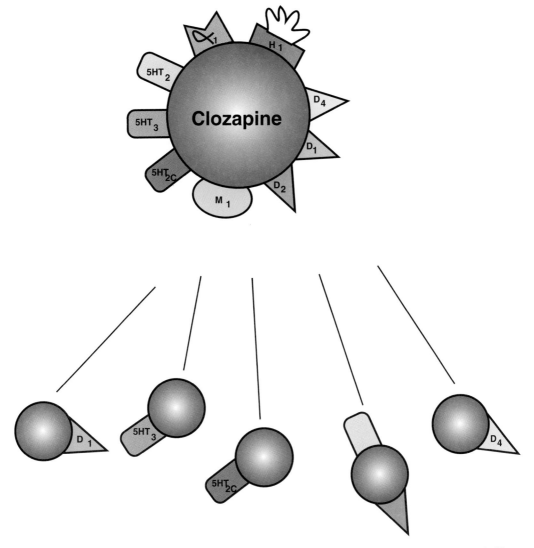

FIGURE 10–13. This figure shows the various pharmacological attempts to capture the special efficacy properties of clozapine without the side-effect profile of clozapine. These attempts include not only the serotonin-dopamine antagonists (SDAs), but also **D1** and **D4** dopamine antagonists, as well as **5HT3** and **5HT2C** antagonists.

ultimately self-defeating, since they simultaneously stimulate the postsynaptic receptors.

One possible therapeutic intervention for reducing excessive dopamine activity is to synthesize an agonist that detects the presynaptic autoreceptor but not postsynaptic dopamine receptors, having the net pharmacological effect of turning off dopamine release and reducing net dopamine activity. One such compound is 3-PPP, which seems to act as an autoreceptor agonist in animal models. Little is yet known about the promise of this approach from published results in clinical trials.

5HT3 antagonists. Blockade of 5HT3 receptors can counter the activity of excessive dopamine in some preclinical models. This has led to the proposal that a novel way of diminishing theoretically increased dopamine activity in schizophrenia would be to block 5HT3 receptors (Fig. 10–13). Preliminary results, largely unpublished, from clinical trials, however, have been disappointing so far.

5HT2C antagonists. Clozapine is, among its many other unique pharmacological properties mentioned above, also a 5HT2C *antagonist*. One theory is that blocking this receptor may not only reduce symptoms in schizophrenia but may possibly also replicate the special efficacy properties of clozapine (Fig. 10–13). Consistent with this notion is the observation that the 5HT2C *agonist* mCPP can cause worsening of schizophrenic symptoms in schizophrenic patients. No serotonin 2C selective antagonists have been tested yet in schizophrenic patients, as the close relationship between 5HT2 receptors (also called serotonin 2A receptors) and 5HT2C receptors means that most drugs antagonize both receptors, and not 5HT2C receptors selectively.

More Speculative Research Strategies for Novel Antipsychotic Agents

Other therapeutic agents in early development include 5HT1A antagonists, combined 5HT1A partial agonists/dopamine-2 antagonists, antagonists of various peptide receptors including cholecystokinin and neurotensin receptors, and even drugs that selectively target various G proteins.

Molecular Approaches to Drug Discovery in Schizophrenia and Other Putative Neurodegenerative Disorders

Another approach to therapeutics is predicated upon the genetics of schizophrenia. Scientists are trying to identify abnormal genes in schizophrenia, and the consequences that such abnormal genes have on molecular regulation in neurons of schizophrenic patients (e.g., see Figs. 4–2, 4–4, 4–5, and 10–14). If a degenerative process is "turned on" genetically at the beginning of the course of the illness (Fig. 10–15), perhaps it could be "turned off" pharmacologically to prevent further progression (Fig. 10–16).

It will not be possible to make a specific therapeutic agent until the site of this abnormal process is discovered within the neuron's DNA and the abnormal gene products clarified. So far there are no specific therapeutic agents that have yet been identified, but one therapeutic approach that can block the expression of an abnormal gene is called "antisense knockout strategy." In this case, a specific bit of DNA is "knocked out" and prevented from being expressed by a molecule to which it binds.

Neurodevelopmental Approaches to Drug Discovery in Schizophrenia and Other Putative Neurodevelopmental Disorders

Studies of neuronal functioning from neuroimaging studies and tests of cognitive functioning of schizophrenic patients suggest that schizophrenia may not actually start when the psychotic symptoms arise. The disease process may actually be the result of abnormal development of the brain from the beginning of life (Fig. 10–

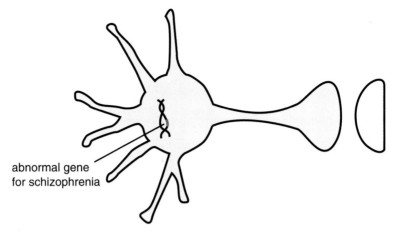

FIGURE 10–14. This figure shows the **postulated abnormal gene for schizophrenia** lying latent in the cell, and not producing abnormal gene products and not causing schizophrenia.

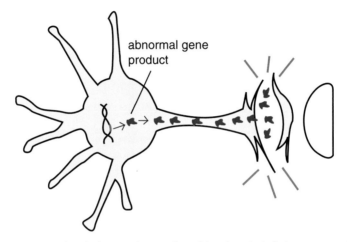

FIGURE 10–15. Here the postulated abnormal gene for schizophrenia is being expressed, leading to an **abnormal gene product** that causes disruption in the functioning of the neurons, leading to psychosis and the other symptoms of schizophrenia.

16), when neurons fail to migrate to the correct parts of the brain, fail to form appropriate connections, and then are subject to breakdown when used by the individual in late adolescence and early adulthood.

If the abnormal disease process is essentially a developmental problem completed very early in brain development, and then "the die is cast," with no further disease process in action, then it may be very difficult indeed to modify such a situation. On the other hand, it is difficult to conceive that a process completed early in life would be entirely asymptomatic until the disease process begins, and that the downhill course and waxing and waning symptomatology of schizophrenia would be due to an entirely static pathophysiological mechanism in the brain. Nevertheless, it may well prove that some neurodevelopmental difficulties are caused in early development

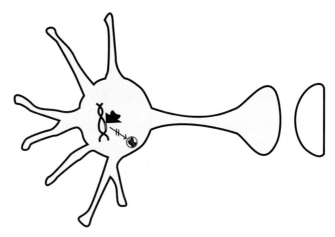

FIGURE 10–16. Genetic approach to therapeutics in schizophrenia based upon molecular neurobiology. If a degenerative process is "turned on" genetically at the beginning of the course of schizophrenia (see Fig. 10–15), perhaps it could be "turned off" pharmacologically by a drug able to prevent the expression of the postulated abnormal gene product in schizophrenia. This theoretically could arrest the disease and prevent it from further progression.

in the schizophrenia disease process. If so, it may very well be extremely difficult to reverse such abnormalities once one is an adult.

On the other hand, there may be rational means to compensate for such postulated neurodevelopmental difficulties by other mechanisms, and to interrupt any ongoing mechanism still present in the symptomatic patient (Fig. 10–17). Therefore, it is critical to learn what possible neurodevelopmental abnormalities exist in schizophrenia and which are present long before the disease symptoms announce themselves in order to learn how to reduce the impact of these in the ultimately symptomatic patient. It may eventually be possible to reawaken neuronal plasticity selectively for therapeutic applications even in the symptomatic adult by using appropriate genetic therapies capable of instructing the genes of the neuron (Fig. 10–17). Such interventions may also stop any ongoing process, and if reversed, may actually have the theoretical capability of repairing the brain and the developmental damage.

These are bold and unsubstantiated theoretical extrapolations based upon the most optimistic therapeutic possibilities that current molecular and neurodevelopmental approaches suggest. Although therapeutic applications may take many years to discover and test, the vision of such therapies is an encouraging possibility to render hope to our patients with schizophrenia today.

Future Combination Chemotherapies for Disorders Associated with Psychosis: Schizophrenia and Cognitive Disorders

Given the economic incentives for being the "cure" and treatment of choice for psychotic disorders, it is not difficult to understand why most drug development activities for the psychoses target a single disease mechanism, with the goal of being the only therapy for that disorder. In reality, it may be overly simplistic to conceptualize disorders with psychotic features as the product of a single disease mecha-

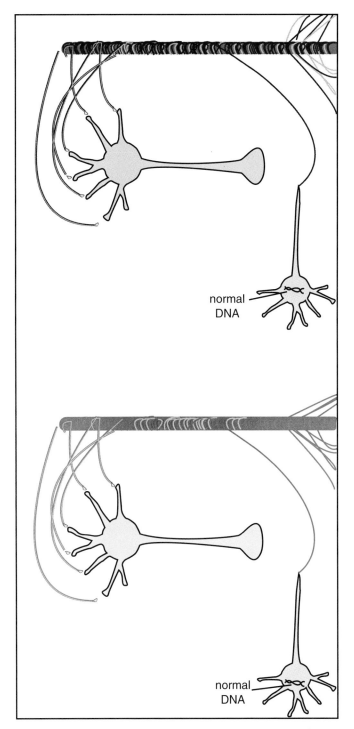

FIGURE 10–17. **Neurodevelopmental theories of schizophrenia** suggest that something goes wrong with the program for the **normal formation of synapses and migration of neurons** in the brain during the prenatal and early childhood formation of the brain and its connections. Depicted here is a concept of how a neuron with normal DNA would develop and form synaptic connections.

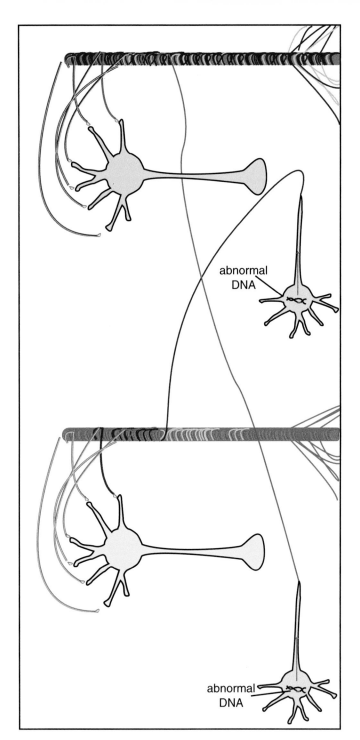

FIGURE 10–18. According to neurodevelopmental theories of schizophrenia, an abnormality in the DNA of a schizophrenic patient may cause the **wrong synaptic connections** to be made during the **prenatal and early childhood formation of the brain and its connections**. Schizophrenia may be the result of abnormal development of the brain from the beginning of life because neurons fail to migrate to the correct parts of the brain, fail to form appropriate connections, and then are subject to breakdown when used by the individual in late adolescence and early adulthood.

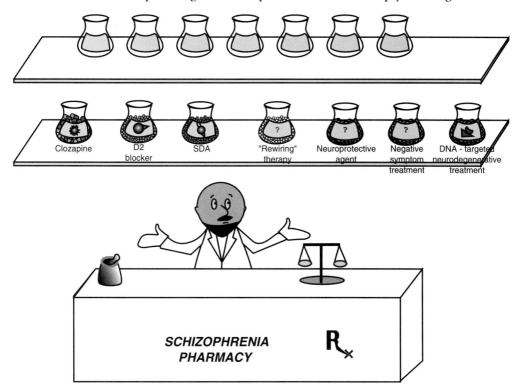

FIGURE 10–19. **Treatments for schizophrenia** are indicated on the left and include the traditional neuroleptic agents (**D2 blockers**) as well as the newer treatments **clozapine** and serotonin-dopamine antagonists (**SDAs**). New treatments are greatly needed and could include those agents shown on the right, including "**rewiring**" **therapies** for neurodevelopmental abnormalities, **neuroprotective agents** for degenerating neurons, improved **negative symptom treatments**, and **DNA-targeted neurodegenerative treatments**. In fact, future treatments may be used in combination to exploit the advantages of all these approaches simultaneously.

nism. Diseases such as schizophrenia and Alzheimer's disease may not only have psychotic features but also various cognitive deficiencies, plus a neurodegenerative component. Also, it takes a leap of faith to believe that such complex disorders could ever be satisfactorily treated with a single entity acting by a single pharmacotherapeutic mechanism.

Indeed, how realistic is it to ask a single therapeutic agent for schizophrenia to treat the positive symptoms of psychosis, the negative symptoms of psychosis, the disorganized symptoms of psychosis; to prevent further neurodegeneration; and to repair neurodevelopmental abnormalities?

Perhaps psychopharmacological treatments for psychotic disorders in the future will need to borrow a chapter out of the book of cancer chemotherapy, where the standard of treatment is to use multiple drugs simultaneously. "Combination chemotherapy" for malignancy utilizes the approach of adding together several independent therapeutic mechanisms. When successful, this results in a total therapeutic response that is greater than the sum of its parts. Usually, this also has the favorable consequence of simultaneously diminishing total side effects, since adverse experiences of multiple drugs are mediated by different pharmacological mechanisms and therefore should not be additive.

Thus, schizophrenia treatments of the future may combine one treatment for positive symptoms (perhaps some sort of dopamine 2 receptor blocking neuroleptic) with another treatment for negative symptoms (possibly a dopamine partial agonist, or an agent working by a combination of actions on dopamine and 5HT receptors) with a neuroprotective agent (e.g., a glutamate antagonist; see Chapter 11). In the long run, some sort of molecular-based therapy to prevent genetically programmed disease progression or to reverse the consequences of aberrant neurodevelopment may also form part of the portfolio of treatments for schizophrenia.

Clinical trials with multiple therapeutic agents working by several mechanisms can be quite difficult to undertake, but as there is a clinical trials methodology that exists in the cancer chemotherapy literature, it may be an approach that should be applied for complex neurodegenerative disorders with multiple underlying disease mechanisms such as schizophrenia.

Summary

This chapter has reviewed the pharmacology of traditional antipsychotic drugs as well as potential antipsychotic treatments of the future. Conventional antipsychotic agents are known as neuroleptics, and these drugs block dopamine-2 receptors in the mesolimbic dopamine pathway in order to reduce positive symptoms of psychosis.

The novel antipsychotic agent clozapine is a unique therapeutic agent for schizophrenia and has a complex pharmacology. Although it is not certain how clozapine mediates its efficacy in patients who fail to respond to conventional neuroleptics, multiple new drugs are in development that attempt to replicate the efficacy of clozapine without the side effects of clozapine. Many such new agents for schizophrenia block one or more receptors for dopamine and serotonin.

In the future, molecular and developmental approaches to drug discovery in schizophrenia may prevent the expression of latent genetically programmed neuronal dysfunctioning, or compensate for abnormal brain development in schizophrenia.

Finally, future treatment of schizophrenia is likely to combine multiple pharmacological mechanisms in order to combat this complex disorder with additive therapeutic approaches utilizing independent pharmacological strategies.

CHAPTER 11

Cognitive Enhancers and Neuroprotective Agents

IV.   Other current research approaches
    A.   Growth factors
    B.   Transplantation
    C.   Benzodiazepine inverse agonists
    D.   Sabeluzole
    E.   Future combination chemotherapies for disorders with cognitive disturbance and memory loss
  V.   Summary

Cognitive enhancement with pharmacological agents is a concept more than a current therapeutic reality. There have been no effective agents for the treatment of cognitive disorders until recently, and those that are used today are frustratingly weak and often transient in their efficacies. Also, the use of various agents as cognitive enhancers differs widely among various countries and even among opinion leaders within a given country.

Neuroprotection is the concept that the neuron dying of a degenerative process can be rescued by a therapeutic drug. It remains largely a theoretical possibility today, rather than a demonstrated therapeutic reality. Until recently, psychopharmacologists did not even conceptualize that it would be possible to interrupt a degenerative neurological illness, since such illnesses have classically been considered to be relentless and irreversible. New advances in psychopharmacology now make it feasible to hypothesize that previously untreatable neurodegenerative disorders such as Alzheimer's disease, amyotrophic lateral sclerosis (ALS; Lou Gehrig's disease), and even stroke can be halted.

Despite the limited success of experimental approaches to date, important inroads into the discovery of cognitive enhancers and neuroprotective agents are being made. It is now an exciting possibility that robust therapeutic agents for cognitive disorders and for neurodegenerative conditions will be developed in the future based upon the pharmacological principles discussed in this chapter.

Clinical Description of Cognitive Disorders

Cognitive disorders are those conditions associated with memory impairment. Many psychiatric and neurological disorders are associated with memory impairment, and a few of the most prominent among these will be discussed here. Such disorders frequently are associated with other impairments, including agitation, psychosis, and neurological dysfunction.

Memory Functioning in Normal Aging

Since complaints of memory decrements are very common in older persons, it has caused a vigorous debate as to what constitutes normal memory as the brain ages. The incidence of dementia certainly increases with advancing age, and it has led some to even pose the question, If we live long enough, will we all be demented?

Although the debate is not yet settled, many experts do not believe that dementia – the profound and often progressive loss of cognitive functioning – is the inevitable consequence of advancing age even though it is clear that with our present lack of preventing the most common dementia, Alzheimer's disease, that more and more of us will certainly decline cognitively as life expectancy increases.

More likely, some kinds of neurochemical changes are related to brain aging in the absence of dementia or depression and may cause mild impairments in cognition known as *age-associated memory impairment* or *age-related cognitive decline*. This condition does not rapidly evolve into dementia. However, in contrast to age-associated memory impairment, there are other kinds of neurochemical changes caused by specific degenerative conditions of the brain, especially those of Alzheimer's disease, which produce a far more progressive and disabling dementia, and which is increasingly common after the age of 65. The specific neurochemical alterations in the brain of demented patients is the subject of intense research scrutiny, and is becoming increasingly differentiated in terms of neuronal and neurochemical functioning from that of the normal aged brain.

Age-Associated Memory Impairment (Age-Related Cognitive Decline)

Over half of elderly residents living in the community complain of memory impairment. They have four common complaints: compared to their functioning of 5 or 10 years ago, they experience a diminished ability (1) to remember names, (2) to find the correct word, (3) to remember where objects are located, and (4) to concentrate. When such complaints occur in the absence of dementia or depression, it is called age-associated memory impairment as well as age-related cognitive decline.

Alzheimer's Disease

Alzheimer's disease is a dementing illness that affects over 10% of persons over the age of 65 residing in the community, and over 50% of residents of nursing homes. It is the fourth leading cause of death in industrialized nations (after heart disease, cancer, and stroke). Currently, about 3 million Americans, or approximately 8% of the elderly population in the United States, suffer from Alzheimer's disease.

Dementia is a *clinical* diagnosis, and is often made based upon clinical features meeting the diagnostic criteria of the *Diagnostic and Statistical Manual of Mental Disorders* (DSM-IV) for the various dementias listed there including dementia of the Alzheimer's type, vascular dementia (formerly multi-infarct dementia), dementia due to other general medical conditions, substance-induced persisting dementia, dementia due to multiple etiologies, and dementia not otherwise specified. In addition, there are DSM-IV diagnostic criteria for amnestic disorders of various types. On the other hand, *Alzheimer's disease* – a specific type of dementia – is defined by *pathological features*, so a definitive diagnosis can only be made at postmortem autopsy. Nevertheless, diagnostic criteria have been developed for *possible* Alzheimer's disease and for *probable* Alzheimer's disease based upon clinical features. These criteria are called the National Institute of Neurological and Communicative Disorders and Stroke/ Alzheimer's Disease and Related Disorders Association (NINCDS/ADRDA) criteria for the clinical diagnosis of Alzheimer's disease, and are the best clinicians can do to make a diagnosis of Alzheimer's disease prior to autopsy or brain biopsy.

The clinical hallmark of Alzheimer's disease is *dementia*, comprised of impairment in *short- and long-term memory*, *abstract thinking*, *judgment*, and *higher cortical functioning* such as language or motor function. However, other features often accompany Alzheimer's disease and add significantly to the overall impairment of the patient, including disordered behavior such as *agitation* and *aggressiveness*, *psychosis*, and *anxiety*.

Another important aspect to Alzheimer's disease is its progressive nature. *Mild Alzheimer's Disease*, the earliest stage at which a diagnosis can be made with confidence, is associated with decreased capacity for complex occupational and social tasks, and often lasts about 2 years. *Moderate Alzheimer's disease* generally causes interference with independent community survival, problems choosing clothing, inability to drive a car, difficulty preparing simple beverages such as coffee or tea, and inability to recall the current year. Moderate Alzheimer's disease can progress to moderately severe Alzheimer's disease in about 18 months.

At the stage of *moderately severe Alzheimer's disease*, patients begin to require assistance with dressing and bathing, the mechanics of toileting, and may have difficulty counting backward from 10, and in participating in sports with slower steps when walking. The magnitude of cognitive and functional decline in moderately severe Alzheimer's disease is often combined with disturbed behavior and makes caregiving especially burdensome to spouses at this stage. This stage often lasts about 2½ years.

When patients become incontinent of urine and feces, begin to scream or cry out frequently, and have speech limited to a few words, they have developed *severe Alzheimer's disease*, which lasts a mean of 1½ years, ending frequently in death from pneumonia.

Other Dementias

There are many other causes of dementia, but none is the subject of such intense interest and research activity as Alzheimer's disease. The clinical features of dementia can be remarkably similar, despite many different causes.

Vascular dementia (formerly multi-infarct dementia) is characterized by dementia that classically has a more stepwise downhill course compared to Alzheimer's disease, which has a more smoothly progressive downhill course. It is caused by multiple strokes, which damage the brain sufficiently to cause dementia and often cause focal neurological signs and symptoms as well. *Normal pressure hydrocephalus* can cause dementia from dilated cerebral ventricles. *Creutzfeldt-Jacob disease* can cause dementia from a "slow" viral infection of the brain. *Depression* can cause a false or "pseudo-dementia" that can be reversed by antidepressants in many cases.

Huntington's disease, Parkinson's disease, and many other neurological disorders can have dementia associated with various neurological signs and symptoms. These dementias are part of a neurodegenerative disorder that destroys various neurons in the brain, including those areas responsible for memory and cognition. Patients with acquired immunodeficiency syndrome (AIDS) often have a dementia resulting from human immunodeficiency virus (HIV) infection of the brain.

Biological Basis of Cognitive Disorders and their Treatments

Understanding of the biological basis of cognitive disorders is undergoing rapid advancement. Here we will emphasize predominantly the research progress and hypotheses about the brain abnormalities underlying Alzheimer's disease.

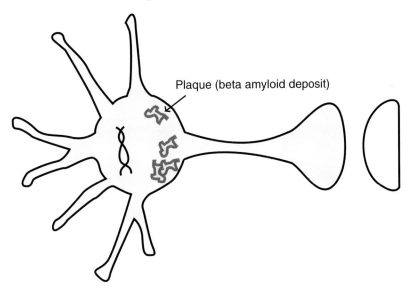

Plaque (beta amyloid deposit)

FIGURE 11–1. Postmortem brain pathology defines what Alzheimer's disease is. Shown here are abnormal degenerative structures called **neuritic plaques** with **amyloid cores**.

Neuropathology of Alzheimer's Disease

The original report of Alzheimer's disease was made by the German neurologist Alois Alzheimer. He described a patient with amnesia, aphasia, and apraxia (disorganized motor movements), as well as delusions and violent behavior who had postmortem brain pathology that today still defines Alzheimer's disease, namely abnormal degenerative structures called *neuritic plaques* with *amyloid cores* (see Fig. 11–1) and *neurofibrillary tangles* of abnormally phosphorylated tau proteins (Fig. 11–2).

Neuritic plaques are extracellular lesions consisting of a substance called beta amyloid. *Neurofibrillary tangles* consist largely of a type of protein wrapped into bundles. These proteins are called tau proteins, which are chemically altered by being abnormally phosphorylated, and then twisted together. Recent research focuses on how these plaques and tangles are formed and how they interfere with neuronal function and cause neuronal cell death (Figs. 11–3 through 11–7).

Amyloid Cascade Hypothesis of Alzheimer's Disease

A leading contemporary theory for the biological basis of Alzheimer's disease centers around the formation of beta amyloid. Perhaps Alzheimer's disease is essentially a disease in which the abnormal deposition of beta amyloid gets to the point that it destroys neurons. This is somewhat analogous to the idea that abnormal deposition of cholesterol may cause atherosclerosis. Thus, Alzheimer's disease may be essentially a problem of too much formation of beta amyloid, or too little removal of it.

One idea is that neurons in some patients destined to have Alzheimer's disease have an abnormality in the DNA that codes for a protein called amyloid precursor protein (APP) (Fig. 11–3). The abnormal DNA starts a lethal chemical cascade in neurons (Figs. 11–4 and 11–5), ultimately resulting in Alzheimer's disease (Figs.

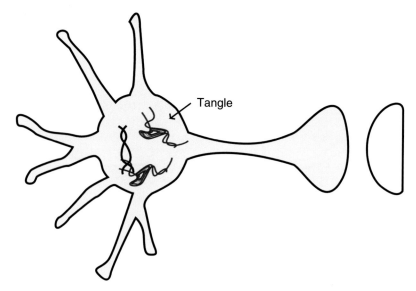

FIGURE 11−2. Another key finding in Alzheimer's disease is the pathological finding of another degenerative structure called **neurofibrillary tangles** made up of abnormally phosphorylated tau proteins.

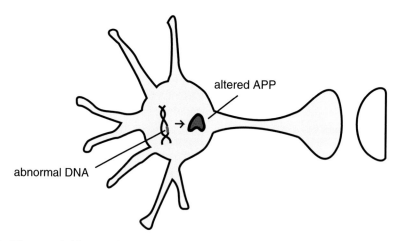

FIGURE 11−3. **The amyloid cascade hypothesis of Alzheimer's disease (part 1).** A leading contemporary theory for the biological basis of Alzheimer's disease centers around the formation of beta amyloid. Perhaps Alzheimer's disease is essentially a disease in which the abnormal deposition of beta amyloid gets to the point that it destroys neurons. Thus, Alzheimer's disease may be essentially a problem of too much formation of beta amyloid, or too little removal of it. One idea is that neurons in some patients destined to have Alzheimer's disease have an **abnormality in the DNA** that codes for a protein called amyloid precursor protein (APP). The abnormal DNA starts a lethal chemical cascade in neurons, beginning with the formation of an **altered APP**.

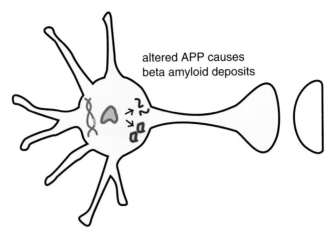

FIGURE 11–4. **The amyloid cascade hypothesis of Alzheimer's disease (part 2).** Once altered amyloid precursor protein (APP) is formed (see Fig. 11–3), it leads to the formation of **beta amyloid deposits**.

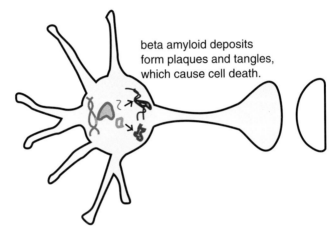

FIGURE 11–5. **The amyloid cascade hypothesis of Alzheimer's disease (part 3).** Once beta amyloid deposits are formed from abnormal amyloid precursor protein (APP), the next step is that beta amyloid deposits form plaques and tangles in the neuron.

11–6 and 11–7). Specifically, the abnormal DNA causes the formation of an altered APP (Fig. 11–3), which instead of being removed from the neuron, causes the formation of beta amyloid deposits (Fig. 11–4). The beta amyloid deposits and fragments go on to form plaques and tangles (Fig. 11–5). The presence of plaques and tangles signals cell damage and cell death (Figs. 11–6 and 11–7). Sufficient cell damage and cell death gives rise to the formation of the symptoms in Alzheimer's disease (Figs. 11–6 and 11–7).

Another version of the amyloid cascade hypothesis is the possibility that something is wrong with a protein that binds to amyloid and removes it (Figs. 11–8 and 11–9). This protein is called apolipoprotein E (APO-E). In the case of "good" APO-E, it binds to beta amyloid and removes it, preventing the formation of Alz-

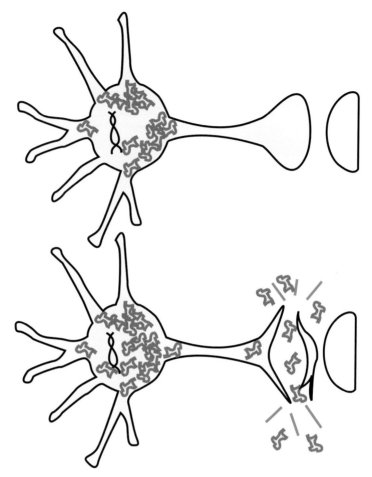

FIGURE 11–6. **The amyloid cascade hypothesis of Alzheimer's disease (part 4).** Formation of numerous neuritic plaques eventually causes the neuron to stop functioning, and even to die.

heimer's disease and dementia (Fig. 1–8). In the case of "bad" APO-E, a genetic abnormality in the formation of APO-E causes it to be ineffective in how it binds beta amyloid. This causes beta amyloid to be deposited in neurons, which goes on to damage the neurons and cause Alzheimer's disease (Fig. 11–9).

Current therapeutics are aimed at the possibility that altering the synthesis of APP (Fig. 11–10) or APO-E (Fig. 11–11) might change the deposition of beta amyloid and prevent the progressive course of Alzheimer's disease. Another possibility is to inhibit the synthesis of beta amyloid, much the same way that lipid-lowering agents act to inhibit the biosynthesis of cholesterol in order to prevent atherosclerosis.

Cholinergic Theories of Alzheimer's Disease

One leading theory for the neurochemical basis of Alzheimer's disease is a "cholinergic deficiency hypothesis," which proposes that the memory disturbance in Alz-

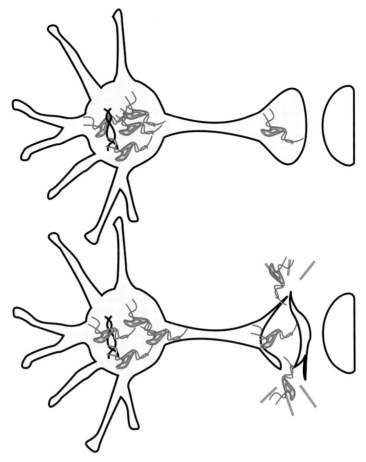

FIGURE 11–7. **The amyloid cascade hypothesis of Alzheimer's disease (part 5).** Formation of numerous neurofibrillary tangles also will eventually cause the neuron to lose its functioning and even to die.

heimer's disease is caused by loss of cholinergic neuronal functioning. Perhaps this is because beta amyloid is deposited in cholinergic neurons and thus destroys them. In order to understand this theory and the therapeutic agents based upon this approach, it is useful to understand the principles of neurotransmission at the cholinergic neuron.

Acetylcholine synthesis. Acetylcholine (ACh) is a prominent neurotransmitter formed in cholinergic neurons from two precursors: choline and acetyl coenzyme A (AcCoA) (Fig. 11–12). Choline is derived from dietary and intraneuronal sources, and AcCoA is made from glucose in the mitochondria of the neuron. These two substrates interact with the synthetic enzyme choline acetyl transferase (CAT) to produce the neurotransmitter ACh.

Acetylcholine destruction and removal. ACh is destroyed by an enzyme called acetylcholinesterase (AChE), which turns ACh into inactive products (Fig. 11–13). ACh's

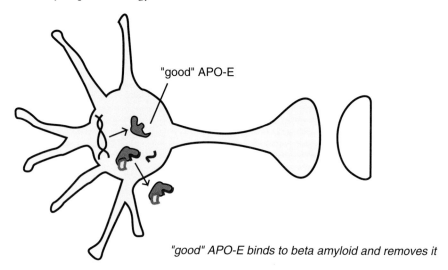

"good" APO-E

"good" APO-E binds to beta amyloid and removes it

FIGURE 11–8. Another version of the amyloid cascade hypothesis is the possibility that something is wrong with a protein that binds to amyloid and removes it. This protein is called APO-E. In the case of "**good**" **APO-E**, it binds to beta amyloid and removes it, preventing the formation of Alzheimer's disease and dementia.

actions can also be terminated by a presynaptic choline transporter similar to the transporters for other neurotransmitters already discussed in relationship to norepinephrine, dopamine, and serotonin neurons.

Acetylcholine receptors. There are numerous receptors for ACh (Fig. 11–14). The major subdivision is between nicotinic and muscarinic cholinergic receptors. There are also numerous subtypes of these receptors, best characterized for muscarinic receptor subtypes. Perhaps the M1 postsynaptic receptor is key to mediating the memory functions linked to cholinergic neurotransmission, but a role for other cholinergic receptor subtypes has not been ruled out.

Cholinergic deficiency hypothesis. Numerous investigations suggest that deficiency of cholinergic functioning may be linked to memory disturbances. Some investigators believe that this underlies the memory disturbance of Alzheimer's disease, while others believe that it may be more related to the memory changes of age-associated memory impairment. At any rate, levels of ACh synthesis and levels of its synthetic enzyme CAT are reduced in brains of Alzheimer's patients. Also, muscarinic antagonists (such as scopolamine) can produce a memory disturbance in normal human volunteers that has some similarity to the memory disturbance in Alzheimer's disease. Procholinergic agents (i.e., agents that enhance cholinergic functioning) can not only reverse scopolamine-induced memory impairments in normal human volunteers but can also enhance memory functioning in Alzheimer's disease.

Cholinergic treatments for Alzheimer's disease. The earliest attempts to boost cholinergic functioning in Alzheimer's disease were made using rather rudimentary cholinergic agents, namely the precursors for ACh synthesis, choline and lecithin (phosphatidyl

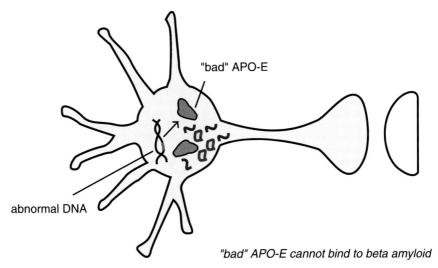

"bad" APO-E

abnormal DNA

"bad" APO-E cannot bind to beta amyloid

FIGURE 11–9. In comparison to Figure 11–8 where "good" APO-E can bind to beta amyloid and remove it, it is possible that patients with Alzheimer's disease have an **abnormality in their DNA** that causes the formation of a **defective or "bad" version of the APO-E protein.** In this case, "bad" APO-E cannot bind to beta amyloid, so the **amyloid is not removed from the neuron.** Consequently, beta amyloid accumulates, forms plaques and tangles, and the neuron loses its function and dies.

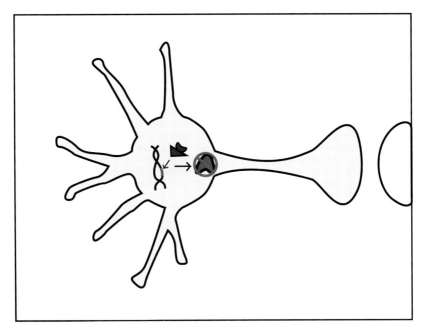

FIGURE 11–10. One current therapeutic approach to preventing the neuronal destruction in Alzheimer's disease is based upon the molecular neurobiology of beta amyloid formation, and the involvement of amyloid precursor protein (APP) in this process. If the **synthesis of APP could be prevented,** it might change the deposition of beta amyloid and prevent the progressive course of Alzheimer's disease. Another possibility is to inhibit the synthesis of beta amyloid itself, much the same way that lipid-lowering agents act to inhibit the biosynthesis of cholesterol in order to prevent atherosclerosis.

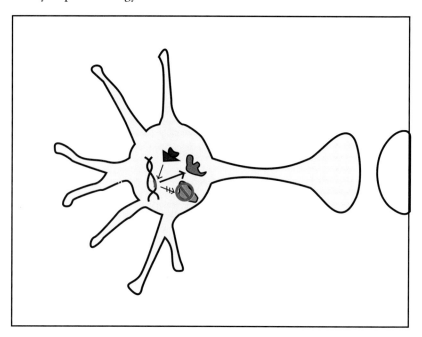

FIGURE 11–11. Another current therapeutic approach to preventing the neuronal destruction in Alzheimer's disease is also based upon the molecular neurobiology of beta amyloid formation, but emphasizes the involvement of APO-E binding protein in this process. If the **synthesis of "good" APO-E could be ensured** or the **synthesis of "bad" APO-E prevented**, possibly amyloid would not accumulate in the neuron. It is hoped that changing the deposition of beta amyloid would prevent the progressive course of Alzheimer's disease.

choline). This was based upon an analogy with Parkinson's disease where neurodegeneration of dopaminergic neurons causes symptoms that can be successfully treated by administering the precursor of dopamine, namely L-DOPA. The hope was that giving the ACh precursors choline and lecithin would enhance ACh synthesis and thereby cause successful treatment of the symptoms of Alzheimer's disease.

Many studies have attempted to show the efficacy of cholinergic precursors in Alzheimer's disease, but this approach has unfortunately not proven to cause clinically significant results. This may be due to the fact that the huge amounts of precursors needed to effect a notable boost in ACh synthesis are not practical to administer. Multiple studies of cholinergic precursors have led to essentially negative results that do not offer meaningful hope for improvement in patients with Alzheimer's disease.

Currently, there are several approaches to boosting ACh functioning that are under investigation and that are attempting to improve memory functioning in Alzheimer's disease. The most powerful and successful to date is to inhibit ACh destruction by inhibiting the enzyme acetylcholinesterase (Fig. 11–15). This causes the buildup of ACh, which is no longer destroyed by acetylcholinesterase. This approach has led to the only therapy approved for treatment of Alzheimer's disease in the United States, namely tetrahydroamino acridine (THA) or tacrine. Other similar agents are in late clinical testing. Since these agents appear to depend upon the presence of intact cholinergic neurons, they may be most effective in the early stages of Alz-

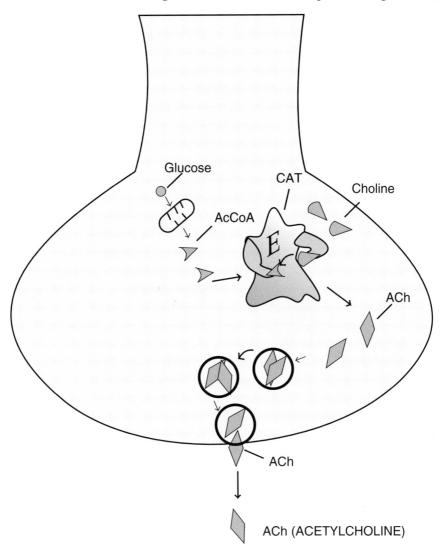

FIGURE 11–12. **Acetylcholine (ACh) is synthesized**. Acetylcholine is a prominent neurotransmitter formed in cholinergic neurons from two precursors: choline and acetyl coenzyme A (AcCoA). Choline is derived from dietary and intraneuronal sources, and AcCoA is made from glucose in the mitochondria of the neuron. These two substrates interact with the synthetic enzyme choline acetyl transferase (CAT) to produce the neurotransmitter ACh.

heimer's disease while cholinergic neurons are still present, since there is no evidence that these agents alter the course of the underlying dementing process.

Although tacrine improves memory and behavioral functioning in Alzheimer's patients as a group, the importance of this improvement in an individual patient can range from very little to a notable short-term improvement. Tacrine can cause liver damage in some patients, and the need to monitor for this and to reduce the dosage or stop the medication limits its use in clinical practice. Also, even in patients with a good immediate effect of THA, the effect does not appear to last much longer

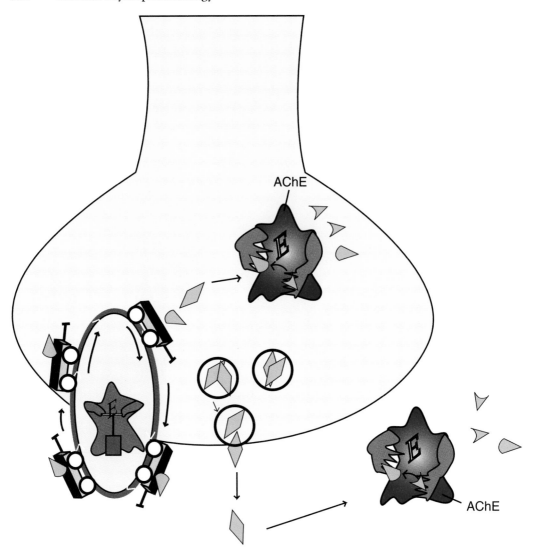

FIGURE 11–13. **Acetylcholine (ACh) destruction and removal.** ACh is destroyed by an enzyme called acetylcholinesterase (AChE), which turns ACh into inactive products. ACh's actions can also be terminated by a presynaptic choline transporter similar to the transporters for other neurotransmitters already discussed in relationship to norepinephrine, dopamine, and serotonin neurons.

than 6 months, since the progress of the disease tends to take away the therapeutic gains over time. As already mentioned, the relentless march of the destructive process underlying Alzheimer's disease is not halted by tacrine, meaning that the improvement in those patients who experience improvement is not sustained.

Another approach that still has only met with limited success is to target cholinergic receptors selectively with a cholinergic agonist. Various agonists are under

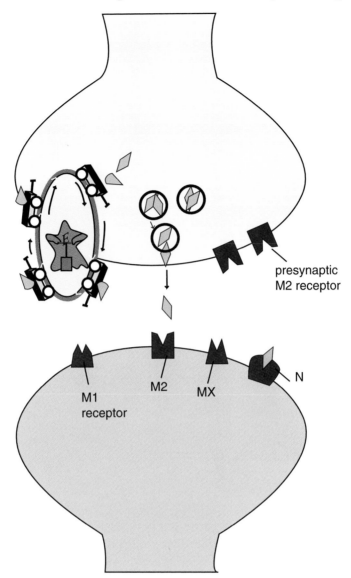

FIGURE 11–14. **Acetylcholine (ACh) receptors**. There are numerous receptors for ACh. The major subdivision is between **nicotinic** (N) and **muscarinic** (M) cholinergic receptors. There are also numerous subtypes of these receptors, best characterized for muscarinic receptor subtypes (M1, M2, Mx). Perhaps the M1 postsynaptic receptor is key to mediating the memory functions linked to cholinergic neurotransmission, but a role for other cholinergic receptor subtypes has not been ruled out.

investigation, especially agonists for the M1 cholinergic receptor (Fig. 11–16). Nicotinic agonists are also being tested (Fig. 11–17). The possible advantage of stimulating nicotinic cholinergic receptors is suggested by several epidemiological studies finding a lower risk for Alzheimer's disease among smokers. In addition, central

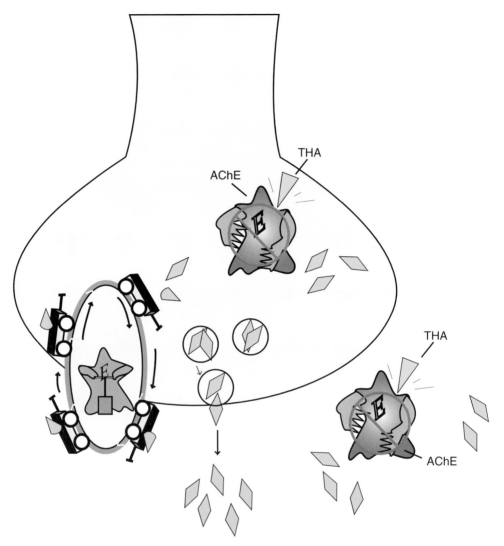

FIGURE 11–15. **Cholinesterase inhibitor treatment for Alzheimer's disease.** Numerous investigations suggest that deficiency of cholinergic functioning may be linked to memory disturbances. Some investigators believe that this underlies the memory disturbance of Alzheimer's disease, while others believe that it may be more related to the memory changes of age-associated memory impairment. At any rate, levels of ACh synthesis and levels of its synthetic enzyme CAT are reduced in brains of Alzheimer's disease patients. A powerful and successful mechanism of boosting ACh in the brain is to inhibit ACh destruction by **inhibiting the enzyme acetylcholinesterase** (AChE). This causes the build-up of ACh, which is no longer destroyed by acetylcholinesterase. This approach has led to the only therapy approved specifically for the treatment of Alzheimer's disease in the United States, namely tetrahydroamino acridine (THA) or tacrine. Other similar agents are in late clinical testing. Since these agents appear to depend upon the presence of intact cholinergic neurons, they may be most effective in the early stages of Alzheimer's disease, while cholinergic neurons are still present, since there is no evidence that these agents alter the course of the underlying dementing process.

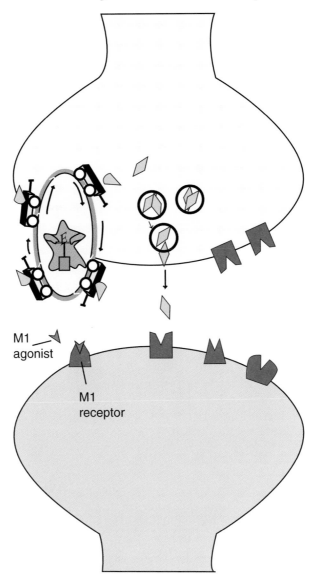

FIGURE 11–16. **Use of agonists for the M1 receptor for the treatment of Alzheimer's disease**. Another approach that still has only met with limited success is to target cholinergic receptors selectively with a cholinergic agonist. Various agonists are under investigation, especially agonists for the M1 cholinergic receptor.

nicotinic receptors are reduced in brains of Alzheimer's patients. To date, no such agents have been licensed for the treatment of Alzheimer's disease.

Yet another possibility is to develop an agent that can release ACh, perhaps through blocking potassium channels. This approach is heavily dependent, however, on the presence of intact remaining presynaptic cholinergic nerve terminals, and may therefore only be effective in the early stages of the disease. Several such agents are under clinical investigation.

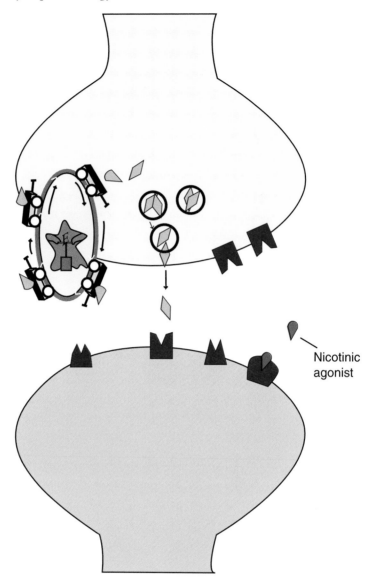

FIGURE 11–17. **Use of agonists for the nicotinic cholinergic receptor for the treatment of Alzheimer's disease**. Nicotinic agonists are also being tested in Alzheimer's disease. The possible advantage of stimulating nicotinic cholinergic receptors is suggested by several epidemiological studies finding a lower risk for Alzheimer's disease among smokers. In addition, central nicotinic receptors are reduced in brains of Alzheimer's disease patients. To date, no such agents have been licensed for the treatment of Alzheimer's disease.

Excitotoxic Hypothesis of Alzheimer's Disease

The excitotoxic hypothesis of Alzheimer's disease proposes that neurons degenerate because of excessive excitatory neurotransmission at glutamate neurons. This process is sometimes also called "excitotoxicity," and is discussed in Chapter 4. Excitotoxicity is not only a hypothesis to explain neurodegeneration in Alzheimer's disease

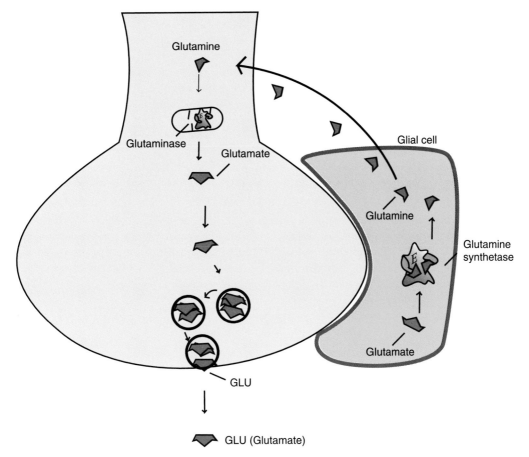

FIGURE 11–18. **Glutamate is produced** (synthesized). Glutamate or glutamic acid (**glu**) is a neurotransmitter that is an amino acid. Its predominant use is not as a neurotransmitter but as a building block amino acid of protein synthesis. When used as a neurotransmitter, it is synthesized from **glutamine**. Glutamine is turned into glutamate by an enzyme in mitochondria called **glutaminase**. It is then stored in synaptic vesicles for subsequent release during neurotransmission. Glutamine itself can be obtained from glia cells adjacent to neurons. Glia cells have a supportive role to neurons, helping to support them both structurally and metabolically. In the case of glutamate neurons, nearby glia can provide glutamine for neurotransmitter glutamate synthesis. In this case, glutamate from metabolic pools in the glia is converted into glutamate use as a neurotransmitter. This is accomplished by first converting glutamate into glutamine in the glia cell via the enzyme **glutamine synthetase**. Glutamine is then transported into the neuron for conversion into glutamate for use as a neurotransmitter.

but has also been invoked as an explanation for neurodegeneration in any number of neurological and psychiatric conditions, including the negative symptoms of schizophrenia, Parkinson's disease, ALS, and even stroke.

In order to understand the hypothesis of excessive excitation of neurons by glutamate, it is necessary to understand glutaminergic neurotransmission.

Glutamate synthesis. Glutamate or glutamic acid is a neurotransmitter that is an amino acid (Fig. 11–18). Its predominant use is not as a neurotransmitter but as a building block amino acid of protein synthesis. When used as a neurotransmitter, it is synthesized from glutamine. Glutamine is turned into glutamate by an enzyme in mitochondria called glutaminase. It is then stored in synaptic vesicles for subsequent release during neurotransmission. Glutamine itself can be obtained from glia cells adjacent to neurons. Glia cells have a supportive role to neurons, helping to support them both structurally and metabolically. In the case of glutamate neurons, nearby glia can provide glutamine for neurotransmitter glutamate synthesis. In this case, glutamate from metabolic pools in the glia is converted into glutamate use as a neurotransmitter. This is accomplished by first converting glutamate into glutamine in the glia cell via the enzyme glutamine synthetase. Glutamine is then transported into the neuron for conversion into glutamate for use as a neurotransmitter.

Glutamate removal. Glutamate's actions are stopped not by enzymatic breakdown, like in other neurotransmitter systems, but by removal by two transport pumps (Fig. 11–19). The first of these pumps is a presynaptic glutamate transporter that works like all the other neurotransmitter transporters already discussed for amine neurotransmitter systems such as dopamine, norepinephrine, serotonin, and acetylcholine. The second transport pump is located on nearby glia, which removes glutamate from the synapse and terminates its actions there.

Glutamate receptors. There are several types of glutamate receptors (Fig. 11–20), including N-methyl-D-aspartate (NMDA), alpha-amino-3-hydroxy-5-methyl-4-isoxazole-propionic acid (AMPA), and kainate, all named after the agonists that selectively bind to them. Another type of glutamate receptor is the metabotropic glutamate receptor, which may mediate long-lasting electrical signals in the brain called long-term potentiation. Long-term potentiation appears to have a key role in memory functions.

NMDA, AMPA, and kainate subtypes of glutamate receptors are probably all linked to an ion channel. The metabotropic glutamate receptor subtype, however, belongs to the G protein–linked superfamily of receptors. The specific functioning of the various subtypes of glutamate receptors is the focus of intense debate. The actions at NMDA receptors will be emphasized here in our discussions on excitotoxicity.

Neuroprotection, excitotoxicity, and the glutamate system in degenerative disorders such as Alzheimer's disease. A major research strategy for the discovery of novel therapeutics in Alzheimer's disease is to target the glutamate system, which might mediate progressive neurodegeneration by an excitotoxic mechanism. Such an excitotoxic mechanism has already been discussed (see Figs. 4–8, 4–9, 4–10, 4–20, and 4–21), and may play a role in various other neurodegenerative diseases such as schizophrenia, Parkinson's disease, Huntington's disease, ALS, and even stroke (Fig. 11–21).

If neurodegeneration is caused by too much glutamate, then antagonists of glutamate could theoretically halt such a neurodegenerative process. The NMDA subtype of glutamate receptor is thought to mediate both normal excitatory neurotransmission (Fig. 11–22) as well as neurodegenerative excitotoxicity in the glutamate excitation spectrum shown in Figure 11–21.

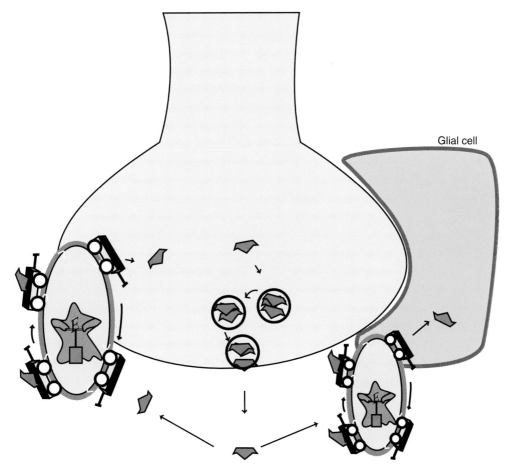

FIGURE 11–19. **Glutamate removal**. Glutamate's actions are stopped not by enzymatic breakdown, like in other neurotransmitter systems, but by removal by two transport pumps. The first of these pumps is a presynaptic glutamate transporter that works like all the other neurotransmitter transporters already discussed for amine neurotransmitter systems such as dopamine, norepinephrine, serotonin, and acetylcholine. The second transport pump is located on nearby glia, which removes glutamate from the synapse and terminates its actions there.

Recall that one form of excitotoxicity may be useful as a pruning mechanism necessary for normal maintenance of the dendritic tree (see Fig. 1–13). Excitotoxicity to an excess, however, is hypothesized to cause various forms of neurodegeneration, ranging from slowly and relentlessly neurodegenerative conditions such as Alzheimer's disease to sudden and catastrophic cell death as occurs in stroke (Fig. 11–21).

The NMDA receptor is a *ligand-gated ion channel*, in the same receptor superfamily as previously discussed for the gamma-amino-butyric acid (GABA) –benzodiazepine receptor complex (see Fig. 11–22). In the case of the GABA receptor, however, the fast transmitting ion channel is an *inhibitory* chloride channel. However, for the NMDA subtype of glutamate receptor, the fast transmitting ion channel is an *excitatory* calcium channel.

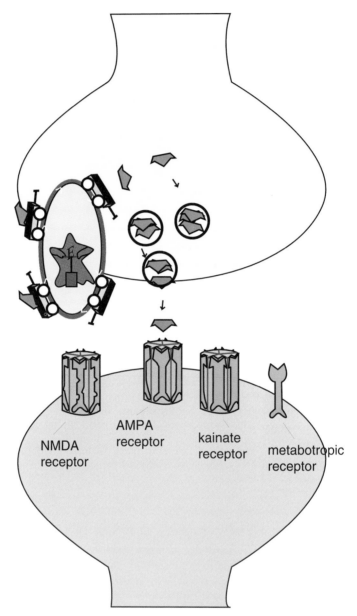

FIGURE 11–20. **Glutamate receptors**. There are several types of glutamate receptors, including three linked to ion channels: *N*-methyl-D-aspartate (**NMDA**), alpha-amino-3-hydroxy-5-methyl-4-isoxazole-propionic acid (**AMPA**), and **kainate**, all named after the agonists that selectively bind to them. Another type of glutamate receptor is the **metabotropic** glutamate receptor, which is a G protein–linked receptor, and which may mediate long-lasting electrical signals in the brain called long-term potentiation. Long-term potentiation appears to have a key role in memory functions.

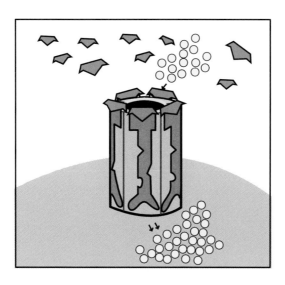

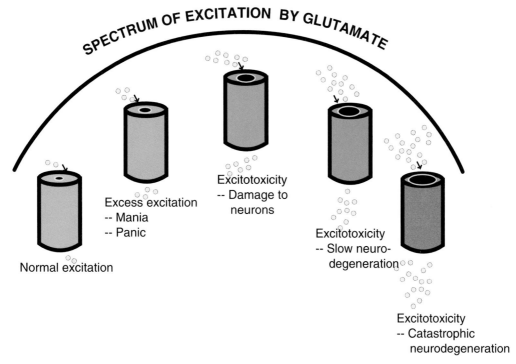

FIGURE 11–21. **Neuroprotection, excitotoxicity, and the glutamate system in degenerative disorders.** A major research strategy for the discovery of novel therapeutics in Alzheimer's disease is to target the glutamate system, which might mediate progressive neurodegeneration by an excitotoxic mechanism. Such an excitotoxic mechanism may play a role in various other neurodegenerative diseases such as schizophrenia, Parkinson's disease, Huntington's disease, ALS, and even stroke. The **spectrum of excitation by glutamate** ranges from **normal neurotransmission**, to excess neurotransmission causing pathological symptoms such as **mania or panic**, to excitotoxicity resulting in **minor damage to dendrites**, to **slow progressive excitotoxicity** resulting in neuronal degeneration such as in Alzheimer's disease, to **sudden and catastrophic excitotoxicity** causing neurodegeneration as in stroke.

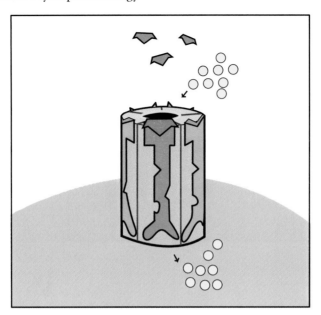

Normal excitatory
neurotransmission

FIGURE 11–22. Shown here is **normal excitatory neurotransmission** at the *N*-methyl-D-aspartate (NMDA) type of glutamate receptor. The NMDA receptor is a **ligand-gated ion channel**. This fast transmitting ion channel is an **excitatory** calcium channel. Occupancy of NMDA glutamate receptors by glutamate causes calcium channels to open and the neuron to be excited for neurotransmission.

Just as is the case for the GABA–benzodiazepine receptor complex, the NMDA glutamate–calcium channel complex also has multiple receptors surrounding the ion channel that act in concert as *allosteric modulators* (Fig. 11–23). One modulatory site is for the neurotransmitter *glycine* (Fig. 11–23A). Another modulatory site is for *polyamines*, and yet another for *zinc* (Fig. 11–23A). The ion *magnesium* can block the calcium channel at yet another modulatory site, presumably inside the ion channel or closely related to it (Fig. 11–23B). Another inhibitory modulatory site is located inside the ion channel, sometime called the *"PCP site,"* since the psychotomimetic agent phencyclidine (PCP) binds to this site (Figure 11–23B).

Antagonists for any of the various modulatory sites around the NMDA–calcium channel complex would possibly restrict the flow of calcium and close the channel and therefore be candidates for neuroprotective agents. Such antagonists are being developed and tested in various disorders hypothesized to be mediated by an excitotoxic mechanism. This therapeutic approach follows in part clinical observations that Alzheimer's disease and other neurodegenerative disorders are not static disorders, but are progressive, suggesting an active and ongoing neurobiological process underlying such disorders.

Excitotoxicity is thus a major current hypothesis for explaining a neuropathological mechanism that could mediate the final common pathway of any number of neurological and psychiatric disorders characterized by a neurodegenerative course. The basic idea is that the normal process of excitatory neurotransmission runs amok, and instead of normal excitatory neurotransmission, things get out of hand, and the neuron is literally excited to death (Fig. 11–21).

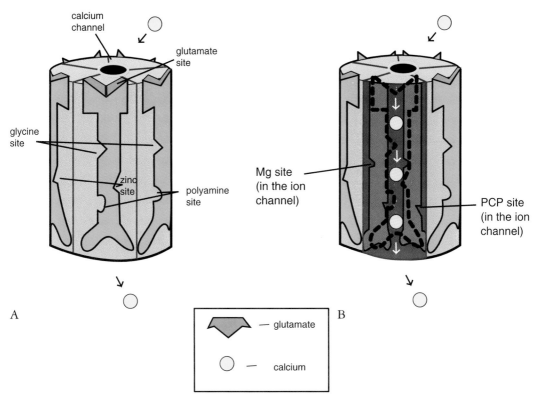

FIGURE 11–23. **Five modulatory sites on the N-methyl-D-aspartate (NMDA) receptor.** The NMDA glutamate–calcium channel complex has multiple receptors in and around it that act in concert as **allosteric modulators.** Three of these modulatory sites are located around the NMDA receptor and are shown in part *A* of this figure. One of these modulatory site is for the neurotransmitter **glycine.** Another modulatory site is for **polyamines,** and yet another for **zinc.** Two of the modulatory sites are located inside of or nearby the ion channel itself, shown in part *B* of this figure. The ion **magnesium** can block the calcium channel at one of these modulatory sites, presumably inside the ion channel or closely related to it. The other inhibitory modulatory site located inside the ion channel is sometimes called the "**PCP site,**" since the psychotomimetic agent phencyclidine (PCP) binds to this site.

We have already mentioned that this process may actually be a normal function of the cell at those times when it needs to revise its synapses and prune out connections that become no longer necessary (as shown earlier in Fig. 1–13). However, if this excitotoxic mechanism is turned on inappropriately, or runs out of control (Fig. 4–7), then it is possible that important and necessary synapses (Figs. 4–20 and 11–21) or even entire neurons could be wiped out by this process, killing them by a neurodegenerative process (Figs. 4–21 and 11–21).

It is possible that the effect of psychosis, panic, mania, or other disease symptoms (Figs. 4–18 and 4–19) are themselves damaging to the brain and that such damage of neurons during the psychotic process could be mediated by excitotoxicity (Figs. 4–20 and 11–21). Psychosis seems to beget psychosis, and uncontrolled psychosis leads to a poorer prognosis than does a course of illness where the number and duration of active psychotic episodes and symptoms are reduced. The same may be

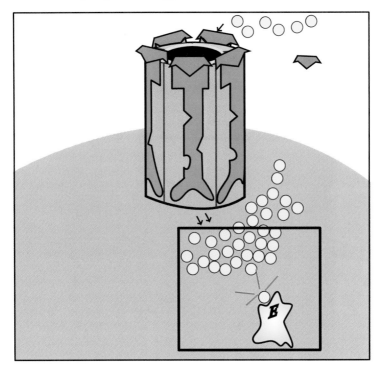

Excess calcium
activates enzyme

FIGURE 11–24. **Cellular events occurring during excitotoxicity (part 1).** Excitotoxicity is a major current hypothesis for explaining a neuropathological mechanism that could mediate the final common pathway of any number of neurological and psychiatric disorders characterized by a neurodegenerative course. The basic idea is that the normal process of excitatory neurotransmission runs amok, and instead of normal excitatory neurotransmission, things get out of hand, and the neuron is literally excited to death. The excitotoxic mechanism is thought to begin with a pathological process that triggers excessive glutamate activity. This causes excessive opening of the calcium channel, shown here, with poisoning of the cell by this excessive calcium.

true for other psychiatric and neurological conditions such as mania, panic, and seizures. These conclusions are based upon data from studies showing that patients who are ill for a shorter time prior to initiating treatment are more likely to respond to therapeutic drugs than those with longer duration of symptoms before treatment was begun. These results suggest that the active phase of certain illnesses like psychosis and dementia may reflect a morbid process that, if allowed to persist, can impair the patient's ability to respond to treatment when finally instituted.

The therapeutic idea underlying the development of neuroprotective agents is that such drugs could stop inappropriate or excessive excitatory neurotransmission and thereby halt the progressive neurodegenerative course of various neurodegenerative disorders. The excitotoxic mechanism is thought to begin with a pathological process that triggers excessive glutamate activity (Figs. 11–21 and 11–24). This causes excessive opening of the calcium channel (Fig. 11–24), with poisoning of the cell by this excessive calcium (Fig. 11–24), resulting in the production of free

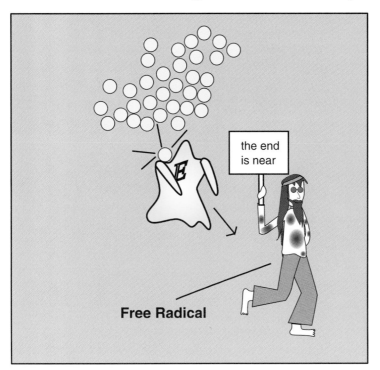

FIGURE 11–25. **Cellular events occurring during excitotoxicity (part 2).** Once excessive gluta-mate causes too much calcium to enter the neuron, the next stage is for the calcium to **activate enzymes that produce free radicals.** Free radicals are chemicals capable of destroying other chemicals and cellular components.

radicals (Fig. 11–25) that overwhelm the cell with toxic actions on its membrane and organelles (Fig. 11–26), ultimately killing it (Fig. 11–27).

There exist various theoretical mechanisms to block the NMDA subtype of glu-tamate receptor, due to the multiple modulatory sites at this receptor complex. First, of course, is the agonist site itself (Fig. 11–28), which could theoretically be blocked by a glutamate antagonist (Fig. 11–29).

Other sites for potential antagonism of glutamate overactivity are the glycine modulatory site (Figs. 11–30 and 11–31), the polyamine modulatory site (Figs. 11–32 and 11–33), and the zinc modulatory site (Figs. 11–34 and 11–35). When agonists occupy these sites, they amplify glutamate actions (Figs. 11–30, 11–32, and 11–34). It is therefore possible that antagonists of these sites would block the ability of glycine (Fig. 11–33), polyamines (Fig. 11–34), or zinc (Fig. 11–35) to amplify glutamate action at their respective modulatory sites.

Other possible drugs would be those that could mimic the blocking actions of magnesium (Figs. 11–36 and 11–37) or phencyclidine (PCP) (Fig. 11–38) at the NMDA glutamate receptor complex. The PCP modulatory site, although a theoret-ical target for a neuroprotective agent, since it is neuroprotective in some animal models, it seems to mediate deep sedation and possibly even psychosis at neuropro-tective doses (Fig. 11–38). This ion channel antagonist site for NMDA-type glu-tamate receptors may therefore not be the optimal site for neuroprotective agents

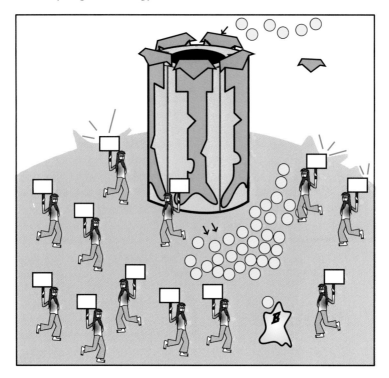

Free radicals begin
destroying the cell

FIGURE 11–26. **Cellular events occurring during excitotoxicity (part 3).** As the calcium accumulates in the cell, and the enzymes produce more and more free radicals, they begin to indiscriminately destroy parts of the cell, especially its membrane and organelles such as energy-producing mitochondria.

for clinical application. In fact, phencyclidine is thought to exert its psychotomimetic actions, and this site is also where dissociative anesthetics are thought to work (see Chapter 12).

We have already discussed that free radicals are generated in this neurodegenerative process (Figs. 11–24 through 11–27). Some drugs (and possibly even vitamin E) are free radical "scavengers," which soak up toxic free radicals like a chemical sponge and remove them (Fig. 11–39). A weak scavenger that has been tested in Parkinson's disease and tardive dyskinesia is vitamin E. A more powerful set of agents, currently available for clinical testing only in intravenous dosage formulations, are the lazaroids (so named because of their putative Lazarus-like actions of raising degenerating neurons from the dead).

One can readily see that there is intense research interest in pharmacological approaches to neurodegeneration, since neurodegenerative excitotoxicity could be a common pathological mechanism underlying a wide range of progressive disorders of the central nervous system (CNS).

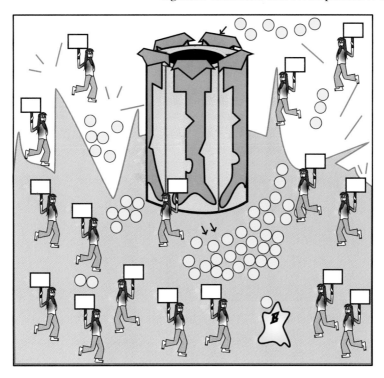

Finally, free radicals destroy the cell

FIGURE 11–27. **Cellular events occurring during excitotoxicity (part 4).** Eventually, the damage is so great that the free radicals essentially destroy the whole neuron.

Various rudimentary "neuroprotective" agents and antioxidant/anti–free radical therapies have already begun clinical testing. Trials of vitamin E, which has some antioxidant/free radical scavenging activity, have already begun in Parkinson's disease, tardive dyskinesia, and even Alzheimer's disease, but without definitive results to date. Vitamin E is not a very potent neuroprotective agent, and may therefore not exhibit sufficient efficacy to show neuroprotective properties in short-term trials.

L-Deprenyl (selegiline) is an irreversible inhibitor of monoamine oxidase (MAO), specifically of the B form. It is currently used in the treatment of Parkinson's disease to boost the effectiveness of dopaminergic agents, and possibly to delay disease progression. It is now being studied in Alzheimer's disease, since it has certain "antioxidant" effects that may prove to be neuroprotective. Some studies suggest that L-deprenyl may have additive effects to those of tacrine, if only short term.

Nimodipine is a calcium channel antagonist, now marketed for cerebrovascular disease, that may normalize cellular calcium levels or possibly affect another mechanism such as calcium-activated enzymes involved in cognition. Nimodipine is in clinical trials to determine its efficacy in improving global measures of memory function. Calcium channel antagonists are already used as possible neuroprotective

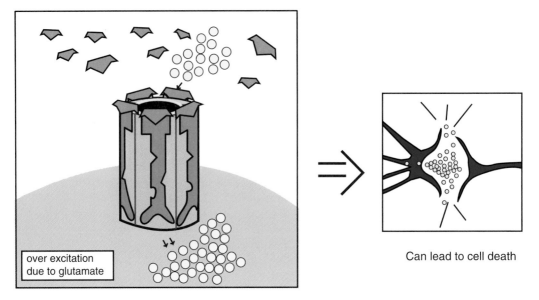

Can lead to cell death

FIGURE 11–28. Excessive glutamate activity is shown here to be mediated by **excesses in the amounts of glutamate itself**. Left to proceed too far, this could lead to cell death from **excitotoxicity**.

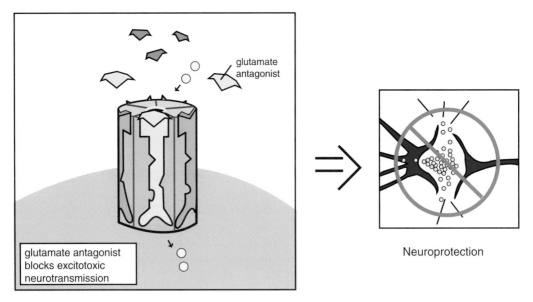

Neuroprotection

FIGURE 11–29. **Antagonists of glutamate** at the agonist site can block excitotoxic neurotransmission, and exert **neuroprotective actions**.

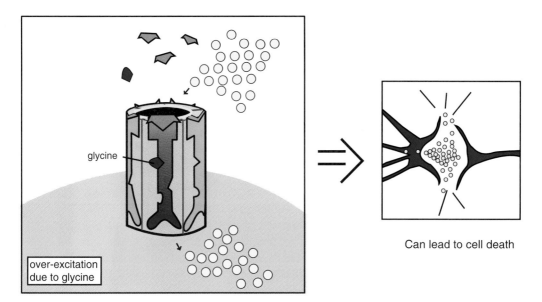

Can lead to cell death

FIGURE 11–30. Excessive glutamate activity is shown here to be mediated by a combination of too much glutamate and **too much glycine**. Here the glycine is helping glutamate mediate overexcitation of the neuron due to excessive opening of the calcium channel. This could lead to **excitotoxicity**.

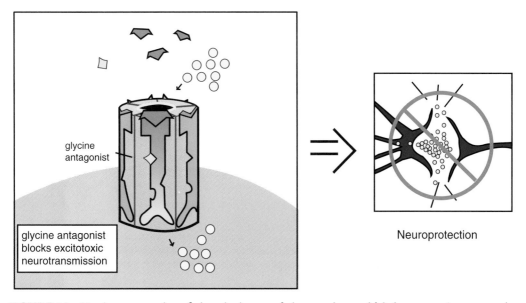

Neuroprotection

FIGURE 11–31. An **antagonist of the glycine modulatory site** could help antagonize excess glutamate neurotransmission and block excitotoxicity. This would be **neuroprotective**.

319

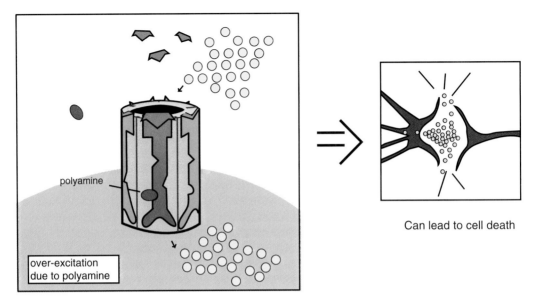

FIGURE 11–32. Excessive glutamate activity is shown here to be mediated by a combination of too much glutamate and **too much polyamine activity**. Here polyamines are helping glutamate mediate overexcitation of the neuron due to excessive opening of the calcium channel. This could lead to **excitotoxicity**.

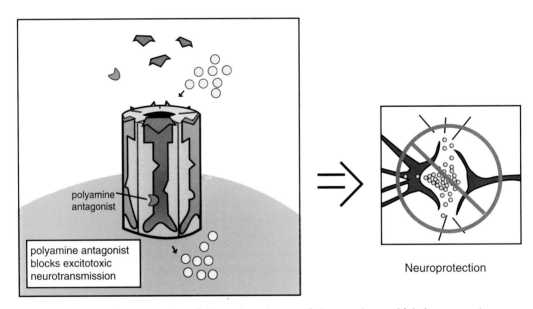

FIGURE 11–33. An **antagonist of the polyamine modulatory site** could help antagonize excess glutamate neurotransmission and block excitotoxicity. This would be **neuroprotective**.

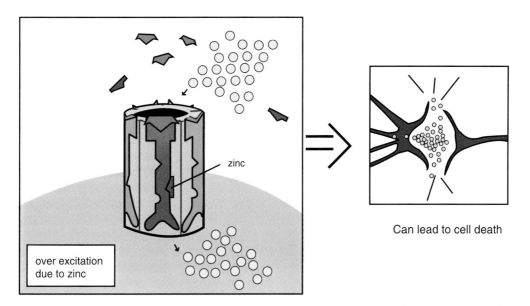

FIGURE 11–34. Excessive glutamate activity is shown here to be mediated by a combination of too much glutamate and **too much activity at the zinc modulatory site**. Here zinc is helping glutamate mediate overexcitation of the neuron due to excessive opening of the calcium channel. This could lead to **excitotoxicity**.

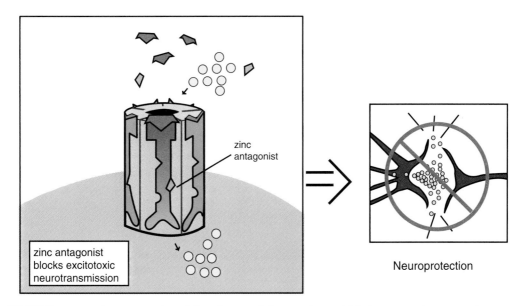

FIGURE 11–35. An **antagonist of the zinc modulatory site** could help antagonize excess glutamate neurotransmission and block excitotoxicity. This would be **neuroprotective**.

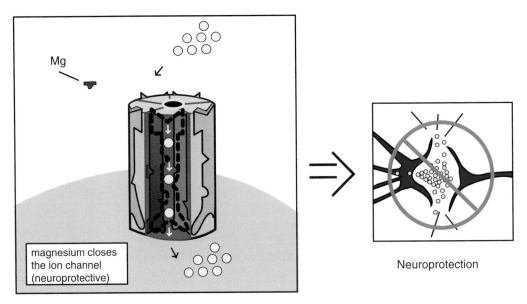

FIGURE 11–36. Magnesium is itself an antagonist to calcium passing through the ion channel. **Magnesium** may therefore be a type of naturally occurring **neuroprotective** chemical.

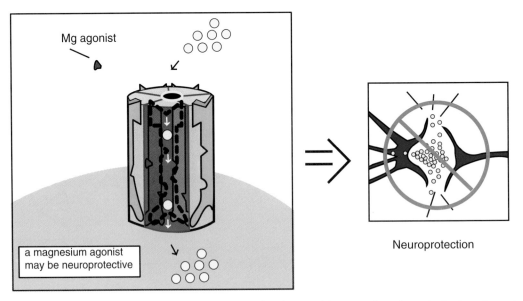

FIGURE 11–37. If the actions of **magnesium** in blocking calcium passing through the ion channel could be **mimicked** by a drug, it could exert **neuroprotective** actions by this mechanism.

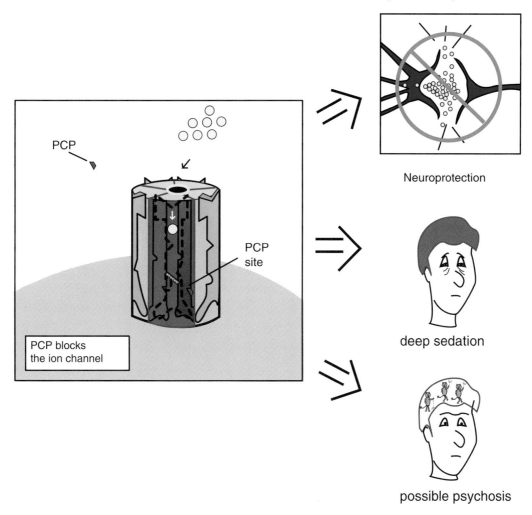

PCP

PCP
site

PCP blocks
the ion channel

Neuroprotection

deep sedation

possible psychosis

FIGURE 11–38. There is a modulatory site near the ion channel at the NMDA glutamate receptor–calcium channel complex that can block this channel and prevent calcium from flowing through it in response to excessive glutamate. This site is sometimes called the "**PCP site**" because it binds to the psychotomimetic drug phencyclidine (PCP). Thus, the PCP modulatory site, although a theoretical target for a neuroprotective agent, since it is **neuroprotective** in some animal models, seems to mediate **deep sedation** and possibly even **psychosis** at neuroprotective doses. So apparently do other drugs that act at this site. This ion channel antagonist site for NMDA-type glutamate receptors may therefore not be the optimal site for neuroprotective agents for clinical application. In fact, phencyclidine is thought to exert its **psychotomimetic actions** by blocking this site on the ion channel at NMDA glutamate receptors.

and/or cognitive enhancing agents, especially in Japan and in some European countries.

Sabeluzole is an agent with some neuroprotective activity in animal models of hypoxia, and also enhances axonal transport and neurite outgrowth in neuronal cells in culture by an uncertain mechanism. It is undergoing clinical testing in Alzheimer's disease at the present time.

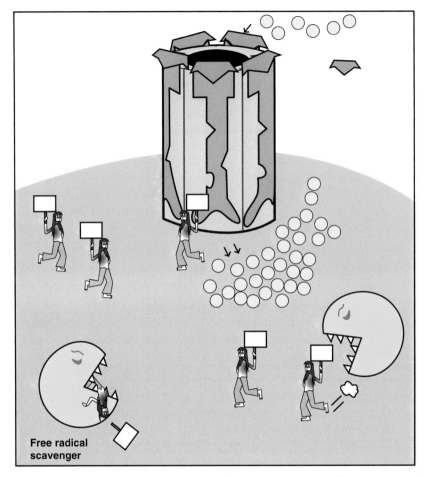

FIGURE 11–39. Free radicals are generated in the neurodegenerative process of excitotoxicity. A drug acting as a free radical "scavenger," soaking up toxic free radicals like a chemical sponge and removing them, would be neuroprotective. Vitamin E is a weak scavenger. Other free radical scavengers, such as the "lazaroids" (so named because of their putative Lazarus-like actions of raising degenerating neurons from the dead) are also being tested.

Cognitive Enhancers and Early Agents of Unproven or Limited Efficacy

Cerebral Vasodilators

Investigation of cerebral vasodilators was originally based upon the hypothesis that dementia is caused by atherosclerosis of cerebral vessels. Over the years, a wide variety of treatment modalities have been proposed to improve cerebrovascular circulation, including carbon dioxide; carbonic anhydrase inhibitors; anticoagulants; nicotinic acid (a vitamin B_6 derivative); pyritinol; meclofenate; vitamin E; hyperbaric oxygen; and vasodilators such as papaverine, cyclandelate, isoxsuprine, vincamine, and cinnarizine. All these modalities were aimed at improving oxygen delivery to the brain. None of these strategies has proved to be effective, however, and the hypothesis that faulty circulation is implicated in the dementia process is no longer tenable.

Nevertheless, there is still some carry-over use of these compounds, which were originally marketed in the era of the "faulty brain circulation hypothesis of dementia." Nafronyl has been used in Europe for elderly confused patients, but improvement is inconsistent. Cinnarizine is a vasodilating and calcium antagonist compound prescribed in Europe for vertigo and dementia related to chronic ischemia with equivocal efficacy. Pentoxifylline is a vasodilator that may improve memory in animals, but not conclusively in patients with dementia.

One of the methodological problems with studies of these earlier drugs is that since they "grew up" during the era when dementia was hypothesized to be solely or largely of cerebrovascular origin, studies of such agents were generally done in a population of dementia patients with a variety of causes of dementia including not only Alzheimer's disease but also vascular (multi-infarct) dementia and dementia of other causes as well. This makes interpretation of studies of such agents very problematic.

Metabolic Enhancers

Hydergine is the brand name of a mixture of ergot alkaloids, and was the first U.S. Food and Drug Administration (FDA) approved drug for the treatment of dementia, although not specifically for memory disturbances in Alzheimer's disease. During the era when Alzheimer's disease and dementia in general were believed to result from vascular disease, Hydergine was marketed as a "cerebral vasodilator" due to its putative but fairly weak alpha adrenergic antagonist actions, which might be expected to cause dilation of blood vessels. Subsequently, the drug was reclassified as a "metabolic enhancer" because of its ability to change second-messenger cyclic adenosine monophosphate (cAMP) levels, and because of the possibility that it acted as a partial agonist at dopamine, serotonin, and norepinephrine receptors. Several studies of higher doses of Hydergine have shown some beneficial effects in dementia, especially when cognitive impairment is mild. Several reports indicate improved mood is more pronounced than change in cognitive status. Currently, there is no consensus on how best to use Hydergine, or other putative "metabolic enhancers" or "cerebral vasodilators," or whether their widespread use is justified.

Vitamins and Hormones

Although vitamin B_{12} and zinc abnormalities have been described in Alzheimer's disease, most studies of replacement therapy with these agents have been negative. Thiamine and estrogen replacement therapies also have equivocal effects upon global assessment of cognitive functioning in trials of Alzheimer's disease patients. Alterations of brain angiotensin renin physiology have been reported in Alzheimer's disease, leading to the testing of angiotensin-converting enzyme (ACE) inhibitors such as captopril, which may have memory-enhancing effects in animals. Data for man, however, remain uncertain. 4-Aminopyridine is a drug that enhances calcium influx into neurons, with possible procholinergic activity, and has been tested in Alzheimer's disease with equivocal results.

Chelation

Speculation regarding the role of aluminum in Alzheimer's disease has prompted clinical and experimental use of chelation therapy to remove aluminum. Trials with chelating agents such as desferrioxamine, however, have been negative and the potential efficacy of future chelation therapy is uncertain. Chelation therapy is now largely considered to be an expensive and elaborate placebo for the treatment of Alzheimer's disease.

Nootropics

Nootropic drugs are a class of psychotropic drugs that enhance learning acquisition and reverse learning impairments in experimental animals. The term "nootropic" was introduced to describe a group of drugs that have the ability to improve certain brain mechanisms postulated to be associated with mental performance. The main features of nootropic agents in addition to the ability to enhance memory and learning are three other hypothesized actions: (1) facilitation of the flow of information between the cerebral hemispheres; (2) enhancement of the resistance of the brain to physical and chemical assault; and (3) lack of sedative, analgesic, or neuroleptic activity.

The naturally occurring agent acetyl-L-carnitine, formed by the acetylation of carnitine in mitochondria, has an analogous structure to ACh, and is sometimes classified as a nootropic agent, or as a weak ACh agonist. Its primary function is to participate in the synthesis of natural chemical products of the cell by facilitating transacetylation. Limited data exist in patients with cerebral ischemia in Japan, some of which suggest improvements in functioning. This has led to speculation that acetyl-L-carnitine may be a nootropic agent. One idea is that it acts by enhancing cellular protection by inhibiting both the formation of damaging lipid peroxides in cellular ischemia and the increased lactate production that follows interrupted blood flow.

The chemical structure of the prototype nootropic, piracetam, is a derivative of GABA. As yet, however, there is no established mechanism of action for nootropics, at GABA neurons or GABA receptors, or elsewhere. However, the toxicity of nootropics appear to be uniformly low. Some scientists hypothesize that nootropics are "metabolic enhancers," by influencing cerebral energy reserves and by increasing energy-containing chemicals such as adenosine triphosphate (ATP) in the brain. The initial nootropic compound was piracetam, but several more have since been developed, including pramiracetam, oxiracetam, and aniracetam. Limited data suggest that nootropics may be useful in improving memory, mood, or behavioral functioning in patients with mild to moderate senile dementia, but not in severely demented patients. These agents are used primarily outside the United States, as no nootropic is approved for any use in the United States. Although it has been difficult to document the ability of nootropics to alleviate symptoms of Alzheimer's disease, nootropics are in general use in some countries, especially in Europe.

More research is clearly needed, however, before one can advocate enthusiastic use of nootropics as cognitive enhancers for Alzheimer's disease.

Psychostimulants and Neurotransmitter Replacement Therapies

Psychostimulants such as methylphenidate may improve mood in depressed demented patients, but do not enhance cognition. Procaine hydrochloride, a local anesthetic that may also act by inhibiting MAO, has similar actions.

Use of agents active at monoamine neurons have been tested in Alzheimer's disease in the hope that modulating these neurons would enhance cognitive functioning. Thus, dopaminergic agents, as well as alpha 2 noradrenergic agonists such as clonidine, have been tested with no clear-cut results.

Neuropeptides

Several neuropeptide neurotransmitter systems are known to be disturbed in Alzheimer's disease, including somatostatin, corticotropin-releasing factor, neuropeptide Y, and substance P. A somatostatin analog tested to date has not been effective.

Arginine vasopressin and several of its analogues were extensively studied because of their role in cognition, and because of their demonstrated effects in animal studies of memory. In Alzheimer's disease patients, their use led to some reports of modest improvements in behavior, with improved energy and mood, but with not much improvement in memory. The same is true of adrenocorticotropic hormone (ACTH) agonists, which appear to affect mood and behavior without clear memory or cognitive effects. Studies of thyrotrophic-releasing hormone (TRH) analogues that have procholinergic effects have been largely negative. The opiate antagonist naloxone does not have consistent effects in improving cognition in Alzheimer's disease.

Treating Ancillary Psychiatric Symptoms

Until a cure or more effective treatments are found for cognitive functions in Alzheimer's disease, treatment of psychiatric symptoms may be the most effective psychopharmacological interventions currently available. Thus, the most treatable symptoms of Alzheimer's disease are not memory and cognitive disturbances, but depression and severe behavior disturbances, especially agitation and disordered thinking. The management of these psychiatric symptoms follows standard psychiatric practice as discussed in the chapters on depression (Chapter 5), antidepressants (Chapter 6), psychosis (Chapter 9), and antipsychotics (Chapter 10).

Thus, antidepressants are useful for treating depression in Alzheimer's disease. However, some antidepressants, particularly the tricyclic antidepressants, can induce delirium and increase the risk of falls. Neuroleptics are useful for treating delusions and hallucinations and can also reduce hostility and irritability. However, neuroleptics induce extrapyramidal side effects. Disturbed sleep is an extremely common component of Alzheimer's disease and one that frequently exhausts caregivers. Low doses of benzodiazepines may help, but should be used cautiously.

Other Current Research Approaches

Growth Factors

Neural regeneration or increased resistance to destructive processes may be achievable with selected neurotrophic factors. Nerve growth factor is the prototype with particular potential to synergize with cholinergic therapy, because its receptors are primarily localized on cholinergic neurons and it is present in relatively high levels in the basal forebrain where cholinergic neurons degenerate in Alzheimer's disease.

There are potential hazards to consider, however, with growth factor treatments. Thus, in addition to cholinergic neural regeneration, there is the possibility of inappropriate "sprouting" and corresponding growth in the wrong fibers. There is also an ominous rise in mRNA for APP, which may actually cause more formation of unwanted beta amyloid, as well as plaques and tangles.

Another growth factor—like substance is GM_1 ganglioside. Gangliosides in the brain are complex lipids associated with developing synapses. GM_1 ganglioside is capable of preventing neuronal degeneration in several animal models, and may also prevent retrograde degeneration of cholinergic neurons in the rat basal forebrain resulting from damage to the cerebral cortex. Although these strategies are in the very earliest stages of development, they represent concrete examples in animal models where endogenous trophic molecules potentially could be used to treat degenerative diseases such as Alzheimer's disease. This is discussed in Chapter 4 and shown in Figures 1–12, 4–14, and 4–15.

Transplantation

The hypothesis that implanting healthy neuronal tissue may promote regeneration and return of function in the diseased brain comes from animal experiments using tissues from fetal CNS, peripheral nerve, paraneural tissue, and cultured cells. When transplanted into the brain, these tissues may exert therapeutic effects via a variety of mechanisms. For example, they may act as a chemical generator (e.g., of growth factors), or as a generator of glial cells, which in turn promote neuronal function. They may also provide the brain with regenerating axons in the transplant material that may innervate other neurons from the diseased brain. At present, this is a highly theoretical area of research without current clinical applications. This is discussed in Chapter 4 and shown in Figure 4–16.

Benzodiazepine Inverse Agonists

Benzodiazepine agonists are a common clinical cause of reversible memory loss. If the opposite of this could be accomplished with an inverse agonist, would this mean that such an agent would actually enhance memory? The pharmacological basis of this speculative possibility is discussed in Chapter 7 and shown in Figure 7–20.

Future Combination Chemotherapies for Disorders Associated with Cognitive Disturbance and Memory Loss

We have already discussed in earlier chapters that there are tremendous economic incentives for developing the "cure" and treatment of choice for Alzheimer's disease. Thus, it is not difficult to understand why most drug development activities for the dementias target a single disease mechanism, just as they do for virtually every other psychiatric disorder. The goal of most ongoing drug development programs in psychopharmacology is to become the single, best, and only therapy for that disorder. In reality, however, it seems overly simplistic to conceptualize disorders with cognitive disturbances as the product of a single disease mechanism. Diseases such as Alzheimer's disease not only have features of cognitive and memory disturbance but may also have various psychotic, mood, and behavioral deficiencies plus a certain neurodegenerative component. Also, it takes a leap of faith to believe that such complex disorders could ever be satisfactorily treated with a single entity acting by a single therapeutic mechanism. This has also been mentioned in Chapter 10 in a similar discussion of the development of new therapies for schizophrenia.

Indeed, how realistic is it to ask a single therapeutic agent for Alzheimer's disease to treat the memory and cognitive symptoms of dementia; to treat the often associated disorganized symptoms of Alzheimer's disease such as psychosis, agitation, and poor impulse control; and to prevent further neurodegeneration.

Perhaps psychopharmacological treatments for cognitive disorders in the future will need to borrow a chapter out of the book of cancer chemotherapy – which we have argued as well for new therapies of schizophrenia. In cancer chemotherapy, the standard of treatment is to use multiple drugs simultaneously. "Combination chemotherapy" for malignancy utilizes the approach of adding together several independent therapeutic mechanisms. When successful, this results in a total therapeutic response that is greater than the sum of its parts. Usually, this also has the favorable consequence of simultaneously diminishing total side effects, since adverse experiences of multiple drugs are mediated by different pharmacological mechanisms and therefore should not be additive.

Thus, Alzheimer's disease treatments of the future may combine one treatment for cognitive and memory symptoms (perhaps some sort of procholinergic agent such as a cholinesterase inhibitor), with another treatment for disturbed, agitated, and violent symptoms of poor impulse control (possibly an atypical neuroleptic, or an agent working by a combination of actions on dopamine and serotonin receptors), with a neuroprotective agent (e.g., a glutamate antagonist) (Fig. 11–40). In the long run, some sort of molecular-based therapy to prevent genetically programmed disease progression will also form part of the portfolio of treatments for Alzheimer's disease (Fig. 11–40).

The reason for this combination medication approach to Alzheimer's disease is that it does not appear to be sufficient merely to replace the deficiencies in acetylcholine activity by drugs that enhance cholinergic function. This approach can boost memory function measurably in some patients, only to have this enhancement eroded by further disease progression within a few months in most patients. The replacement of cholinergic deficiencies by various pharmacological strategies may help memory; correcting other neurotransmitter imbalances (e.g., of dopamine and serotonin) may treat behavioral disorders; neuroprotective and genetic strategies may halt the degenerative process and replace the functions of degenerated nerves (Fig. 10–40).

Clinical trials with multiple therapeutic agents working by several mechanisms can be quite difficult to undertake, but as there is a clinical trials methodology that exists in the cancer chemotherapy literature, it may be an approach that should be applied for complex neurodegenerative disorders with multiple underlying disease mechanisms.

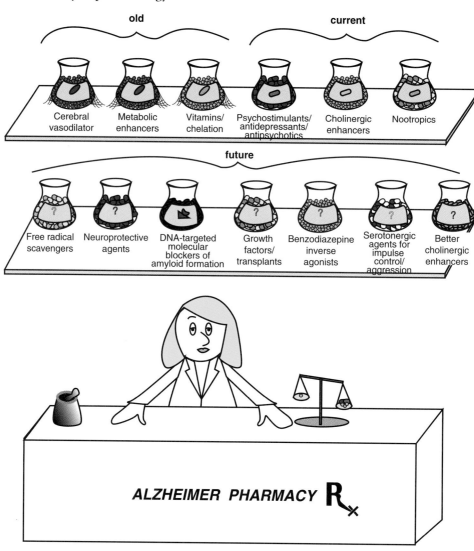

FIGURE 11–40. The Alzheimer pharmacy. A few years ago this pharmacy was entirely empty, or included only agents of unproven or limited efficacy.

Summary

In this chapter, we have provided a simple description of some of the *clinical features of dementia* as well as memory complaints that may be a part of the *normal aging process*. We have described the clinical and pathological features of *Alzheimer's disease*, emphasizing the formation of *amyloid plaques and neurofibrillary tangles* in this disorder. The *amyloid cascade hypothesis* is a leading theory to explain the neurodegeneration of Alzheimer's disease, perhaps by deposition of neurotoxic amyloid protein. This could be due to the formation of amyloid from abnormal precursors, or the failure to remove amyloid because of abnormal binding proteins that cannot get rid of amyloid.

Neurotransmitter-based therapies for Alzheimer's disease include various mechanisms to *enhance cholinergic functioning*. The pharmacology of cholinergic neurons was presented, as well as various approaches to enhancing it in Alzheimer's disease. The pharmacology of glutamate neurotransmission was also presented, including hypotheses that *excessive glutamate neurotransmission* could be excitotoxic and cause neurodegeneration in Alzheimer's disease and other neurological disorders including stroke. We have discussed the various theoretical targets within the glutamate system that might be able to block excitotoxically mediated neurodegeneration.

Finally, various other approaches to the treatment of Alzheimer's disease, past and future, were discussed here. This includes older agents of unproven or limited efficacy as well as future therapies based upon contemporary knowledge of the neurobiological basis of Alzheimer's disease.

CHAPTER 12

DRUGS OF ABUSE

Psychopharmacology is defined in this text as the study of drugs that affect the brain. The previous chapters of this book have addressed how psychotropic drugs affect the brain when they are used by experts for therapeutic purposes. Unfortunately, psychotropic drugs are all too commonly misused. This can be either misuse of prescription drugs by poorly informed medical professionals or abuse by individuals for nontherapeutic purposes. Most who abuse psychotropic drugs get their supply from sources outside the medical profession, either legal (e.g., alcohol and cig-arettes) or illegal.

Misuse and abuse of psychotropic agents are major public health problems throughout the world. Such problems lead not only to multiple medical and psychiatric complications but also to a myriad of social problems. Society has turned to psychopharmacology to explain how abuse of psychotropic agents affects the brain. Thus, the task of psychopharmacology in the area of drug abuse is to answer the question: How do psychotropic drugs affect the brain when they are misused or abused for nontherapeutic purposes? We will attempt to answer this question for the major classes of psychotropic agents that are abused.

Our approach to this problem is to discuss how nontherapeutic use, short-term abuse (intoxication), and the complications of long-term abuse affect chemical neurotransmission in the brain. We will not discuss the many other important aspects of psychoactive substance abuse, leaving it to other experts to explore such issues as the relationship of drug abuse to economics, criminal behavior, and violence.

Explanation of Terms

Before exploring the neurochemical mechanisms related to psychoactive substance abuse, it is useful to define several terms as they will be used here (Table 12–1). Because drug abuse has become such a prominent social problem, the various terms used in this field have been increasingly employed by those outside this field, including the lay public and those with political or social agendas. These latter individuals often do not mean the same thing when using a given term as does a psychopharmacologist, whose perspective is limited to the mechanism of action of a drug upon chemical neurotransmission. Thus, it is necessary first to define these terms as they will be used here from a psychopharmacological perspective before applying them to specific agents. Whenever available, DSM-IV definitions will be used for all terms.

Reinforcement

Reinforcement is the term that explains in part the reason why individuals repeatedly abuse a drug: namely, drugs of abuse have various *reinforcing properties* that are rewarding to the individual. This leads to repeated self-administration in order to produce these pleasurable effects over and over again. The neurochemical basis of reinforcement (or reward) is thought to depend upon the specific mechanisms of action of the various drugs of abuse upon neurotransmission. The possible mechanism for each individual drug is discussed below, and a unifying hypothesis based upon the mesolimbic dopamine system and the psychopharmacology of pleasure is discussed at the end of this chapter.

Two Types of Misuse: Intoxication versus Abuse

Sanctioned uses of drugs have always been defined within a culture, and therefore differ across cultures and are prone to change as cultures change over time. One consequence of drug misuse is *intoxication*, a reversible drug-specific syndrome characterized by clinically significant maladaptive behavior or psychological changes that

Table 12−1. *Key terms and their definitions*

Intoxication − the development of a reversible clinical syndrome of maladaptive behavioral or psychological changes due to taking a recent dose of a drug acting on the central nervous system (see Table 12−2 for the official DSM-IV definition of substance intoxication).

Abuse − self-administration of any drug in a culturally disapproved manner that causes adverse consequences specifically defined in DSM-IV (see Table 12−3 for the official definition of substance abuse).

Addiction − a behavioral pattern of drug abuse characterized by overwhelming involvement with the use of a drug (compulsive use), the securing of its supply, and a high tendency to relapse after discontinuation (not defined in DSM-IV).

Dependence − the physiological state of neuroadaptation produced by repeated administration of a drug, necessitating continued administration to prevent the appearance of the withdrawal syndrome. DMS-IV requires that at least three out of a list of seven items occur within a 12-month period (see Table 12−4 for the official definition of substance dependence).

Reinforcement − the tendency of a pleasure-producing drug to lead to repeated self administration (not specifically defined in DSM-IV).

Tolerance − tolerance has developed when after repeated administration, a given dose of a drug produces a decreased effect, or, conversely, when increasingly larger doses must be administered to obtain the effects observed with the original use (see Table 12−4 for DSM-IV definition).

Cross-tolerance and cross-dependence − the ability of one drug to suppress the manifestations of physical dependence produced by another drug and to maintain the physically dependent state (not specifically defined in DSM-IV).

Withdrawal − the psychological and physiological reactions to abrupt cessation of a dependence-producing drug (see Table 12−5 for the official DSM-IV definition of substance withdrawal).

Relapse − the reoccurrence upon discontinuation of an effective medical treatment, of the original condition from which the patient suffered (not specifically defined in DSM-IV).

Rebound − the exaggerated expression of the original condition sometimes experienced by patients immediately after cessation of an effective treatment (not specifically defined in DSM-IV).

are due to the psychopharmacological actions of the drug upon neurotransmission. The symptoms of intoxication range from belligerence, to changes in mood, to cognitive impairment or impaired judgment, to impaired social or occupational functioning (see Table 12−2 for the official DSM-IV definition of intoxication).

Another form of drug misuse occurs when a drug has been taken over a 12-month period of time and in a manner that produces clinically significant impairment or distress; this is called *abuse* (see Table 12−3 for the official DSM-IV definition of substance abuse).

Our culture has difficulty defining misuse not only for illicit drugs but also for "legal" drugs such as alcohol and cigarettes, and even for prescription drug use supervised by experts. On the one hand, our society clearly disapproves of and has criminalized the obtaining and selling drugs from "the street" rather than from a

Table 12–2. *DMS-IV criteria for substance intoxication*

A. The development of a reversible substance-specific syndrome due to recent ingestion of (or exposure to) a substance. NOTE: Different substances may produce similar or identical syndromes.

B. Clinically significant maladaptive behavioral or psychological changes that are due to the effect of the substance on the central nervous system (e.g., belligerence, mood lability, cognitive impairment, impaired judgment, impaired social or occupational functioning) and develop during or shortly after use of the substance.

C. The symptoms are not due to a general medical condition and are not better accounted for by another mental disorder.

Table 12–3. *DSM-IV criteria for substance abuse*

A. A maladaptive pattern of substance use leading to clinically significant impairment or distress, as manifested by one (or more) of the following, occurring within a 12-month period:
    1. Recurrent substance use resulting in a failure to fulfill major role obligations at work, school, or home (e.g., repeated absences or poor work performance related to substance use; substance-related absences, suspension, or expulsions from school; neglect of children or household).
    2. Recurrent substance use in situations in which it is physically hazardous (e.g., driving an automobile or operating a machine when impaired by substance use).
    3. Recurrent substance-related legal problems (e.g., arrests for substance-related disorderly conduct).
    4. Continued substance use despite having persistent or recurrent social or interpersonal problems caused or exacerbated by the effects of the substance (e.g., arguments with spouse about consequences of intoxication, physical fights).

B. The symptoms have never met the criteria for substance dependence for this class of substance.

licensed medical practitioner. This applies especially to opiates, stimulants, and hallucinogens, but there is less strong disapproval of other illicit drugs, such as marijuana.

There is also debate on the line between use and misuse of prescription agents such as amphetamines, sleeping pills, and anxiolytics, even when used within the prescribing guidelines of an expert. For example, some members of our society believe that benzodiazepine use should be disapproved even if sanctioned by a physician for an anxiety disorder. These critics would call such use of drugs "abuse" due to inappropriate diagnosing and "overmedication" to the detriment of existential being, self-actualization, and personal growth. On the other hand, another medical professional may see the same clinical situation as a medically sanctioned use of a drug for a medical illness (i.e., standard medical care requiring the use of a benzodiazepine, a sleeping pill, or a stimulant). Thus, the use of the term abuse can vary quite widely. For our discussion, we will use the DSM-IV definition.

Table 12-4. *DSM-IV criteria for substance dependence*

A maladaptive pattern of substance use, leading to clinically significant impairment or distress, as manifested by three (or more) of the following, occurring at any time in the same 12-month period:

1. Tolerance, as defined by either of the following:
   (a) A need for markedly increased amounts of the substance to achieve intoxication or desired effect
   (b) Markedly diminished effect with continued use of the same amount of the substance

2. Withdrawal, as manifested by either of the following:
   (a) The characteristic withdrawal syndrome for the substance defined for each specific substance in DSM-IV
   (b) The same (or a closely related) substance is taken to relieve or avoid withdrawal symptoms

3. The substance is often taken in larger amounts or over a longer period than was intended

4. There is a persistent desire or unsuccessful efforts to cut down or control substance use

5. A great deal of time is spent in activities necessary to obtain the substance (e.g., visiting multiple doctors or driving long distances), use the substance (e.g., chain-smoking), or recover from its effects

6. Important social, occupational, or recreational activities are given up or reduced because of substance use

7. The substance use is continued despite knowledge of having a persistent or recurrent physical or psychological problem that is likely to have been caused or exacerbated by the substance

Addiction and Dependence

Addiction and dependence are frequently confused. Addiction is hard to define, with little consensus on what it means among many who use the term, and is not defined as a condition in DSM-IV. Dependence is easier to define and will be emphasized in our discussions here (see Table 12–4 for the official DSM-IV definition of substance dependence).

Thus, the term *addiction* is frequently employed by those who are not experts in psychopharmacology when *dependence* is what they mean. That is, *addiction* is a behavioral pattern of drug abuse characterized by overwhelming involvement with the use of a drug (compulsive use), the securing of its supply, and a high tendency to relapse after discontinuation; whereas *dependence* is the physiological state of neuroadaptation produced by repeated administration of a drug, necessitating continued administration to prevent the appearance of a withdrawal syndrome. The terms "addiction" and "addict" often evoke negative emotional reactions that can contribute to difficulties in communicating scientific concepts.

Several things can occur when a drug causes dependence and the individual continues taking it: namely, *cross-dependence, tolerance,* and *cross-tolerance.* Several other things can occur when a drug causes dependence and the individual abruptly stops

Table 12–5. *DSM-IV criteria for substance withdrawal*

A.	The development of a substance-specific syndrome due to the cessation of (or reduction in) substance use that has been heavy and prolonged
B.	The substance-specific syndrome causes clinically significant distress or impairment in social, occupational, or other important areas of functioning
C.	The symptoms are not due to a general medical condition and are not better accounted for by another medical disorder

taking it; namely, *withdrawal* and *rebound*. Each of these will now be defined. Later, in relationship to specific drugs, the various neuroadaptive mechanisms that mediate each of these will also be discussed in terms of the impact they have on chemical transmission of specific neurotransmitters.

Tolerance and Cross-Tolerance

Tolerance has developed when after repeated administration, a given dose of a drug produces a decreased effect, or, conversely, when increasingly larger doses must be administered to obtain the effects observed with the original use (see Table 12–4 for DSM-IV definition of tolerance). Related to this are *cross-tolerance* and *cross-dependence*, which are the ability of one drug to suppress the manifestations of physical dependence produced by another drug and to maintain the physically dependent state, respectively.

Withdrawal

Withdrawal is the term for the adverse psychological and physiological reactions to abrupt cessation of a dependence-producing drug (see Table 12–5 for the official DSM-IV definition of substance withdrawal). It is very important to distinguish withdrawal from rebound, as these are frequently confused, even by psychopharmacologists, because both are related to the neurochemical changes that mediate dependence. *Rebound* is what happens when dependence occurs in patients who have taken a drug for a medically sanctioned use, and then that drug is suddenly stopped (i.e., their symptoms come back in an exaggerated fashion). *Withdrawal*, on the other hand, is what happens when tolerance occurs in those who have abused a drug and then that drug is suddenly stopped (i.e., they develop withdrawal symptoms, often craving, dysphoria, and signs of sympathetic nervous system overactivity).

Dependence is a term that is not frequently used outside of psychopharmacology, but in fact is a key feature of many antihypertensive medications, hormones, and other treatments throughout medicine. Thus, several antihypertensives can produce *rebound* hypertension, worse than the original blood pressure elevation, when suddenly discontinued. These patients are not "addicted" to their blood pressure medications, although they are dependent upon them. Such hypertensive patients who suddenly discontinue these antihypertensive drugs do not experience withdrawal effects, since their symptoms are an exaggerated manifestation of their original condition, and not a new set of symptoms such as craving or dysphoria.

It is interesting to note that by analogy, a panic disorder patient who suddenly stops a benzodiazepine and gets rebound panic attacks may sometimes be incorrectly accused of being addicted to benzodiazepines. As in the case of the patient discontinuing antihypertensives, this panic patient is dependent upon his medication, and is experiencing rebound, not withdrawal or addiction. These distinctions among dependence, addiction, rebound, and withdrawal should be kept in mind when educating patients about their medications associated with these actions.

Detoxification

Detoxification is the slow tapering of a drug that has caused dependence and would cause withdrawal if stopped too suddenly. Detoxification can be accomplished either by slowly withdrawing the dependence-forming drug itself, or by substitution with a cross-dependent drug that has a similar pharmacological mechanism of action. In either case, detoxification is done by slowly tapering the dependent or cross-dependent drug so that the neuroadaptational mechanisms of dependence can readapt during dose tapering and thus prevent the emergence of withdrawal symptoms.

Tapering of a drug treatment for a medical condition (such as hypertension or panic) that has caused dependence can also prevent the emergence of rebound. In this case, it is not called detoxification, but tapered discontinuation. Detoxification generally implies a method to prevent withdrawal, not to prevent rebound.

Rebound and Relapse

Another important distinction to make is that of *rebound* from *relapse*, as these two terms are constantly confused. The term *relapse* was already introduced in our discussion of depression in Chapter 5. Relapse refers to the reoccurrence of disease symptoms upon discontinuation of an effective medical treatment. Relapse assumes an underlying medical condition for which the drug was administered, and which therefore constituted a medically sanctioned use.

Thus, in the case of diabetes mellitus, if a patient requires insulin, he is generally referred to as "insulin-dependent," not "addicted to insulin." If such a patient suddenly stops his insulin, his glucose levels will generally return to pretreatment levels (i.e., *relapse* of diabetes, not *rebound* to a worse state of diabetes).

In the case of panic disorder, we have already mentioned that if a patient requires benzodiazepines to suppress panic attacks, he can be referred to as "benzodiazepine-dependent," not "addicted to benzodiazepines." Moreover, if such a patient suddenly stops benzodiazepines, he may experience *rebound* panic attacks (i.e., panic attacks that are more frequent and severe than the original panic disorder). Upon discontinuation of benzodiazepines, especially if they are tapered over a long period of time, this patient may very well experience the return of his usual panic attacks (i.e., *relapse* of panic disorder).

This patient has not developed withdrawal symptoms if he experiences panic attacks after discontinuing benzodiazepines. However, if the patient develops insomnia, irritability, seizures, and agitation – none of which were symptoms of his original panic attacks – he *has* developed symptoms of *withdrawal*. This anecdote thus demonstrates the distinctions among rebound, relapse, and withdrawal in a panic disorder patient dependent upon benzodiazepines.

In summary, there are many important terms in the field of psychotropic drug abuse that are frequently used differently not only by lay persons, patients, politicians, and social scientists but also by psychopharmacologists. We have attempted to define how the terms will be used here, recognizing that the field is constantly defining the "correct" or possibly "politically correct" definitions, and that those proposed here may only be useful within the context of this chapter.

Benzodiazepines

Pharmacology of Benzodiazepine Abuse

We have already discussed extensively the mechanism of therapeutic actions of benzodiazepines in Chapter 7 as anxiolytics as well as anticonvulsants, muscle relaxants, and sedative-hypnotics. Namely, benzodiazepines act as allosteric modulators of gamma-amino-butyric acid type A (GABA A) receptors (Fig. 12–1). This causes a net boosting of chloride conductance through a chloride channel, enhancing inhibitory neurotransmission and causing anxiolytic actions. Such actions are also thought to underlie the production of the reinforcing properties of euphoria or a sedating sort of tranquility that causes some individuals to abuse these drugs. Excessive actions of benzodiazepines at the same receptors that mediate their therapeutic actions is thought to be the psychopharmacological mechanism of euphoria, drug reinforcement, and at an extreme, overdose.

When benzodiazepines are used or abused chronically, they may cause adaptive changes in benzodiazepine receptors such that they become less powerful in modulating GABA A receptors in response to a benzodiazepine as time goes on (Fig. 12–2). Incidentally, it is this very same shift in benzodiazepine receptor sensitivity that is postulated to occur as the cause of panic disorder (see Fig. 8–13). It is not surprising, therefore, that patients who abuse anxiolytics experience anxiety and even panic attacks when they stop taking the drugs (Fig. 12–3).

This shift in benzodiazepine receptor sensitivity in benzodiazepine abusers to a desensitized receptor (Fig. 12–2) may become manifest as the need to take higher doses of benzodiazepines in order to get "high." This receptor desensitization is especially uncovered once chronic abusive benzodiazepine administration is discontinued, and particularly if discontinuation is sudden (Fig. 12–3).

In the case of sudden benzodiazepine discontinuation in a chronic benzodiazepine abuser, the presence of desensitized benzodiazepine receptors actually worsens the impact of benzodiazepine discontinuation. The brain, which is used to too much benzodiazepine being at its receptors, is suddenly starved for benzodiazepine. Therefore, the brain experiences the reverse of benzodiazepine intoxication, namely dysphoria and depression instead of euphoria; anxiety and agitation instead of tranquility and lack of anxiety; insomnia instead of sedation and sleep; muscle tension instead of muscle relaxation, and at worst, seizures instead of anticonvulsant effects (see also Fig. 7–20).

These actions continue either until benzodiazepine is replaced or until the receptors readapt to the sensitivity they had prior to excessive use of the benzodiazepines. Alternatively, one can reinstitute benzodiazepines, but taper them slowly, so that the receptors have time to readapt during dosage reduction, and withdrawal symptoms are prevented.

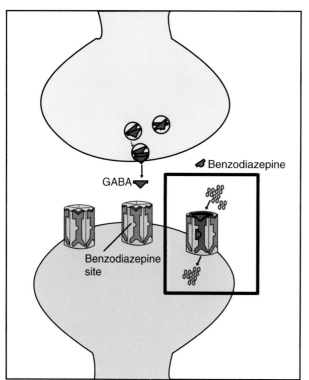

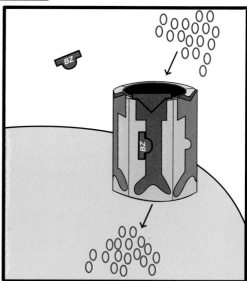

If benzodiazepine is given
to a drug-naive patient, there
is an acute benzodiazepine effect,
and the channel opens a lot.

FIGURE 12–1. **Acute administration of a benzodiazepine to a nondependent individual.** Benzodiazepines act as allosteric modulators of GABA A receptors. If a benzodiazepine is given to a drug-naive patient, there is an acute benzodiazepine effect, opening the chloride channel maximally. This causes a net boosting of chloride conductance through a chloride channel, enhancing inhibitory neurotransmission and causing anxiolytic actions. Such actions are also thought to underlie the production of the reinforcing properties of euphoria or a sedating sort of tranquility that causes some individuals to abuse these drugs. Excessive actions of benzodiazepines at the same receptors that mediate their therapeutic actions is thought to be the psychopharmacological mechanism of euphoria, drug reinforcement and, at an extreme, overdose.

340

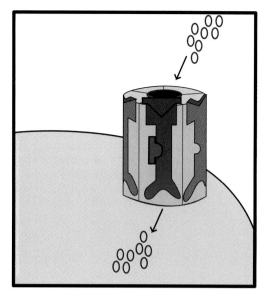

If benzodiazepine is given
to a patient who is tolerant to the drug,
the channel opens a little (still enough
to have an anxiolytic effect)

FIGURE 12–2. **Chronic administration of a benzodiazepine to an individual who has developed tolerance and dependence**. When benzodiazepines are used or abused chronically, they may cause **adaptive changes** in benzodiazepine receptors such that they become less powerful in modulating GABA A receptors in response to a benzodiazepine as time goes on. Administration of a benzodiazepine to such an individual causes the chloride channel to open less than before, but still enough to give an anxiolytic or perhaps euphoric and drug-reinforcing effect. That effect may be diminished, however, compared to acute administration prior to the development of this desensitization and tolerance.

In summary, benzodiazepine dependence is thought to be mediated by adaptive changes in benzodiazepine receptors to a state of diminished sensitivity. Withdrawal symptoms are produced when desensitized receptors plus benzodiazepine deficiency work together to produce essentially the opposite clinical effects as experienced during benzodiazepine intoxication. Readaptation of the receptors reverses dependence and stops symptoms of withdrawal.

Clinical Aspects of Benzodiazepine Abuse

One area of psychopharmacology where it has been particularly difficult to establish the difference between *use* and *abuse* is the case of benzodiazepines. Some believe that benzodiazepines are overused because of naive assumptions by physicians and patients about the safety of these agents. Others may discount criticism of benzodiazepine abuse as hysterical "benzo bashing."

Use of benzodiazepines shortly after they were marketed in the 1960s did lead to a certain euphoria about them as the pendulum swung past appropriate use at times to indiscriminate use both by patients and by physicians. Claims eventually arose that the benzodiazepines were not only overprescribed for minor degrees of anxiety (the "overmedicated society"), but also that their real problems were overlooked just because such problems were much less when compared to the barbitu-

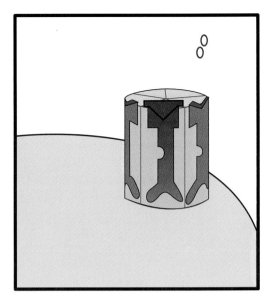

If benzodiazepine is suddenly stopped for a patient who is tolerant to the drug, the channel closes, creating anxiety

FIGURE 12–3. **Acute withdrawal of benzodiazepines in a benzodiazepine-dependent individual**. If benzodiazepines are suddenly stopped in a patient who is tolerant to them and dependent upon them, benzodiazepine receptors will experience this as an **acute deficiency** at their binding sites. Thus, the presence of desensitized benzodiazepine receptors actually worsens the impact of benzodiazepine discontinuation. The brain, which is used to too much benzodiazepine being at its receptors, is suddenly starved for benzodiazepine. Therefore, the brain experiences the reverse of benzodiazepine intoxication, namely dysphoria and depression instead of euphoria; anxiety and agitation instead of tranquility and lack of anxiety; insomnia instead of sedation and sleep; muscle tension instead of muscle relaxation; and at worst, seizures instead of anticonvulsant effects. These actions continue either until benzodiazepine is replaced or until the receptors readapt to the sensitivity they had prior to excessive use of the benzodiazepines. Alternatively, one can reinstitute benzodiazepines, but taper them slowly, so that the receptors have time to readapt during dosage reduction, and withdrawal symptoms are prevented.

rates they replaced. Valium and eventually Xanax became some of the most widely prescribed drugs in the world, and a part of everyday vocabulary.

A backlash against the benzodiazepines developed when it came to be recognized that some patients indeed have difficulties discontinuing these drugs, particularly after long-term use. Thus, *withdrawal* effects were described due to *dependency* on the benzodiazepines. *Rebound* anxiety and rebound insomnia were noted, and even cases of frank drug abuse with severe withdrawal reactions when the benzodiazepines were withdrawn.

The surprise that the benzodiazepines were associated with some unexpected and previously ignored difficulties created a popular era of "benzo bashing," where the problems of the benzodiazepines were not just recognized but were overstated as the pendulum began to swing back in the direction of disillusionment. Benzodiazepine adversaries began to call these agents the "opium of the masses" and to misuse the terms *addiction and abuse* when the real problems were *dependence and withdrawal*. This plays exceedingly well in the popular press. So strong has the backlash against benzodiazepines become that many patients fear taking these drugs altogether.

A Happy Median

The truth about the benzodiazepines now seems to be settling out as the pendulum is coming back to the center. The original Pollyanna attitude that the drugs can do no harm is no more accurate than irrational fears overstating benzodiazepines as dangerous drugs that do more harm than good. The informed psychopharmacologist must know the definition of the key terms discussed above, and know how to use them with precision if one is to know the scientific basis for the risks and the benefits of the benzodiazepines.

Discontinuation of Benzodiazepines

The long-term use of benzodiazepines – as well as any other drug class discussed here that has the potential to produce tolerance – obliges the psychopharmacologist to have expertise in recognizing and managing long-term complications. *Dependence and withdrawal* problems can often be prevented if benzodiazepines can be withdrawn after short-term use prior to the completion of the neuroadaptive mechanisms that produce tolerance (see Figs. 12–1, 12–2, and 12–3).

If benzodiazepine use causes dependence because of the necessity of long-term use, when the time comes to discontinue treatment, one must know how to withdraw these agents. Ignorance of how to do this as well as aborted attempts to successfully withdraw the benzodiazepines are often key reasons for long-term inappropriate use of these agents. In some cases it may just seem easier to continue the agent than to go through the hassle and discomfort of an appropriate withdrawal program, especially if the patient has had a bad experience previously with attempts at withdrawal and is resistant to stopping medication. This situation is a too frequent perception by patients and their physicians and can sabotage efforts to discontinue any dependence-forming drug.

Discontinuation of benzodiazepines is more complex in patients with an underlying anxiety disorder than in patients who abused them but had no underlying anxiety disorder. In the case of a patient with an anxiety disorder, in addition to treating or preventing withdrawal symptoms, there is the need to anticipate rebound symptoms of anxiety, and relapse of anxiety, possibly necessitating reinstitution of some other form of therapy as benzodiazepines are being tapered. In cases where alternative treatments are not effective, continued administration of benzodiazepines may be necessary even though the patient is dependent upon them because the risk/benefit calculation weighs in favor of continuing treatment.

The first step in benzodiazepine discontinuation is to consider the problem being treated (Table 12–6). Specifically, does the problem justify continued treatment with a benzodiazepine? Has the patient significantly benefitted from treatment with a benzodiazepine? If not, benzodiazepine treatment may not be justified at all. If so, benzodiazepine discontinuation may not be justified. If the patient has benefitted, but is stable and ready for a trial off medication, discontinuation would generally be justified. Often, assessment of patients on benzodiazepines reveals a marginal justification for the original prescription of these agents and discontinuation is definitely indicated in such cases.

The second step in the decision process for benzodiazepine discontinuation is to ask whether the patient's use of the benzodiazepine has remained within the pre-

Table 12—6. *Key considerations in discontinuing benzodiazepines*

Step 1.   Consider the problem being treated. Does the problem justify continued treatment with a benzodiazepine? Has the patient significantly benefitted from treatment with a benzodiazepine?

Step 2.   Ask whether the patient's use of the benzodiazepine has remained within the prescribed limits and duration of treatment. Also, has the patient avoided the use of other prescribed or nonprescribed agents?

Step 3.   Determine whether the patient has been free of any signs of intoxication or impairment from the use of benzodiazepine medication, either alone or in combination with other agents.

Step 4.   Does a family monitor of the patient confirm that there have been no problems with the benzodiazepine use and that the patient has benefitted from the use of the medication?

Table 12—7. *Patient readiness to begin benzodiazepine tapering*

Patient feeling ready and confident
Patient educated about anxiety and medication discontinuation
Patient back to premorbid functioning
Patient no longer preoccupied with anxiety
Major conflicts and stressors resolved
No foreseeable stressors during tapering

scribed limits and duration of treatment (Table 12—6). Has the patient also avoided the use of other prescribed or nonprescribed agents?

The third step in proceeding with benzodiazepine discontinuation is to determine whether the patient has been free of any signs of intoxication or impairment from the use of benzodiazepine medication, either alone or in combination with other agents (Table 12—6). Patients who do not stay within the guidelines of dosage given to them by their prescribing physician are not as likely to comply with dosage reduction efforts to taper medication to the point of discontinuation. Also, patients who purposely take more medication than required to reduce symptoms of anxiety in order to purposely produce euphoric or other subjective feelings of intoxication are not good candidates for successful compliance with a tapering program.

Finally, does a family monitor of the patient confirm that there have been no problems with the benzodiazepine use and that the patient has benefitted from the use of the medication (Table 12—6)? The use of a family monitor can allow the clinician to collect more objective data than the patient may be willing or able to offer him/herself.

Implementing a Successful Benzodiazepine Tapering Program

Successful tapering involves proper *timing* for the start of taper (Table 12—7). It is most helpful but not absolutely necessary that the patient be generally free of the anxiety symptoms for which the medication was originally prescribed. Also, the patient should be in a stable set of life circumstances, free from current significant stressors such as divorce, bankruptcy, etc.

The patient should also be *prepared* for the taper well in advance of its implementation. It may be useful to mention in fact that the patient will be tapered at a specific time in the future when the patient receives the first prescription of medication. Follow-up visits may reinforce that taper will begin when symptoms have been under control for a certain length of time. As that time approaches, it will not be a surprise to the patient that tapering is part and parcel of the use of benzodiazepines for the treatment of anxiety. It may be useful to prepare a written taper schedule for the patient in advance of actually beginning this, so that the patient may study it and understand the taper program, have input to it, and work with the prescribing clinician to tailor it uniquely to the individual's needs.

Physicians and patients should both be ready to *handle anticipated problems* during the taper, such as what to do if withdrawal symptoms develop, or if anxiety symptoms reemerge (Table 12–8). This generally will require an adjustment of dose, and perhaps a lengthening of the originally planned taper schedule.

The most frequent error made by patients and prescribers alike is to be too aggressive in the rate of taper (Table 12–8). Chronic use of benzodiazepines may require many months (or even more than a year) of tapering in some cases, and usually many weeks of tapering in the typical case. It is often better to err on the side of tapering too slow than tapering too fast (Table 12–8).

These general principles of managing benzodiazepine use, abuse, tolerance, dependence, and withdrawal can be usefully applied to *any* drug that has the capability of causing dependence. The specific issues for managing patients who abuse and/or are dependent upon the other drugs discussed in this chapter (e.g., sedative-hypnotics, opiates, stimulants, tobacco, alcohol, and others) will not be addressed in this chapter in order to emphasize psychopharmacological mechanisms rather than clinical management. The reader is referred to standard psychiatric textbooks to learn about the many details of appropriate psychological and psychiatric management of patients who abuse and become dependent upon drugs.

Sedative-Hypnotics and Depressants

Pharmacology of Sedative-Hypnotic Depressant Abuse

The pharmacological mechanisms of these drugs are basically the same as those described above for the benzodiazepines, and have been already introduced in Chapter 7. However, these drugs are much less safe in overdose, cause dependence more frequently, are abused more frequently, and produce much more dangerous withdrawal reactions. Apparently, the receptor mediating the pharmacological actions of these agents – presumably an allosteric modulator at GABA A ligand gated chloride channels – is even more readily desensitized with even more dangerous consequences than the benzodiazepine receptor (Fig. 12–4). It must also mediate a more intense euphoria and a more desirable sense of tranquility than the benzodiazepine receptor.

Since benzodiazepines are frequently an adequate alternative therapy for these drugs, physicians can help minimize abuse of these agents by prescribing them rarely

Table 12–8. *Factors involved in problems
tapering benzodiazepines*

Taper too rapid
Dosage decrease too large
Fear of tapering
Relapse of underlying anxiety disorder
Caffeine use
Alcohol use
Illicit drug use
Premenstrual syndrome (PMS) symptoms
Life stressors
Medical conditions

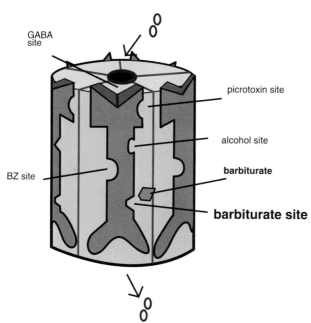

FIGURE 12–4. **Pharmacology of sedative-hypnotic depressant abuse.** The pharmacological mechanism of action of these drugs is not yet proven but is thought to be basically the same as that described for the benzodiazepines, namely allosteric modulators at GABA A ligand gated chloride channels.

if ever. In the case of withdrawal reactions, reinstituting and then tapering the offending agent under close clinical supervision can assist the detoxification process.

The various agents used as sedative-hypnotics other than benzodiazepines are discussed in Chapter 7. They get more attention as drugs of abuse than as drugs prescribed for use as sedative-hypnotics because of the presence of reasonable alternatives to them, and to the historical abuse of these agents. Thus, some agents are obtained from unscrupulous or uninformed physicians, but many of these are obtained by abusers from illicit sources of materials never intended for prescription use. These agents include barbiturates and related compounds such as ethchlorvynol and ethinamate; chloral hydrate and derivatives; and piperidinedione derivatives such as glutethimide and methyprylon.

Opiates

Pharmacology of Opiates: Use and Abuse

Since we have not discussed the use of opiates as legitimate treatments for pain, it will be useful at this point to explain some of the pharmacological principles underlying opiate use in pain.

Opiates act upon a variety of receptors, called opiate receptors. There are several subtypes of opiate receptors in the central nervous system (CNS), and the three most important subtypes thought to be related to the mediation of the analgesic effects of opiates are the mu, delta, and kappa opiate receptors (Fig. 12–5).

The brain, as is now well known, makes its own endogenous opiate-like substances, sometimes referred to as the "brain's own morphine." More and more types of endogenous opiates are being discovered. They are peptides derived from a precursor proteins called pro-opiomelanocortin (POMC), proenkephalin, and prodynorphin. Parts of these precursor proteins are cleaved off to form endorphins or enkephalins, stored in opiate neurons, and presumably released during neurotransmission to mediate endogenous opiate-like actions (Fig. 12–5). However, the precise number and function of endogenous opiates and their receptors, and their role in pain relief and in other CNS actions remain largely unknown.

Exogenous opiates in the form of pain relievers (such as codeine or morphine) or drugs of abuse (such as heroin) are also thought to act at mu, delta, and kappa opiate receptors (Fig. 12–6). Acute actions of opiates cause relief of pain by acting as agonists at opiate receptor subtypes. At and above pain-relieving doses, the opiates induce euphoria, which is the main reinforcing property of the opiates. In sufficient doses, opiates induce a very intense but brief euphoria sometimes called a "rush" followed by a profound sense of tranquility that may last several hours, followed in turn by drowsiness ("nodding"), mood swings, mental clouding, apathy, and slowed motor movements. In overdose, these same agents act as depressants of respiration, and can also induce coma. The acute actions of opiates can be reversed by synthetic opiate antagonists such as naloxone and naltrexone, which compete for the opiate agonists at opiate receptors and reverse their actions there.

When given chronically, the opiates readily cause both tolerance and dependence. Apparently, adaptation of opiate receptors occur quite readily after chronic opiate administration (see analogous process for benzodiazepine receptors in Fig. 12–2). The first sign of this is the need of the patient to take a higher and higher dose of opiate in order to relieve pain or to induce the desired euphoria. Eventually, there may be little room between the dose that causes euphoria and that which produces toxic effects of an overdose.

Another sign that dependence has occurred and that opiate receptors have adapted by decreasing their sensitivity to agonist actions is the production of a withdrawal syndrome once the chronically administered opiate wears off. The opiate antagonists such as naloxone can precipitate a withdrawal syndrome in opiate-dependent persons. The opiate withdrawal syndrome is characterized by the patient feeling dysphoria; craving another dose of opiate; being irritable; and having signs of autonomic hyperactivity such as tachycardia, tremor, and sweating. Piloerection ("goose-bumps") is often associated with opiate withdrawal, especially when the drug is stopped suddenly ("cold turkey"). This is so subjectively horrible that the opiate abuser will

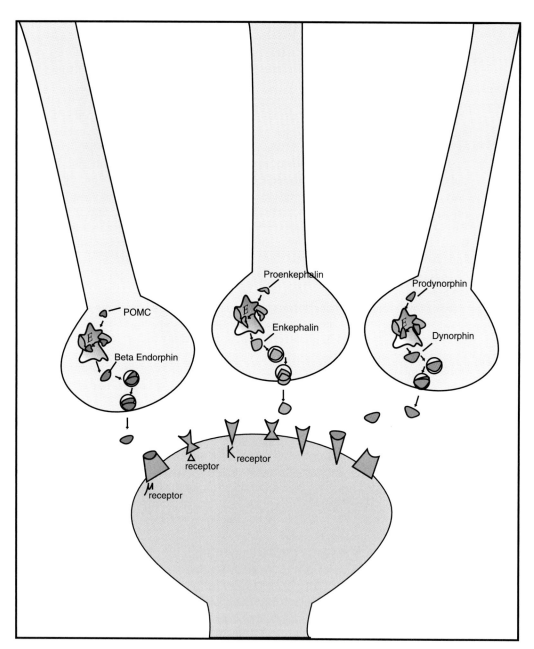

FIGURE 12–5. **Pharmacology of the endogenous opiate systems**. The brain makes its own endogenous opiate-like substances, sometimes referred to as the "brain's own morphine-like molecules." They are peptides derived from precursor proteins called pro-opiomelanocortin (POMC), proenkephalin, and prodynorphin. Parts of these precursor proteins are cleaved off to form endorphins or enkephalins, stored in opiate neurons, and presumably released during neurotransmission to mediate endogenous opiate-like actions. However, the precise number and function of endogenous opiates and their receptors and their role in pain relief and in other CNS actions remain largely unknown.

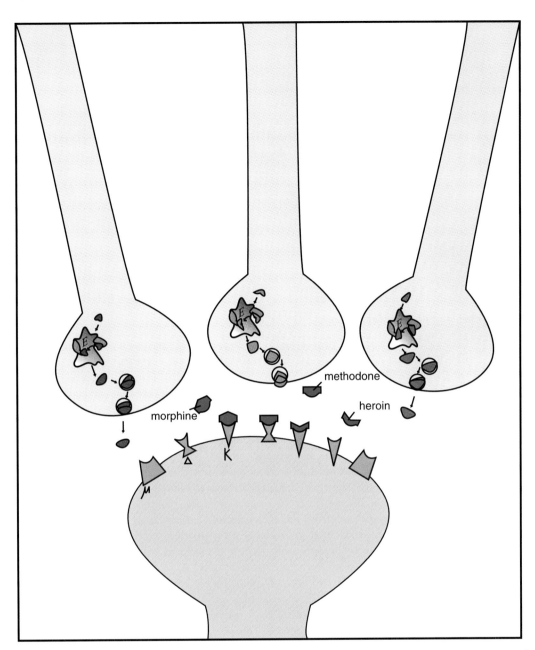

FIGURE 12–6. **Pharmacological actions of opiate drugs.** Opiate drugs act upon a variety of receptors, called opiate receptors. There are several subtypes of opiate receptors in the central nervous system, and the three most important subtypes thought to be related to the mediation of the analgesic effects of opiate drugs are the mu, delta, and kappa opiate receptors. Exogenous opiate drugs in the form of pain relievers (such as codeine or morphine) or drugs of abuse (such as heroin or methadone) are also thought to act at mu, delta, and kappa opiate receptors. Acute actions of opiate drugs cause relief of pain by acting as agonists at opiate receptor subtypes. At and above pain-relieving doses, the opiate drugs induce euphoria, which is the main reinforcing property of the opiates. In sufficient doses, opiates induce a very intense but brief euphoria sometimes called a "rush" followed by a profound sense of tranquility that may last several hours, followed in turn by drowsiness ("nodding"), mood swings, mental clouding, apathy, and slowed motor movements. In overdose, these same agents act as depressants of respiration, and can also induce coma.

often stop at nothing in order to get another dose of opiate to relieve symptoms of withdrawal. Thus, what may have begun as a quest for euphoria may end up as frantic efforts to avoid withdrawal.

In the early days of opiate use/abuse/intoxication, and prior to the completion of the neuroadaptive mechanisms that mediate opiate receptor desensitization, opiate intoxication alternates with normal functioning. Later, after the opiate receptors adapt and the person becomes dependent, the abuser may experience very little euphoria, but mostly the state of lack of withdrawal alternating with the presence of withdrawal.

Opiate receptors can readapt to normal if given a chance to do so in the absence of additional intake of an opiate. This may be too difficult to tolerate, so reinstituting another opiate, such as methadone, which can be taken orally and then slowly tapered, may assist in the detoxification process.

Stimulants: Cocaine and Amphetamine

Pharmacology of Cocaine Abuse

Cocaine has two major properties: it is both a local anesthetic and an inhibitor of the dopamine transporter (Fig. 12–7). Cocaine's local anesthetic properties are still used in medicine, especially by otolaryngologists. Freud himself exploited this property of cocaine to help dull the pain of his tongue cancer. He may have also exploited the second property of the drug, which is to produce euphoria, reduce fatigue, and create a sense of mental acuity due to inhibition of dopamine reuptake at the dopamine transporter. Cocaine also has similar but less important actions at the norepinephrine and the serotonin transporters.

At higher doses, cocaine can produce undesirable effects, including tremor, emotional lability, restlessness, irritability, paranoia, panic, and repetitive stereotyped behavior. At even higher doses, cocaine can induce intense anxiety, paranoia, and hallucinations, with hypertension, tachycardia, ventricular irritability, hyperthermia, and respiratory depression. In overdose, cocaine can cause acute heart failure, stroke, and seizures. Acute intoxication with cocaine produces these various clinical effects depending upon the dose, and is mediated by inhibition of the dopamine transporter, and in turn by the effects of excessive dopamine activity in dopamine synapses.

Repeated intoxication with cocaine may produce complex adaptations of the dopamine neuronal system, including both tolerance and indeed the opposite phenomenon, called sensitization or "reverse tolerance." One example of reverse tolerance may be what happens to some abusers upon repeated intoxication with cocaine at doses that previously only induced euphoria. In these cases, cocaine causes a behavioral reaction that can take the form of an acute paranoid psychosis virtually indistinguishable from paranoid schizophrenia (Fig. 12–8).

This should not be surprising, because the major hypothesis for the etiology of the positive symptoms of psychosis discussed in Chapter 9 on schizophrenia is an excess of dopamine activity, especially in the mesolimbic dopamine pathways. In fact, research studies indicate that the reinforcing properties of cocaine are also mediated predominantly via dopamine-2 (D2) receptors in the mesolimbic dopamine pathways. Too much of a "good" thing (i.e., the compulsive quest for euphoria and pleasure through pleasurable stimulation of mesolimbic D2 receptors) apparently

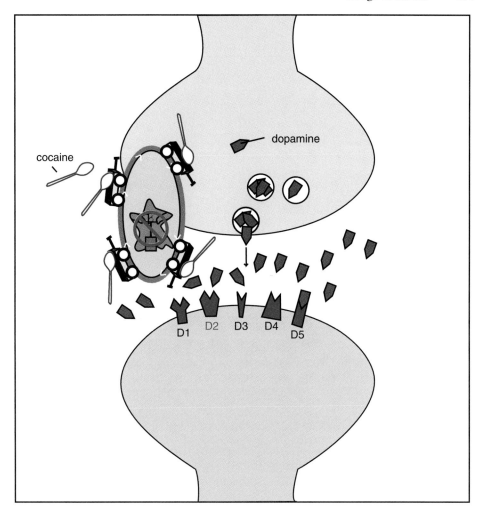

FIGURE 12–7. **Pharmacology of cocaine.** Cocaine is a powerful inhibitor of the dopamine transporter. Blocking this transporter acutely causes dopamine to accumulate, and this produces euphoria, reduces fatigue, and creates a sense of mental acuity. Cocaine has similar but less important actions at the norepinephrine and the serotonin transporters.

will in some cases spill over into an unwanted *over*activity of this pathway. This undesirable overactivity reproduces the psychopharmacological pathophysiology underlying the positive symptoms of schizophrenia (see Fig. 9–1).

This complication of cocaine abuse seems to require chronic use and sensitization of the mesolimbic dopamine system, which eventually releases progressively more and more dopamine until repetitive cocaine abuse may eventually cause an eruption into frank psychosis. How the dopamine synapse becomes sensitized to cocaine so that this effect can be produced upon repeated administration is unknown. Interestingly, treatment with dopamine receptor blocking neuroleptics can also relieve the symptoms of cocaine intoxication and cocaine psychosis, as would be expected from the analogy with schizophrenia (see Figs. 9–2 and 9–4).

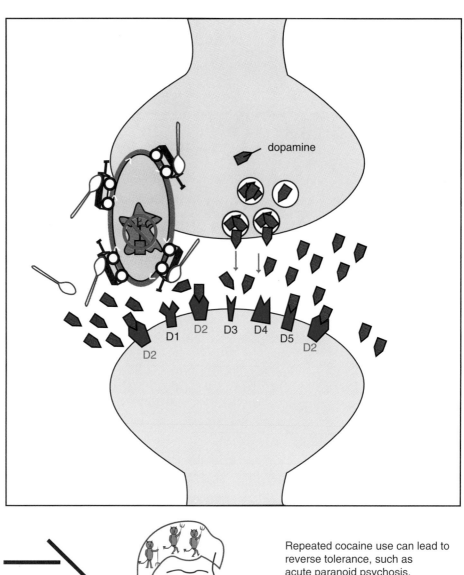

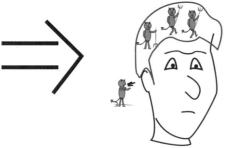

Repeated cocaine use can lead to
reverse tolerance, such as
acute paranoid psychosis.

FIGURE 12–8. **Production of reverse tolerance in a cocaine abuser**. Repeated intoxication with cocaine may produce complex adaptations of the dopamine neuronal system, such as sensitization or "reverse tolerance." Thus, in repeated users, cocaine releases more and more dopamine. In such cases, doses of cocaine that previously only induced euphoria can create an acute paranoid psychosis virtually indistinguishable from paranoid schizophrenia.

In addition to the acute intoxicating effects and the chronic reverse tolerance effects of cocaine, all of which are mediated by increasing dopamine levels and its release at dopamine synapses, there are also longer term effects of cocaine, possibly due to other adaptations of dopamine receptors. As abusers use cocaine for longer and longer periods of time, their dopamine receptors adapt and, following an episode of intoxication, mediate an increasingly bothersome withdrawal (abstinence) syndrome. There is the subjective experience following the euphoria of a sense of "crashing" characterized by craving more cocaine; agitation; and anxiety giving way to fatigue, depression, exhaustion, hypersomnolence, and hyperphagia. After several days, if another dose of cocaine is not taken, the chronic abuser may experience other signs of withdrawal including anergy, decreased interest, anhedonia, and increased cocaine craving.

Since dopamine neurotransmission via D2 receptors in the mesolimbic dopamine pathway is thought to mediate in large part the psychopharmacology of pleasure, and therefore the reinforcing properties of many drugs of abuse, it is not surprising that cocaine abusers describe their highs as more intense and pleasurable than orgasm, and their lows as the inability to experience pleasure (anhedonia). These latter complaints are somewhat reminiscent of symptoms of depression, and it is not surprising that a condition that acts to mobilize and deplete dopamine and then to desensitize dopamine receptors could create a condition that mimics some of the signs of major depressive disorder.

Interventions aimed at repleting dopamine stores and readapting dopamine receptor sensitivity would be theoretically useful for the cocaine abuser dependent – with both tolerance and reverse tolerance – upon cocaine. However, the most useful intervention often is to allow the dopamine system to restore itself with time alone, provided that the abuser can remain abstinent long enough for the system to recover. This, of course, is often not feasible or even desired by the abuser.

Pharmacology of Amphetamine Abuse

Amphetamine also has potent pharmacological effects on the dopamine neuron. Unlike cocaine, its predominant action is to release dopamine (Figs. 12–9 and 12–10), but once released, it does have secondary effects on inhibiting dopamine reuptake and metabolism. Amphetamine and derivatives of amphetamines also have weaker releasing actions at noradrenergic synapses, and some amphetamine derivatives also release serotonin. The net effect of amphetamine and its derivatives is very similar to cocaine, although the euphoria it produces may be less intense if longer lasting.

Signs of amphetamine intoxication, toxicity, overdose, sensitization by production of an acute paranoid psychosis, and withdrawal syndrome are all similar to those described above for cocaine.

Hallucinogens and Designer Drugs

Pharmacology of Hallucinogen Abuse

The hallucinogens are a group of agents that produce intoxication, sometimes called a "trip" associated with changes in sensory experiences, including visual illusions

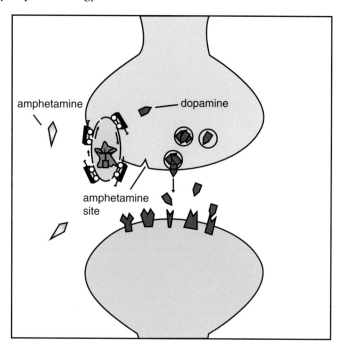

FIGURE 12–9. **Pharmacology of amphetamine (part 1).** Amphetamine's predominant action is to release dopamine. At the dopamine neuron, there is a presynaptic site where amphetamine acts to release dopamine. In this figure, dopamine neurotransmission is proceding normally, and amphetamine is yet to act (see Fig. 12–10).

and hallucinations, an enhanced awareness of external stimuli, and an enhanced awareness of internal thoughts and stimuli. These hallucinations are produced with a clear level of consciousness and a lack of confusion and may be both *psychedelic* and *psychotomimetic*.

Psychedelic is the term for the subjective experience that, due to heightened sensory awareness, one's mind is being expanded or that one is in union with mankind or the universe and having some sort of a religious experience. *Psychotomimetic* means that the experience mimics a state of psychosis (see Table 9–3), but the resemblance between a trip and psychosis is superficial at best. As previously discussed, the stimulants cocaine and amphetamine much more genuinely mimic psychosis.

Hallucinogen intoxication includes visual illusions; visual "trails" where the image smears into streaks of its image as it moves across a visual trail; macropsia and micropsia; emotional and mood lability; subjective slowing of time; the sense that colors are heard and sounds are seen; intensification of sound perception; depersonalization and derealization; yet retaining a state of full wakefulness and alertness. Other changes may include impaired judgment, fear of losing one's mind, anxiety, nausea, tachycardia, increased blood pressure, and increased body temperature.

Not surprisingly, given the list of symptoms above and comparing them to the list of symptoms for a panic attack in Chapter 8 (see Table 8–3), hallucinogen intoxication can cause what is perceived as a panic attack but often called a "bad

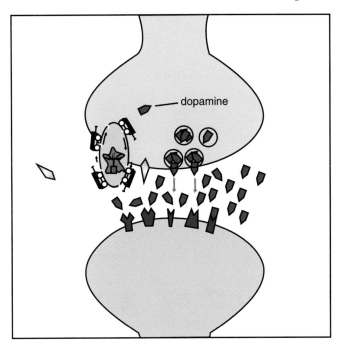

FIGURE 12–10. **Pharmacology of amphetamine (part 2).** Here amphetamine is acting at its pre-synaptic site to release dopamine from the dopaminergic neuron, which then floods the postsynaptic dopamine receptors. Amphetamine also has some secondary effects on inhibiting dopamine reuptake and metabolism. Amphetamine and derivatives of amphetamines also have weaker releasing actions for norepinephrine at noradrenergic synapses, and some amphetamine derivatives also release serotonin from serotonin synapses. The net effects of amphetamine and its derivatives are very similar to cocaine, although the euphoria it produces may be less intense if longer lasting.

trip." As intoxication escalates, one can experience an acute confusional state called delirium, where the abuser is disoriented and agitated. This can evolve further into frank psychosis with delusions and paranoia.

Common hallucinogens include two major classes of agents. The first class of agents resemble serotonin (indole alkylamines) and includes the classical hallucinogens lysergic acid diethylamide (LSD), psilocybin, and dimethyltryptamine (DMT). The second class of agents resembles norepinephrine and dopamine and are also related to amphetamine (phenylalkylamines) and include mescaline, 2,5-dimethoxy-4-methylamphetamine (DOM), and others. More recently, synthetic chemists have come up with some new "designer drugs" such as 3,4-methylene-dioxymethamphetamine (MDMA).

These are neither stimulants nor hallucinogens in the classical sense, but produce a complex subjective state sometimes referred to as "ecstacy," which is also what abusers call MDMA itself. MDMA produces euphoria, disorientation, confusion, enhanced sociability, and a sense of increased empathy and personal insight.

Hallucinogens have rather complex interactions at neurotransmitter systems, but one of the most prominent is a common action as agonists at 5HT2A receptors sites

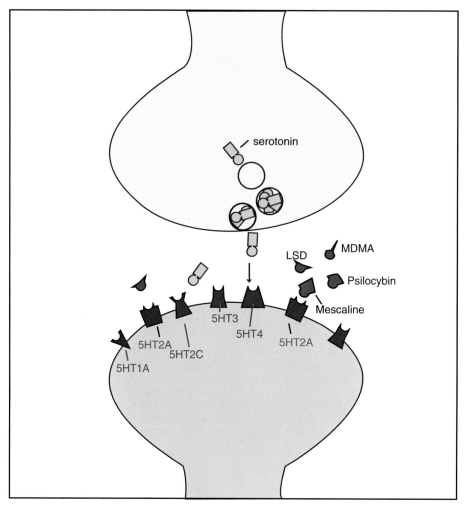

FIGURE 12–11. **Pharmacology of hallucinogens**. Hallucinogenic drugs such as LSD, mescaline, and psilocybin – as well as the "designer drugs" such as MDMA – act as **agonists at 5HT2 receptors**.

(Fig. 12–11). These agents certainly have additional effects at other 5HT receptors (especially 5HT1A somatodendritic autoreceptors) and also at other neurotransmitter systems, especially norepinephrine and dopamine, but the relative importance of these other actions is less well known. MDMA also appears to be a powerful releaser of 5HT, and it and several drugs structually related to it may even destroy serotonin axon terminals. However, the action that appears to explain a common mechanism for most of the hallucinogens is the stimulation of 5HT2A receptors.

Hallucinogens can produce incredible tolerance, sometimes after a single dose. Desensitization of 5HT2A receptors is hypothesized to underlie this, but the mechanism of this rapid desensitization remains unproven. Another unique dimension of hallucinogen abuse is the production of "flashbacks," namely the spontaneous recurrence of some of the symptoms of intoxication that lasts from a few seconds to several hours but in the *absence* of recent administration of the hallucinogen. This occurs days to months *after* the last drug experience, and can apparently be precipitated by a number of environmental stimuli.

The psychopharmacological mechanism underlying flashbacks is unknown, but its phenomenology suggests the possibility of some sort of neurochemical adaptation, perhaps of the serotonin system and its receptors, that is related to reverse tolerance and which must be incredibly long lasting. Flashbacks are superficially analogous to another complication of psychotropic drug administration, namely tardive dyskinesia in which neurochemical adaptations occur following drug administration that are very long lasting and perhaps irreversible (see Chapters 9 and 10 and Fig. 9–5). However, the neurochemical mechanism of hallucinogen flashbacks is still very poorly understood.

Phencyclidine

Pharmacology of Phencyclidine Abuse

Phencyclidine (PCP) was originally developed as an anesthetic but proved to be unacceptable for this use because it induces a unique psychotomimetic/hallucinatory experience. Its structurally related and mechanism-related analog ketamine is still used as an anesthetic, but causes far less of the psychotomimetic/hallucinatory experience. PCP causes intense analgesia, amnesia, delirium, stimulant as well as depressant actions, staggering gait, slurred speech, and a unique form of nystagmus (vertical nystagmus). Higher degrees of intoxication can cause catatonia (excitement alternating with stupor and catalepsy), hallucinations, delusions, paranoia, disorientation, and lack of judgment. Overdose can include coma, extremely high temperature, seizures, and muscle breakdown (rhabdomyolysis).

We have already discussed the mechanism of action of PCP in Chapter 11 in our discussion on neuroprotective agents. PCP acts as an allosteric modulator of the *N*-methyl-D-aspartate (NMDA) subtype of glutamate receptor (Fig. 12–12). It specifically acts to block this receptor and to decrease the flux of calcium into the cell. PCP and other agents that act at the PCP receptor have been proposed as possible neuroprotective agents (see Chapter 11). However, neuroprotection is apparently attainable only at the expense of anesthesia and psychosis (see Fig. 11–38). Also, PCP could potentially disrupt normal and necessary excitatory neurotransmission at NMDA receptors.

Marijuana

Pharmacology of Marijuana Abuse

Cannabis preparations are smoked in order to deliver their psychoactive substances, cannabinoids, to the blood and eventually the brain. The major psychoactive cannabinoid in marijuana is delta-9-tetrahydrocannabinol (THC). Marijuana can have both stimulant and sedative properties. In usual intoxicating doses, it produces a sense of well-being and relaxation, a sense of friendliness, a loss of temporal awareness including confusing the past with the present, slowing of thought processes, im-

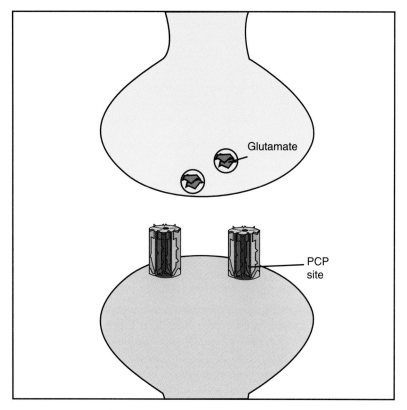

FIGURE 12–12. **Pharmacology of phencyclidine (PCP).** PCP is an **antagonist of N-methyl-D-aspartate (NMDA) glutamate receptors** at a site probably closely associated with the ion channel for calcium there.

pairment of short-term memory, and a feeling of achieving special insights. At high doses, marijuana can induce panic, toxic delirium, and rarely psychosis.

One complication of long-term use is the "amotivational syndrome" in frequent users. This syndrome is seen predominantly in heavy daily users and is characterized by the emergence of decreased drive and ambition, thus "amotivational." It is also associated with other socially and occupationally impairing symptoms, including a shortened attention span, poor judgment, easy distractibility, impaired communication skills, introversion, and diminished effectiveness in interpersonal situations. Personal habits may deteriorate, and there may be a loss of insight, and even feelings of depersonalization.

The pharmacological mechanism underlying the actions of THC are very poorly understood. It is possible that there are "THC" receptors in the brain, and that the brain makes its own cannabinoid-like neurotransmitters ("the brain's own marijuana"). Since even the mechanism of acute use and intoxication with THC is poorly understood, it is only conjecture how the tolerance, dependence, and amotivational state of chronic use might be mediated.

Nicotine

Pharmacology of Nicotine Abuse

Cigarette smoking is a nicotine delivery system. Nicotine acts directly upon nicotinic cholinergic receptors (see discussion of cholinergic neurons in Chapter 11 and Figs. 11–14 and 11–17). Beyond this, the pharmacological mechanisms associated with nicotine use, dependence, and withdrawal are not well known.

One major line of evidence suggests that the reinforcing actions of nicotine have some similarities to those of cocaine and amphetamine, since dopaminergic cells in the mesolimbic dopamine pathway appear to receive cholinergic input onto nicotinic receptors that are stimulated by cigarette smoking (Fig. 12–13). This may mediate the pleasure experienced by smokers. Occupancy of nicotinic cholinergic receptors on mesolimbic dopaminergic neurons may also mediate the other reinforcing actions of smoking such as elevating mood, enhancing cognition, and decreasing appetite.

The psychopharmacological and behavioral actions of nicotine, however, appear to be much more subtle than those of cocaine. Whereas cocaine blocks the dopamine transporter and causes a flood of dopamine to act at the dopamine synapse, nicotine may shut down the nicotinic receptor shortly after binding to it (Fig. 12–14) so that neither it nor acetylcholine (ACh) itself can stimulate the nicotinic receptor any further. Thus, dopaminergic stimulation of mesolimbic dopamine receptors stops after a short period and small amount of nicotinic stimulation. Instead of the longer and much more intense euphoria of cocaine, the pleasure of nicotine is a desirable but small boost in the sensation of pleasure (mini-"rush") followed by a slow decline until the nicotinic receptors switch back on and the smoker takes the next puff or smokes the next cigarette. Nicotine's psychopharmacological effects, therefore, may be somewhat self-regulating, which may explain why its effects on behavior are more limited than the effects of cocaine or amphetamine.

Both stimulant users and smokers may down-regulate their dopamine receptors because of excessive dopamine stimulation. However, nicotine users may up-regulate their nicotinic cholinergic receptors to help compensate for the fact that nicotine keeps turning them off (Fig. 12–15). These possible changes in dopamine and nicotine receptors may be related to the psychopharmacological mechanisms underlying nicotine's profound ability to produce dependence and withdrawal.

Dependence on nicotine causes a withdrawal syndrome characterized by craving and agitation, reminiscent of a less severe version of a stimulant abuser in withdrawal. Recent availability of a nicotine delivery system through a transdermal patch is popular as an adjunct to assist patients detoxify from smoking. The pulsatile delivery of nicotine through smoking (Fig. 12–16) can be substituted by a continuous delivery through a transdermal skin patch acting similarly to a constant intravenous infusion (Fig. 12–17). The idea is that the nicotine and dopamine receptors are allowed to readapt more gradually to normal than happens if the smoker is suddenly abstinent. The hope is that the withdrawal syndrome is prevented or blunted when nicotine is delivered transdermally. In addition, the nicotine dose can be progressively decreased depending upon how much nicotine dose reduction the abstinent smoker can tolerate. This is increased in a slow stepwise fashion until the patient is able to tolerate complete abstinence from smoking and complete discontinuation of transdermal nicotine delivery. The success of this approach depends upon

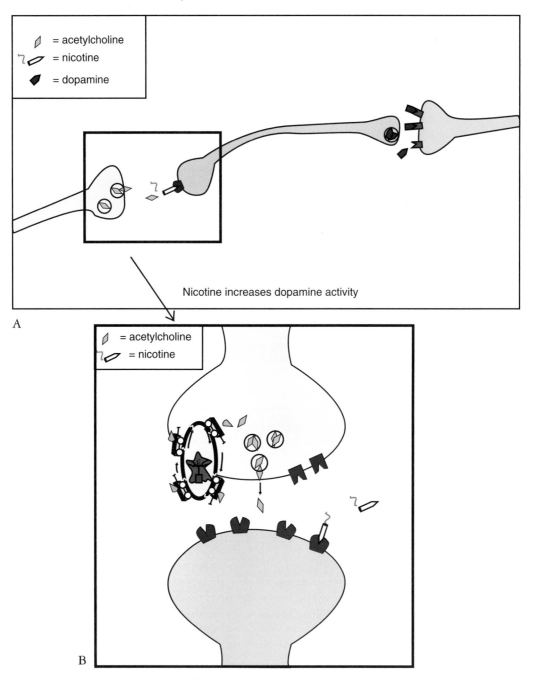

FIGURE 12–13. **Pharmacology of nicotine (part 1).** Nicotine acts directly upon nicotinic cholinergic receptors. These nicotinic cholinergic receptors are themselves located in part upon mesolimbic dopamine neurons. When nicotine stimulates these receptors (*A*), it causes the release of dopamine from the mesolimbic neurons (*B*), and thereby a sense of pleasure.

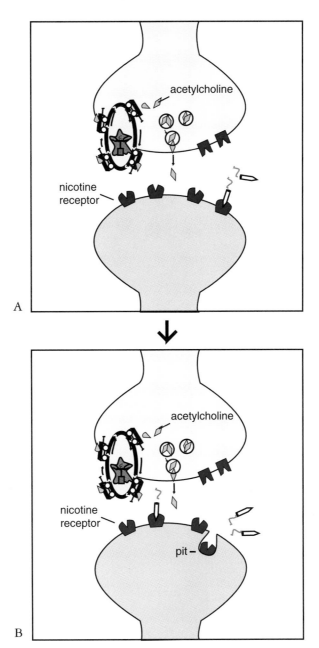

FIGURE 12–14. **Pharmacology of nicotine (part 2).** Although Figure 12–13 suggests that the pharmacology of nicotine shares similarities to the pharmacology of cocaine, the actions of nicotine appear to be much more subtle than those of cocaine. Whereas cocaine blocks the dopamine transporter and causes a flood of dopamine to act at the dopamine synapse, nicotine may shut down the nicotinic receptor (B) shortly after binding to it (A) so that it cannot stimulate the nicotinic receptor any further for a time. Thus, dopaminergic stimulation of mesolimbic dopamine receptors stops after a short period and small amount of nicotinic stimulation. Instead of the longer and much more intense euphoria of cocaine, the pleasure of nicotine is a desirable but small boost in the sensation of pleasure (mini-"rush") followed by a slow decline until the nicotinic receptors switch back on and the smoker takes the next puff or smokes the next cigarette. Nicotine's psychopharmacological effects, therefore, may be somewhat self-regulating, which may explain why its effects on behavior are more limited than the effects of cocaine or amphetamine.

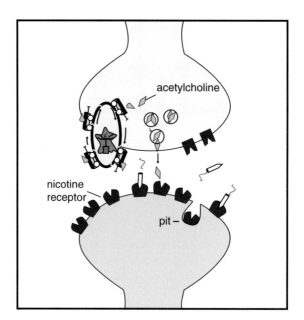

FIGURE 12–15. **Pharmacology of nicotine (part 3)**. Over time, smokers may eventually up-regulate their nicotinic cholinergic receptors to help compensate for the fact that nicotine keeps turning them off. These changes in nicotine receptors may be related to the psychopharmacological mechanisms underlying nicotine's profound ability to produce dependence and withdrawal.

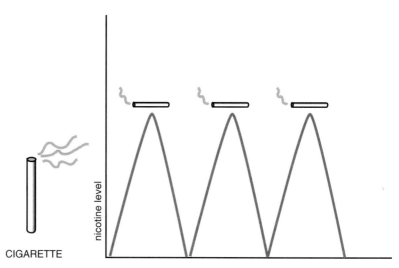

FIGURE 12–16. Cigarette smoking is a **pulsatile nicotine delivery system**. Dependence on nicotine causes a withdrawal syndrome between cigarettes as the nicotine level leaves the blood and the brain. If allowed to progress without smoking another cigarette, withdrawal from nicotine is characterized by craving and agitation, reminiscent of a less severe version of a stimulant abuser in withdrawal.

362

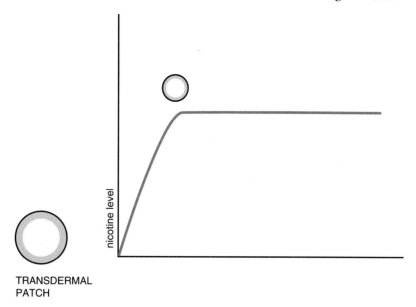

TRANSDERMAL
PATCH

FIGURE 12–17. **Transdermal nicotine administration** for the **treatment of nicotine withdrawal**. Recent availability of a nicotine delivery system through a transdermal patch is popular as an adjunct to assist patients detoxify from smoking. The pulsatile delivery of nicotine through smoking (Fig. 12–16) can be substituted by a continuous delivery through a transdermal skin patch acting similarly to a constant intravenous infusion. The idea is that the nicotine and dopamine receptors are allowed by readapt more gradually to normal than happens if the smoker is suddenly abstinent. The hope is that the withdrawal syndrome is prevented or blunted when nicotine is delivered transdermally. In addition, the nicotine dose can be progressively decreased depending upon how much nicotine dose reduction the abstinent smoker can tolerate. This is increased in a slow stepwise fashion until the patient is able to tolerate complete abstinence from smoking and complete discontinuation of transdermal nicotine delivery. The success of this approach depends upon the motivation of the smoker to quit, and the use of adjunctive psychological support and information programs to help the smoker cope better with abstinence.

the motivation of the smoker to quit, and the use of adjunctive psychological support and information programs to help the smoker cope better with abstinence.

Alcohol

Pharmacology of Alcohol Abuse

The pharmacology of alcohol is poorly characterized and relatively nonspecific. On the one hand, some evidence, already discussed in Chapter 7, suggests that the brain may have some type of "alcohol receptor" that acts as an allosteric modulator of GABA A receptors (see Figs. 7–14 and 12–18). This is probably overly simplistic, as alcohol has numerous effects on a wide variety of neurotransmitter systems, receptors, membranes, and enzymes. Neither the acute actions of alcohol in mediating intoxication nor the chronic actions of alcohol in mediating dependence, tolerance, and withdrawal are understood very well. However, various research studies do suggest possible psychopharmacological mechanisms for the actions of alcohol on neurotransmission.

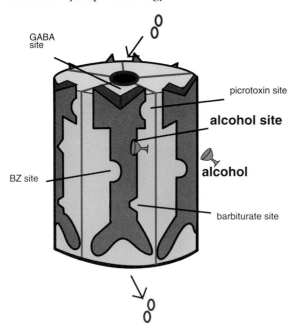

GABA
site

picrotoxin site

alcohol site

BZ site

alcohol

barbiturate site

FIGURE 12–18. **Pharmacology of alcohol**. Alcohol may mediate some of its pharmacological effects at the GABA A receptor complex as an allosteric modulator of the inhibitory chloride channel.

In addition to alcohol's ability to enhance inhibitory neurotransmission at GABA A receptor ligand gated chloride channels as already discussed, it also reduces excitatory neurotransmission at the NMDA subtype of glutamate receptor, which serves as a ligand gate to calcium channels. That is, alcohol enhances inhibition and reduces excitation, and this may explain its characterization as a depressant of CNS neuronal functioning. These effects of alcohol on ion fluxes may thus explain some of its intoxicating, amnestic, and ataxic effects.

Alcohol's reinforcing effects, on the other hand, may be mediated predominantly through the release of dopamine in the mesolimbic dopamine system (Fig. 12–19). Alcohol may also release serotonin, and this serotonin release may also cause indirect actions upon dopamine neurons in the mesolimbic dopamine system. A role for the opioid system in the dependence caused by alcohol is suggested by the fact that the opioid antagonist naltrexone has recently been approved in the United States for the treatment of alcohol dependence, since it has been shown to decrease craving and to increase abstinence rates in alcohol-dependent subjects. Also, alcohol may cause the release of endogenous opioids, particularly upon mesolimbic dopaminergic neurons, suggesting yet another manner in which alcohol manages to stimulate the pleasure-mediated dopamine neurons in the brain.

In summary, although there are many provocative research leads for explaining the mechanism of action of alcohol use, abuse, intoxication, tolerance, dependence, withdrawal, and treatment, our knowledge of the psychopharmacology of alcohol is still in its infancy.

The subject of how to treat alcohol abuse and dependence is complex, and most of the effective interventions have been based upon empiric psychological and psychiatric therapies. The reader is referred to standard texts in psychiatry and psychology for a discussion of these treatments, as they are beyond the scope of this text.

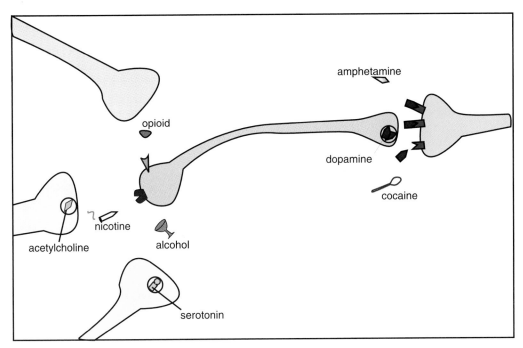

FIGURE 12–19. **Mesolimbic dopamine pathway and the psychopharmacology of pleasure.** Since the subjective experience of pleasure may be profoundly influenced if not mediated by stimulating mesolimbic dopamine receptors, it is not surprising that so many of the drugs of abuse that we have discussed may have a net impact upon this neuronal system. This includes the stimulants cocaine and amphetamine, which act presynaptically to directly cause an increase in dopamine availability. It also includes several other drugs of abuse that appear to act through inputs to the mesolimbic dopamine neuron at its dendrites. Thus, alcohol, opiates, serotonin, and nicotine may all impact this neuron through synaptic input to the mesolimbic dopaminergic cell bodies and dendrites. Shown here, therefore, is a neurobiological model for the psychopharmacology of pleasure. When dopamine release is enhanced from this pathway by any of a number of mechanisms, pleasure is experienced. This is reinforcing to the use of the drug, causes repeated use of the drug, and eventually in some cases, dependence upon the drug. Furthermore, since the dopamine system may desensitize itself to too much input, it may essentially "desensitize" pleasure. This could lead to unpleasurable feelings once the effects of the drug wear off or is withdrawn.

Mesolimbic Dopamine Pathway and the Psychopharmacology of Pleasure

Since the subjective experience of pleasure may be profoundly influenced if not mediated by stimulating mesolimbic dopamine receptors, it is not surprising that so many of the drugs of abuse we have discussed may have a net impact upon this neuronal system. Shown in Figure 12–19 is a neurobiological model for the psychopharmacology of pleasure. When dopamine release is enhanced from this pathway by any of a number of mechanisms, pleasure is experienced. This is reinforcing to the use of the drug, causes repeated use of the drug, and eventually in some cases, dependence upon the drug. Furthermore, since the dopamine system may desensitize itself to too much input, it may essentially "desensitize" pleasure. This could lead to unpleasurable feelings once the effects of the drug wear off or the drug is withdrawn.

Summary

In this chapter we have attempted to emphasize the psychopharmacological mechanisms of actions of drugs of abuse, and have used these mechanisms to describe drug dependence as well.

We have attempted to define some of the terms frequently used in describing drug abuse and dependence, including abuse, addiction, dependence, reinforcement, tolerance, cross-tolerance and cross-dependence, withdrawal, relapse, and rebound.

We have specifically emphasized the mechanism of action of classes of agents including benzodiazepines, barbiturate-type sedative-hypnotics, opiates, the stimulants cocaine and amphetamine, hallucinogens, phencyclidine, marijuana, nicotine, and alcohol. The role of the mesolimbic dopamine pathway in the psychopharmacology of pleasure was discussed as a unifying hypothesis whereby many of the drugs of abuse could mediate their reinforcing properties, which may ultimately lead to their abuse.

Suggested Reading

Ancill, R., Holliday, S., and Higenbottam, J. (1994) *Schizophrenia: exploring the spectrum of psychosis.* Chichester, John Wiley & Sons.

Barlow, D.H. (Ed.) (1993) *Clinical handbook of psychological disorders.* New York, Guilford Press.

Bloom, F.E. and Kupfer, D.J., (Eds.) (1995) *Psychopharmacology: the fourth generation of progress.* New York, Raven Press.

Bloom, F.E. and Lazerson, A. (1988) *Brain, mind and behavior,* 2nd edition. New York, W.H. Freeman and Company.

Cooper, J.R., Bloom, F.E., and Roth, R.H. (1996) *The biochemical basis of neuropharmacology,* 7th edition. New York, Oxford University Press.

den Boer, J.A. (Ed.) (in press) *Clinical management of anxiety: theory and practical applications.* New York, Marcel Dekker, Inc.

Depression in primary care, volume 1, detection and diagnosis; clinical practice guideline, number 5, U.S. Department of Health and Human Services, AHCPR Publication No. 93-0551, Public Health Service, Agency for Health Care Policy and Research, Rockville, MD, April, 1993.

Depression in primary care, volume 2, treatment of major depression; clinical practice guideline, number 5, U.S. Department of Health and Human Services, AHCPR Publication No. 93-0551, Public Health Service, Agency for Health Care Policy and Research, Rockville, MD, April, 1993.

Diagnostic and statistical manual of mental disorders, 4th edition (DSM-IV), American Psychiatric Association Press, Washington, DC, 1994.

Dollery, C. (1991) *Therapeutic drugs.* New York, Churchill Livingstone.

Drachman, D.A. (1994) If we live long enough, will we all be demented? *Neurology,* 44, 1563–5.

Foa, E.B. and Wilson, R. (1991) *Stop obsessing! How to overcome your obsessions and compulsions.* New York, Bantam Books.

Freedman, D.X. and Stahl, S.M. (1992) Pharmacology: policy implications of new psychiatric drugs. *Health Affairs,* 11(3), 157–63.

Games, D., et al. (1995) Alzheimer-type neuropathology in transgenic mice overexpressing V717F beta-amyloid precursor protein. *Nature*, **373**, 523–7.

Gelenberg, A.J., Bassuk, E.L., and Schoonover, S.C. (1991) *The practitioner's guide to psychoactive drugs*, 3rd edition. New York, Plenum Medical Book Company.

Gilman, A.G., Rall, T.W., Nies, A.S. and Taylor, P. (1996) *The pharmacological basis of therapeutics*, 9th edition. New York, Pergamon Press.

Groves, P.M. and Rebec, G.V. (1992) *Introduction to biological psychology*, 4th edition. Dubuque, IA, Wm. C. Brown Publishers.

International classification of diseases, 10th edition (ICD-10) classification of mental and behavioral disorders: clinical descriptions and diagnostic guidelines. World Health Organization, Geneva, 1993.

Iversen, L.L. (1986) Chemical signalling in the nervous system. In Hokfelt, T., Fuxe, K., and Pernow, B. (Eds.) *Progress in brain research*, Vol. 68. San Diego, Academic Press, pp. 15–21.

Jenike, M.A. (1989) *Geriatric psychiatry and psychopharmacology: a clinical approach.* Chicago, Yearbook Medical Publishers, Inc.

Kaplan, H.I, Freedman, A.M., and Sadock, B.J. (1995) *Comprehensive textbook of psychiatry*, 6th edition. Baltimore, Williams & Wilkins.

Kaplan, H.I. and Sadock, B.J. (1993) *Pocket handbook of psychiatric drug treatment.* Baltimore, Williams and Wilkins.

Katon, W. (1989) *Panic disorder in the medical setting.* National Institute of Mental Health, U.S. Dept. of Health and Human Services Publication no. ADM 89-1629, Washington, DC, U.S. Government Printing Office.

Kunovac, J.L. and Stahl, S.M. (in press) Serotonin-specific anxiolytics: now and in the future. In Montgomery, S. and Halbreich, U. (Eds.) *Pharmacotherapy of mood and cognition.* Washington, DC, American Psychiatric Press, Inc.

Kunovac, J.L. and Stahl, S.M. (1995) Future directions in anxiolytic pharmacotherapy. *Psychiatric Clinics of North America*, **18**, 4-1–4-15.

Leonard, B.E. (1992) *Fundamentals of psychopharmacology.* Chichester, John Wiley & Sons.

Lowinson, J.H., Ruiz, P., Milman, R.B., and Langrod, J.G. (1992) *Substance abuse: a comprehensive textbook*, 2nd edition. Baltimore, Williams & Wilkins.

Martindale, W. (1993) *The extra pharmacopoeia*, 30th edition. London, The Pharmaceutical Press.

McKhann, G., Drachman, D., Folstein, M., et al. (1984) Clinical diagnosis of Alzheimer's disease. *Neurology*, **34**, 939–44.

Meltzer, H.Y. (Ed.) (1987) *Psychopharmacology: the third generation of progress.* New York, Raven Press.

Meltzer, H.Y. and Stahl, S.M. (1976) The dopamine hypothesis of schizophrenia: a review. *Schizophrenia Bulletin*, **2**(1), 19–76.

Michels, R. (1995) *Psychiatry.* Philadelphia, J.B. Lippincott Company.

Montgomery, S. and Halbreich, U. (Eds.) (in press) *Pharmacotherapy of mood and cognition.* Washington, DC, American Psychiatric Press, Inc.

O'Malley, S.S., Jaffe, A.J., and Chang, G. (1992) Naltrexone and coping skills therapy for alcohol dependence: a controlled study. *Archives of General Psychiatry*, **49**, 881–7.

Paniccia, G.S. and Rapaport, M.H. (1995) Serotonin receptors, social phobia and panic disorder. *International Review of Psychiatry*, **7**, 131–40.

Physician's desk reference, 49th edition. (1995) Montvale, NJ, Medical Economics Data Production Company.

Pollack, M.H. (Ed.) (1995) Anxiety disorders: longitudinal course and treatment. *Psychiatric Clinics of North America*, **18**.

Practice guidelines for major depressive disorder in adults; American Psychiatric Association, Washington, DC, 1993.

Prien, R.F. and Robinson, D.S. (Eds.) (1994) *Clinical evaluation of psychotropic drugs: principles and guidelines*. New York, Raven Press.

Preskorn, S.H. (1994) *Outpatient management of depression*, Caddo, OK, Professional Communications Inc.

Robins, L.N. and Regier, D.A. (1991) *Psychiatric disorders in America: the epidemiologic catchment area study*. New York, The Free Press (Macmillan, Inc.).

Robinson, J.H. and Prichard, W.S. (1992) The role of nicotine in tobacco use. *Psychopharmacology*, **108**, 897–407.

Schatzberg, A.F. and Cole, J.O. (1991) *Manual of clinical psychopharmacology*, 2nd edition. Washington, DC, American Psychiatric Press.

Schatzberg, A.F. and Nemeroff, C.B. (Eds.) (1995) *Textbook of psychopharmacology*. Washington, DC, American Psychiatric Press, Inc.

Schuckit, M.A. (1995) Drug and alcohol abuse: a clinical guide to diagnosis and treatment, 4th edition, New York, Plenum Publishing Corporation.

Siegel, G., Agranoff, B., Albers, R.W., and Molinoff, P. (1989) *Basic neurochemistry*, 4th edition. New York, Raven Press.

Sinha, S. and Lieberburg, I. (1992) Review article. Normal metabolism of the amyloid precursor protein (APP). *Neurodegeneration*, 1, 169–75.

Sprouse, J.S. and Wilkinson, L.O. (1995) Innovative therapeutic actions by targeting serotonin 1A receptors selectively. *International Review of Psychiatry*, 7, 5–16.

Stahl, S.M. (1987) Needs and opportunities for innovation in psychopharmacology. *Journal of the Royal Society of Medicine*, 80(7), 413–17.

Stahl, S.M. (1988) Basal ganglia neuropharmacology and obsessive-compulsive disorder: the obsessive compulsive disorder hypothesis of basal ganglia dysfunction. *Psychopharmacology Bulletin* 24, 370–4.

Stahl, S.M. (1992) Serotonin neuroscience discoveries usher in a new era of novel drug therapies in psychiatry. *Psychopharmacology Bulletin*, 28(1), 3–9.

Stahl, S.M. (1994) Is serotonin receptor down regulation linked to the mechanism of action of antidepressant drugs? *Psychopharmacology Bulletin*, 30(1), 39–43.

Stahl, S.M. (1994) New therapeutic advances in schizophrenia. In Ancill, R., Holliday, S., and Higenbottam, J. (Eds.) *Schizophrenia: exploring the spectrum of psychosis*. Chichester, John Wiley & Sons, pp. 137–52.

Stahl, S.M. (Ed.) (1995) Serotonin receptor subtypes in psychiatry. *International Review of Psychiatry*, 7, 1–144.

Stahl, S.M. (in press) Diagnostic dilemmas in anxiety disorders. In den Boer, J.A. (Ed.) *Clinical management of anxiety: theory and practical applications*, New York, Marcel Dekker, Inc.

Stahl, S.M. (1996) Phenomenology of anxiety disorders: clinical heterogeneity and comorbidity. In Westenberg, H.G.M., Den Boer, J.A., and Murphy, D.L. (Eds.) *Advances in the neurobiology of anxiety disorders*. Chichester, John Wiley & Sons, pp. 21–38.

Stahl, S.M., Judd, L.L., and Kunovac, J.L. (in press) Overview of new anxiolytics. In Montgomery, S. and Halbreich, U. (Eds.) *Pharmacotherapy of mood and cognition*. Washington, DC, American Psychiatric Press, Inc.

Stahl, S.M. and Soefje, S. (1995) Panic attacks and panic disorder: the great medical imposters. *Seminars in Neurology*, 15, 126–32.

Stahl, S.M. and Wets, K. (1988) Recent advances in drug delivery technology for neurology. *Clinical Neuropharmacology*, 11, 1–17.

Stolerman, I.P. and Jarvis, M.J. (1995) The scientific case that nicotine is addictive. *Psychopharmacology*, 117, 2–10.

Swerdlow, N. (1995) Serotonin, obsessive compulsive disorder and the basal ganglia. *International Review of Psychiatry*, 7, 115–30.

Volpicelli, J.R., Alterman, A.I., and Hayashida, M. (1992) Naltrexone in the treatment of alcohol dependence. *Archives of General Psychiatry*, 49, 876–80.

Wells, K.B., Stewart, A., Hays, R.D., Burnam, M.A., Rogers, W., Daniels, M., Berry, S., Greenfield, S., and Ware, J. (1989) The functioning and mental well-being of depressed patients: results from the medical outcomes study. *Journal of the American Medical Association*, 262, 914–19.

Yamamura, H.I., Enna, S.J., and Kuhar, M.J. (1985) *Neurotransmitter receptor binding*, 2nd edition. New York, Raven Press.

Index

Note: page numbers followed by f indicate illustrations, page numbers followed by t indicate tables.